Important Telephone Numbers

Emergency Room _____

_____

Poison Control Center _____

_____

Ambulance _____

_____

Family Doctor _____

_____

Specialist _____

_____

Specialist _____

_____

Dentist _____

_____

Dentist's Emergency No. _____

_____

Hospital No. _____

_____

Take Care of Yourself

A CONSUMER'S GUIDE TO MEDICAL CARE

Revised Edition

Donald Vickery, M.D.
James Fries, M.D.

Addison-Wesley Publishing Company

Reading, Massachusetts

Menlo Park, California • London • Amsterdam • Don Mills, Ontario • Sydney

Library of Congress Cataloging in Publication Data

Vickery, Donald M.
  Take care of yourself.

  Includes index.
  1. Medicine, Popular.   2. Self-care, Health.
I. Fries, James F.   II. Title.
RC81.V5 1981   616.02′4   81-10768

ISBN 0-201-08197-0   AACR2
ISBN 0-201-08198-9 (pbk.)

ISBN 0-201-08197-0 hc
ISBN 0-201-08198-9 paperback
ISBN 0-201-08199-7
IJ-DO-8987654

ABCDEFGHIJK-DO-8987654

Preface

Au revoir, auf wiedersehen, take care of yourself. With these traditional parting phrases, we express our feelings for our friends. When I see you again, be healthy. Keep your priceless health. We show our priorities with the parting salutation we use. Not money, and not fame. Take care of yourself.

This book is about how to take care of yourself. For us the phrase has four meanings. First, "take care of yourself" means taking care of the habits that lead to vigor and health. Your lifestyle is your most important guarantee of lifelong vigor, and you can postpone most serious chronic diseases by the right preventive health decisions. Second, "take care of yourself" means periodic monitoring for those few diseases that can sneak up on you without advance warning, such as high blood pressure, cancer of the breast or cervix, glaucoma, or dental decay. In such cases, taking care of yourself may mean going to a health professional for assistance. Third, "take care of yourself" means responding decisively to new medical problems that arise. Most often, your response should be self-care, and you can be your own doctor. But at other times you need professional help. Responding decisively means that you pay particular attention to the decision about going, or not going, to see the doctor. This book is particularly directed at helping you make that decision.

Many people think that all illness must be treated at the doctor's office, clinic, or hospital. In fact, over 80 percent of new problems are treated at home, and an even larger number could be. The public has had scant instruction in determining when outside help is needed and when it is not. In the United States, the average person sees a doctor slightly more than five times a year. Over 1.5 billion prescriptions are written each year, about 8 for each man, woman, and child. Medical costs now average over $1,000 per person per year—over 9.1 percent of our gross national product. Among the billions of different medical services used each year, some are life-saving, some result in great health improvement, and some give great comfort. But there are some that are totally unnecessary and some that are even harmful.

In our national quest for a symptom-free existence, as many as 70 percent of all visits to doctors for new problems have been termed unnecessary. For example, 11 percent of such visits are for uncomplicated colds. Many others are for minor cuts that do not require stitches, for tetanus shots despite current immunizations, for minor sprains of the ankle, and for the other problems discussed in this book. But, while you don't need a doctor to treat most coughs, you do for some. For every ten or so cuts that do not require stitches there is one that does. For every type of problem, there are some instances in which you should decide to see the doctor and some for which you should not.

Consider how important these decisions are. If you delay a visit to the doctor when you really need it, you may suffer unnecessary discomfort or have an illness untreated. On the other hand, if you go to the doctor when you don't need to, you waste time, often lose money, and may lose dignity. In a subtle way your confidence in your own ability and in the healing power of your own body begins to be eroded. You can even suffer physical harm if you receive a drug that you don't need or a test that you don't require. Your doctor is in an uncomfortable position when you come in unnecessarily and may feel obligated to practice "defensive medicine" just in case you have a bad result and a good lawyer. This book, above all else, is intended to help you with these decisions. It provides you with a "second opinion" within easy reach on your bookshelf. It contains information to help you make sound judgments about your own health.

There is a final intended meaning in the title of our book. Your health is your responsibility; it depends upon your decisions. There is no other way. You have to decide how to live, whether to see a doctor, which doctor to see, how soon to go, whether to take the advice offered. No one else can make these decisions, and they profoundly direct the course of future events. To be healthy, you have to be in charge.

Take Care of Yourself.

Reston, Virginia, D.M.V.
Stanford, California, J.F.F.
July 1981

Acknowledgments

We are grateful to many people for their help with this second edition, including the thousands of readers who have written with suggestions and encouragement and the hundreds of health workers who have used the first edition in their programs and practices.

In particular, we would like to thank Dr. William Bremer, Dr. William Carter, Dr. Grace Chickadonz, Dr. Peter Collis, Charlotte Crenson, Ann Dilworth, William Fisher, Sarah Fries, Dr. Halsted Holman, Dr. Robert Huntley, Dr. Kenneth Larsen, Dr. Kate Lorig, Prof. Nathan Maccoby, Florence Mahoney, Lawrence McPhee, Dr. Dennis McShane, Dr. Eugene Overton, Charles L. Parcell, Clarence Pearson, William Peterson, Dr. Robert Quinnell, Dr. Robert Rosenberg, Dr. Ralph Rosenthal, Lloyd Schieferbein, Dr. Douglas Solomon, Dr. Michael Soper, John Staples, Judy Staples, Warren Stone, Dr. Richard Tompkins, Shelley Vickery, Dr. William Watson, and Dr. Craig Wright for their advice and support.

Manuscript preparation would not have been possible without the efforts of Louise Davies, Sharon Joseph, Ann Nachman, Bonnie Obrig, Diana Pfeiffer, and Scip Wylbur, and we gratefully acknowledge their help.

To Our Readers

This book is strong medicine. It can be of great help to you. The medical advice is as sound as we can make it, but it will not always work. Like advice from your doctor, it will not always be right for you. This is our problem: if we don't give you direct advice, we can't help you. If we do, we will sometimes be wrong. So here are some qualifications: If you are under the care of a physician and receive advice contrary to this book, follow the physician's advice; the individual characteristics of your problem can then be taken into account. If you have an allergy or a suspected allergy to a recommended medication, check with your doctor, at least by phone. Read medicine label directions carefully; instructions vary from year to year, and you should follow the most recent. And if your problem persists beyond a reasonable period, you should usually see a doctor.

Contents

Contents

CHAPTER 8

Reducing Your Medication Costs 57

CHAPTER 9

The Home Pharmacy 61

CHAPTER 10

Avoiding Medical Fraud 85

Contents

xiv

Introduction

You can do more for your health than your doctor can. We introduced the first edition of *Take Care of Yourself* in 1976 with this phrase. The concept that health is more a personal responsibility than a professional responsibility was controversial at that time. These ideas did not originate with us; they can be found in the earlier writings of Rene Dubos, Victor Fuchs, and John Knowles, among others. But the concept remained strange and awkward to a society that was heavily dependent upon experts of every kind and seemingly addicted to ever more complex gadgetry and medications. Most people seemed to feel that American ingenuity could cure any disease. We could proclaim war on cancer, or on any other problem, and in a few years the problem would be solved. We would hire the experts, and they would find the cure.

What a difference a few years can make. The surgeon general of the United States recently released a carefully worded report, *Health Promotion and Disease Prevention*, with these words: "You, the individual, can do more for your own health and well-being than any doctor, any hospital, any drugs, any exotic medical device." The report goes on to detail a strategy for improved national health based upon personal efforts. The strategy of *Take Care of Yourself* is now a nationally accepted one.

In 1976 we warned against dependence upon annual physical examinations and narrowly conceived screening programs. We urged caution in influenza vaccination on the eve of release of the Swine Flu vaccine. We spoke strongly against routine use of the popular tranquilizers and suggested that the best home medicine cabinet should contain only six items. We promoted regular vigorous exercise, including jogging, for all age groups. We suggested that people with sore throats try to obtain a throat culture without a visit to the doctor, and that people might call their doctor first about some problems rather than going directly to the office or emergency room. Most importantly, we suggested that most visits to doctors for new problems were not necessary and that people could learn to recognize such problems. Now, in 1981, it is hard to remember that these issues were controversial just five years ago. The controversies have now been largely resolved, and we are proud to feel that *Take Care of Yourself* has played a role in the changing national perception of health.

The first edition of *Take Care of Yourself* included fourteen printings totaling nearly 1.5 million copies. It was distributed widely through health plans and institutions, notably through Blue Cross plans in many states. Acceptance by professional review panels was testimony to the soundness of the medical advice in *Take Care of Yourself*, but it was also a testament to farsighted panels and program directors who saw the need for new approaches to health problems. The success of the first edition was possible only because of the support of these many people.

But, does it work? Can you improve your health with the aid of a book? Can you use the doctor less, use health services more wisely, save money? Could it be dangerous to rely on advice from a book? How much change could you reasonably expect? We do not have the final answers to these questions, but we do have some good approximations. *Take Care of Yourself* has been more carefully evaluated by critical scientists than any health book ever written. The largest studies are still in progress, but results from five types of early studies are already very encouraging.

First, the indications for seeking medical care given in *Take Care of Yourself* have been checked against the conditions of patients as they came to their family doctor or the local emergency room. About one-half of all visits for new problems could have been avoided had patients read the book and followed the instructions. Naturally, not all people would refer to a book, and many would not follow the advice it provided. Still, this finding confirms a number of other studies that indicate that many visits to doctors are not necessary.

Second, people who were given *Take Care of Yourself* have been asked what use they made of it. In Middlebury, Vermont, responses to a questionnaire were tabulated for 359 people. Of these, 342 found *Take Care of Yourself* to be a good reference book, and 349 had used it for a problem at least once. Five out of every six felt that it improved the effectiveness and appropriateness of their medical care, and over half felt that they had saved money. In Woodland, California, a telephone survey of 295 families indicated that 89 percent had read at least some of the book and 40 percent had used it for one or more problems. Of those who used the book, approximately three times as many people decided not to go to the doctor than those who did go to the doctor. Two people reported that as a result of the book they had delayed a visit to the doctor that later turned out to be necessary. No negative results from using the book were reported. Asked about their feelings, 55 percent said that they were more personally confident about their health care. None reported loss of confidence.

Third, in a Seattle study an attempt was made to see how the decision charts of *Take Care of Yourself* might be used in the home for new medical problems. The study indicated that people who used the book would have been directed to the doctor slightly more often than once a year. The particular group studied went to the doctor less than one-third as often as the national average, and the authors of the study concluded that under some circumstances the book might increase visits to doctors. We hope that this is so. *Take Care of Yourself* has been developed to improve appropriate use of physician services, and only secondarily to reduce visits to doctors. So if you are one of the relatively few people in our society who almost never go to the doctor, you may find us urging you to go to the doctor more often.

Fourth, in certain studies some people (drawn by lot) were given *Take Care of Yourself* and the rest were not. In Woodland, California, 460 families were given the book and 239 families were not. The number of visits to doctors by those who were given *Take Care of Yourself* was reduced by 7.5 percent more than those who were not given the book. Visits to doctors decreased 14 percent for upper respiratory tract infections (colds). In San Jose, California, Blue Cross sponsored a larger study and reinforced the use of the book through seminars in the workplace and a monthly newsletter. Preliminary analysis shows a major decrease in visits to doctors by those persons receiving the book. None of these studies are conclusive, and some studies are still in progress. Nevertheless, we are greatly encouraged by what seems to be a very large effect for a very small investment. Every study has shown benefits. Even in the study showing the smallest effects, the decrease in national health costs, if generalized, would be over $8 billion each year.

Finally, *Take Care of Yourself* has been used as one part of a comprehensive program encouraging personal responsibility for health. The best-studied program of this kind, in Palo Alto, California, has resulted in a decrease in use of physicians of over one-half (2.2 visits per year compared with 5.0) and a proportionately larger decrease in the number of days spent in the hospital. These programs are never entirely typical of all communities, but they illustrate the potential benefits that can accrue for motivated individuals.

New dimensions have been added to this edition of *Take Care of Yourself*. We have provided wider ranging and more comprehensive information and have introduced several new concepts. More health problems are discussed, and the sections on exercise and lifestyle have been expanded, reflecting new knowledge in these areas. After receiving suggestions from literally thousands of doctors and patients, we have reviewed and improved the decision charts. Chapters discussing new information about aging and vitality and the special problems of the elderly have been added.

Perhaps the largest change in the book is a subtle one; we are now talking less about sickness and how to prevent it and more about health and how to maintain it. Health and the slowing of the aging process are now known to be greatly influenced by the same factors that increase illness. A vigorous life style, a continuing sense of adventure and excitement, continued exercise of personal will, individual responsibility, and laughter are essential to the healthy person. Ultimately we cannot prevent death at the end of our appointed span, but we can preserve our vigor and joy until that time.

Section I SKILLS FOR THE MEDICAL CONSUMER

1 Your Habits and Your Health

For the most part, your health is up to you. You can do much more than any physician to maintain your health and well-being. To do this, you have to get in the habit of health. At the age of fifty, individuals with good health habits are physically thirty years younger than individuals with poor health habits; you can have a physical age of sixty-five or a physical age of thirty-five. It's up to you.

Your doctor's examination of your heart will not prevent a heart attack, but you can greatly decrease chances of a heart attack by maintaining a good diet and exercising, and by not smoking cigarettes. You don't really need a physician to remind you that alcohol acts to destroy the liver and stomach lining, or that you can avoid lung diseases if you quit smoking tar-laden cigarettes, or that fat people have more health problems than slim people. You already know these things, and your destiny is controlled by your decisions.

In contrast, surprisingly few diseases can be prevented by actions of the physician. On occasion, the physician may detect an illness, such as high blood pressure or cancer, at an early stage, and appropriate medical treatment can contribute significantly to your long-term health. Unfortunately, at the present time there is no way that your doctor can halt the progression of our major chronic diseases such as atherosclerosis, diabetes, osteoarthritis, emphysema, cirrhosis, and cancer of the lung. Perhaps it would be nice if the doctor could do it and you could avoid the responsibility, but this is not possible.

If we could eliminate all unhealthy habits, what would happen? Lung cancer and emphysema would almost completely disappear, death due to all cancers as a group would decrease by almost one-half, cirrhosis of the liver would become a rare disease. Peptic ulcers and gastritis would decrease greatly, massive upper GI bleeding (bleeding from the stomach) would become unusual, pancreatitis (inflammation of the pancreas) would be rare. High blood pressure would be less common, and there would be fewer strokes and heart attacks. Atherosclerosis (hardening of the arteries)

3

would occur less frequently. We could eliminate one-half of the hospital beds now available. The cost of medical care would decrease, the price paid for the expensive bad habits would be saved, and the consumer would have more pocket money. The number of sick days would decrease by over one-half, and the national productivity would rise. An incredible set of possibilities!

Without the help of the patient, medicine can make no such promises. It is up to each of us. Here we review some of the habits that directly affect our health.

FITNESS

Probably the most important lifetime habit is active exercise. Body parts need to be used to work well; use them or lose them. Our organs tend to rust out more quickly than they wear out.

Without exercise the muscles get flabby. The bones become brittle. The sex drive decreases. The heart muscle becomes soft; in medical terms "cardiac reserve" is lost. The weakened heart muscle is less able to respond to the needs of stressful situations. The body cells cannot use oxygen as efficiently. The reflexes decay, and falls and accidents become more likely.

Exercise is the key to many of the health risk factors. It helps with weight control, decreases cholesterol, lowers pulse and blood pressure, helps counter stress, and helps prevent depression. It increases physical reserve, improves stamina during the working day, and promotes personal confidence.

Your exercise program should be pleasurable, and almost all people obtain deep satisfaction from their exercise program after it has become a habit. It is the initial undertaking and perseverance that are difficult. You don't have enough time? Exercise is the activity that adds time to your day by increasing your stamina, and it adds vigorous years to your life.

Exercise should be regular, at least four days a week. It should be "aerobic," so that it conditions the heart and the oxygen-utilization mechanisms; this means steady exercise for at least fifteen minutes that is sufficient to raise the heart rate and break a sweat.

Exercise should be undertaken gradually, to allow the body to prepare for the next level of activity. You may require many months or even several years to develop your full program. Be gentle in the beginning, increasing your activity slowly as you feel the ability and the desire. If your activity is causing discomfort, you are progressing too rapidly.

The particular activity matters little and can be freely chosen. Jogging is currently the most popular, but it has no particular advantages over other forms of exercise. We have been regular runners for many years and enjoy the solitude of the fields and hills. Other people like to run on a track, swim, bicycle, walk, or jump rope. Some sports, such as basketball and soccer, can give aerobic exercise. Your particular choice is much less important than choosing an activity that gives you pleasure, one you can anticipate continuing for a long period of time. Schedule the activity into your routine: an early morning or lunchtime or cocktail-hour run, bicycling to work, a time for swimming, a brisk walk after breakfast.

Even if your work is physical, you need an exercise program; you will find that it helps you to maintain your energy level at work. Very few physical jobs require aerobic exercise, and lifting and pushing at intervals throughout the day, while tiring, is not good conditioning. Then too, there are psychological benefits from exercise programs that are freely undertaken, from the voluntary decision to take personal responsibility.

People who exercise tend to become intolerable converts, and their new euphoria is often translated into missionary zeal. Many overly detailed exercise formulas have been promoted, but in fact, common sense is your best guide. The body was designed for a less pampered life than we have given it over recent decades, and it works better if used more. You need to decide how to translate this general principle into your own life.

COFFIN NAILS

Cigarette smoking, it says on the pack, may be hazardous to your health. This is the most harmful of the personal vices, and is fortunately becoming less socially acceptable. Physicians rate smokers by their number of "pack-years," which is the number of packs per day multiplied by the number of years that you have smoked. For example, if you have smoked two packs per day for five years, you are a ten pack-year smoker. For each pack-year that you smoke, you decrease your life expectancy by about one month. You greatly increase your chance of sudden death. A heavy smoker, smoking two packs daily for thirty years, or sixty pack-years, has decreased his or her life expectancy by five years.

THE CIGARETTE SMOKER
More Heart Attacks	(x2)
More Strokes	(x4)
More Lung Cancer	(x300)
More Emphysema	(x300)
More Skin Wrinkles	(x4)
More High Blood Pressure	(x2)

Other bad things happen too. The physical reserve of the cigarette smoker is decreased. Smokers are less healthy, less vigorous, have less active sex lives, and appear to develop skin wrinkles at earlier ages. They spend twice as much time in the hospital as nonsmokers.

Just as important, the last years of a cigarette smoker are not a period of grace and beauty. Tortured wheezing, swollen purple lips, and the feeling of suffocation mark these years. In medical slang, the late-stage cigarette smoker is termed a "blue bloater." Fortunately, present evidence suggests that the ex-cigarette smoker can regain much lost function and improve life expectancy, although not back to that of the nonsmoker. Pipe and cigar smoke, when not inhaled, is less hazardous and accounts for only a fraction of the problems created by inhaled cigarette smoke, but smoking a pipe or cigar can also certainly decrease your social acceptability. The militant nonsmoker ("Would you mind putting out that cigarette?") is a constructive new social phenomenon, and the smokers are being packed into smaller and smaller spaces in the back of the airplane. The hazards of "second-hand smoke" are real, although relatively small, and many people feel that forced exposure to the smoke of others is deeply offensive. Give up your cigarettes and avoid the hassles.

THE TWO-MARTINI LUNCH

The drinking of alcoholic beverages is a social custom for the great majority of adults in the United States. In moderation this custom may improve circulation, reduce blood pressure, and act as a relatively mild and safe tranquilizer. However, 10 percent of our population have serious drinking problems. These people constitute over 20 percent of all hospitalized patients. They typically suffer from one or more of a set of related serious problems; cirrhosis of the liver, ulcer disease, bleeding from the bowel, premature senility, and vitamin deficiencies are among the most frequent. Sometimes they show signs of severe mental psychosis, and they may exhibit the spectacular "delirium tremens"—the "DT's" or "the shakes." They drive automobiles into immovable objects or innocent folks with a frequency that is truly alarming; deaths related to alcohol represent nearly one-half of all deaths in young adult life. Suicide and homicide are frequently related to alcohol use.

Alcohol is high in calories. It may increase obesity, as in a "beer belly," and it thereby increases other health problems related to obesity. People who drink heavily tend to eat less nutritional food. This can result in a variety of nutritional problems as well as cirrhosis of the liver.

Treatment of the alcoholic continues to be a frustrating, often unsuccessful venture. Within the medical community, enthusiasm for a wide variety of treatment methods waxes and wanes. Nonmedical organizations, especially Alcoholics Anonymous, enjoy a success rate that is at least equal to that of any "medical" treatment. Associated organizations, such as Al Anon, which work with the families of alcoholics, also show considerable promise. The key elements of these treatments are that they deal with motivated people who truly wish to change, and the treatments continually reinforce the subject's desire to remain free of alcoholic influence.

When should you seek help? Everyone has a different definition of how much alcohol is too much, and the amount probably is different for different people. You should seek help if you have problems with alcohol, and you should not make excuses for the problems. Face up to them. Here are some of the frequent signals that you need help: a drunken driving citation, an automobile accident after two or more drinks, missing work because of feeling poorly from drinking the night before, a pattern of work absences on Monday mornings, a hospitalization for an alcohol-related problem such as gastritis or upper bowel hemorrhage, inability to function at top efficiency in the afternoon because of a two-martini lunch or its equivalent. If you develop the insight that you have these serious problems and that your situation must be changed, you are a good candidate for successful treatment.

THE DRUG SCENE

All drugs can be used to excess, with harmful consequences. The major drugs of our society are alcohol, nicotine, and caffeine, and each has its well-known problems. But there are two other categories of drugs whose consequences are more easily ignored: the illegal or "street" drugs, and the various "happiness pills" obtained with a doctor's prescription.

Marijuana is a rather mild drug with a soothing effect. However, experiments indicate that large amounts of marijuana administered over a long period of time may cause genetic damage in animals. Heavy use is associated with loss of motivation in many individuals. Marijuana has been used extensively by young people and has adversely affected their early life decisions regarding further schooling and choice of occupation. Its medical consequences are presently not well known. Marijuana users are fond of saying that their drug is not as hazardous as alcohol or cigarette smoking; this statement will probably prove to be false, but even if it were true, it is a very naive kind of argument. Armed robbery is not as bad as murder, but this is a rather weak justification for armed robbery.

Amphetamines and "speed" stimulate the body, creating an illusion of extra energy, but they almost certainly increase some forms of heart disease by constricting the small blood vessels. It is now generally agreed that they have almost no medical use, their prescription is much more tightly controlled than it was five years ago, and tragedies such as that which occurred to Elvis Presley have increased public awareness of the problems posed by these agents.

The "hard" drugs and narcotics (such as heroin, cocaine, morphine, demerol, and methadone) have potential for fatal overdose, and addiction invariably leads to social degeneration of the user. A large fraction of crimes, both violent and nonviolent, are related to these drugs; not because the user is directly crazed by the drug but because money must be obtained to buy more. Recently, there has been some "fashionable" use of cocaine in social circles noted more for their high income and personal idiosyncracies than for their good sense. Cocaine is a highly dangerous drug, and do not let anyone tell you differently. Stay away from it!

Legal drugs are no less hazardous than illegal drugs, but because they are "respectable," we forget their hazards. The number of prescriptions for these drugs is going down, and we hope that *Take Care of Yourself* has had something to do with the decline in their sales. These drugs hinder your taking care of yourself. During the period of peak use, more than one out of every six people in the United States were regularly using a pre-scribed mood-changing drug. Even now, such drugs are in first and second place of all drugs prescribed and hold eight positions in the top twenty prescription drugs used—a truly shocking indictment.

Tranquilizers, in the language of the street, are "downers." These have been the most popular mood-changing drugs and include Valium, Librium, Equanil, Miltown, and others. They used to be prescribed when a patient reported "nervousness" or "anxiety," or as a quick and satisfactory method of getting the patient out of the office. That is, they were given for symp-toms reflecting difficulty in coping; but "downers," like alcohol, further im-pair one's ability to cope with the immediate environment. One standard tablet of the stronger of these medications (such as Librium or Valium) is roughly equivalent, as a sedative, to one alcoholic drink. Most would agree that taking one or two drinks three times a day is not the best way to solve life's problems.

Sedatives may also be given to "help" patients sleep. Insomnia, while a troublesome complaint, is not often helped by sleeping pills. The body's in-stinct for sleep is extremely powerful; sleep is demanded by the body when it is needed. Many adults require only six hours of sleep, and this amount appears to decrease with age. A feeling of poor sleep one night often leads to an early bedtime the next night; this leads to a restless night with pe-riods of wakefulness, causing the patient to think sleep has been inade-quate, and a vicious cycle begins. True insomnia requiring medical care is unusual. Sedatives, which do not simulate natural sleep very closely, are seldom needed.

If you do use sedatives, you or your child may die of an overdose of them. They affect enzymes in the liver, and can lead to complications when other drugs are used at the same time. They may carry over into a morning hangover, and they increase the chance that your children won't listen to you when you tell them about the evils of their drugs.

"Uppers," usually amphetamines, used to be prescribed in a misguided attempt to help patients lose weight. They do not assist in weight reduc-tion, except very temporarily, and many studies have demonstrated the fu-tility of weight reduction programs based on the use of these agents. They cause severe mood changes, tightening of the small arteries, and impose an extra strain on the heart. Amphetamines were once used in the athletic arena by trainers and players because they create the illusion of physical prowess. However, careful studies in track-and-field events, where direct measurement of performance is possible, indicate that amphetamines nei-ther help nor hinder performance at events such as the hundred-yard dash or the mile run but have a tendency to impair performance in such events as the hurdles or pole vault which require close coordination.

Drugs are chemicals. The drugs you swallow react in the bloodstream, with other drugs or with various chemicals already made by your body. If several drugs are taken together, the complexity of their interactions is such that no physician or scientist can adequately analyze the situation. Almost any medical symptom can represent a side effect of a drug or a combination of drugs. Between 10 and 20 percent of all hospital admissions ae now felt to represent complications of prescription drugs. The great majority of the drugs that have caused these reactions were medically optional and were not required to maintain the health of the patient. Medications sometimes help to eliminate disease, but they do not make you healthy; do not look for health in a pill bottle.

THE FAT OF THE LAND

Once you are ten pounds over your ideal weight each additional pound costs you a month of your life. Each pound slows you down, makes you less effective in personal encounters, and often lowers your self-image. Fat people are hospitalized more frequently than people of normal weight; they have more gallbladder problems, more surgical complications, more cases of breast cancer, more high blood pressure, heart attacks, and strokes. They also develop atherosclerosis (hardening of the arteries) at earlier ages. These facts are well-known.

It is less commonly known that the fat person cannot even eat much more than his or her thin counterpart. A day's food represents about one pound of body weight: if you fast, on average you lose a pound a day; if you eat double, you gain a pound. Thus, if you gain ten pounds each year, you will be very fat, but this weight gain represents only an additional ten-days worth of food over the year, or approximately 3 percent. The fat person can eat only 1 to 5 percent more than a thin person.

We respect the difficulty of this problem, and we share these difficulties with you. But the solutions are personal, not medical. A few people have glandular illnesses that cause their weight problem, but for most of us the problem is not a medical one. As with the other habits that change health, management of the problem begins with its recognition as a problem. Weight control requires lifelong discipline and vigilance. It is not easy.

There are generally two phases to weight control: the weight reduction phase and the weight maintenance phase. The method you use to lose weight doesn't matter too much (although liquid-protein diets are somewhat dangerous), and you can choose from any of a number of sound diets. Diets usually have a gimmick of some kind which encourages you and helps you remember the diet. Most people have some success with losing weight; if you set a target, tell people what you are trying to do, and stick with it for a while you can probably lose weight.

Weight maintenance at your new weight is more difficult. Weigh yourself regularly and record the weight on a chart. Draw a red line at three pounds over your desired weight and maintain your weight below the line, using whatever method you need. Accept no excuses for increasing weight; it is easier and healthier to make frequent, small adjustments in what you eat than to try to counteract binges of overeating with dieting. Keep yourself off the roller coaster. You have to choose between calories and complications, early diet and early demise.

THE ERRANT VEHICLE

Fastening an automobile seat belt doesn't seem like medical treatment, but it is very powerful preventive medicine. Trauma now accounts for 74 percent of all deaths between the ages of fifteen and twenty-five, and accidents are the fourth most important cause of death at all ages.

Seat belts, interlock devices, speed limits, and drunken driving programs are often considered to be annoying interferences with our personal freedoms. Yet, attention to safety measures is the easiest of all of the personal health habits. Because accidents kill often in youth, the total health impact in terms of years of life lost is even greater than statistics suggest. Young people forget the importance of good health habits because they do not feel threatened by cancer, heart disease, and strokes. But poor driving habits, such as not using seat belts, showing off, and drinking before driving, can kill just as surely as cigarettes, and even more quickly. Young Americans who die on the highway usually perish at the hand of another young American.

SELF-DESTRUCTION
SYNDROMES

Cigarette smoking, inactivity, alcohol abuse, obesity, drug use, and accidents all represent a form of suicide or self-destruction. These factors combine to be the most important determinants of your present and future health. You can live longer and feel better by employing enjoyable disciplines in your life-style. Get back in control. Remember that the effects of each bad health habit are cumulative. The probability of early death or disability increases the longer you continue to smoke, the longer you are obese, the longer you lack exercise, and the percentage of time that you ignore your seatbelt. Stopping bad habits at any time is beneficial. And for most of these problems, moderation, rather than total elimination, is the crucial health element.

Avoid making excuses: "Everyone is overweight in my family." "I just wish I had the time to exercise." "It's easy to give up smoking, I've done it fifty times." "I never drink before lunchtime." "I can handle it." "I don't smoke cigarettes all the way." "Diets just don't work for me." It is embarrassing to hear such statements offered by apparently intelligent people. First you need insight; then change is possible.

How can you conquer a habit? This is accomplished only by hard work. We have given most of the principles above. Avoid self-deception. Set goals and write them down. Chart your progress. Work with others who have the same problems. Plan to work at it the rest of your life. Tell others what you are doing. Discover the pleasant dividends of your change of habit and remind yourself of them: a better sex life, better physical reserve during the day, admiring looks from others, more energy, more money, a clear mind, less illness.

Decide to make permanent changes in your life. Crash diets, periods of time "on the wagon," and spurts of physical activity are all poor practice. When you exercise beyond your conditioning, you stress muscles, ligaments, and the heart. When your weight bounces from high to low to high like a yo-yo it is just as harmful to your heart and arteries as if you had kept the initial high weight. The spree drinker adds additional social and medical problems to those of the steady alcoholic. These issues are for a lifetime, and there are no short-term solutions.

You are the patient. It is your life and your responsibility. Define for yourself those health goals which are important to you and your family. Define a solid and workable program to approach these goals, and plan to maintain that program for the rest of your life. You will live longer, feel better, and have more energy to share with your family and friends.

2 An Ounce of Prevention

An ounce of prevention, it is said, is worth more than a pound of cure. Medicine in recent years has been oriented to "cure" rather than prevention, even though many of the greatest medical successes, such as eradication of smallpox and control of paralytic polio, have been achieved through preventive measures. We have been "crisis-oriented": our approach has been to wait for a consequence to appear and then try to treat it. Now, interest is appropriately focusing upon preventive medicine. The most important part of preventive medicine, moderating health habits, was discussed in the first chapter. The idea of preventive medicine also includes the following four strategies, and it is important to understand both their strengths and their limitations:

- the checkup or periodic health examination
- multiphasic screening
- early treatment
- immunizations and other public health measures

THE MYTH OF THE ANNUAL CHECKUP

The "annual checkup" is still recommended by some schools, camps, employers, and the army. Curiously enough doctors seldom go to each other for routine checkups, nor do they send their families. The complete "executive physical," made popular a few years ago by large corporations that wished to insure the health of their most critical employees, is slowly being discontinued. Even these elaborate checkups, involving several days in the hospital, do not detect early and treatable diseases with any regularity, and they raise false confidence to some degree. That is, they encourage the false belief that if you are regularly checked you do not need to concern yourself as much about personal health maintenance, the theme of this book.

The organization requesting a medical checkup may well have a different purpose than you do. Sometimes, their purpose may be to detect diseases that could affect your future performance so that they can avoid hiring, insuring, or depending upon you. The checkup may indeed help in these respects. But your interest is more in finding conditions about which something can be done, and for this the checkup is not very successful. If you heed the warnings of Chapter 1 and attend to new symptoms as discussed in Part 2, there are very few advantages to be gained from the "annual checkup." Nearly everyone now agrees that an annual physical examination is not indicated; decreases in screening have recently been recommended by a national Canadian task force and by the American Cancer Society.

There are a few areas in which periodic screening is necessary, and it is important to keep them in mind:

• High blood pressure is a significant medical condition that gives little warning of its presence. During adult life it is advisable to have your blood pressure checked at least every year or so. This measurement can easily be done by a nurse, physician's assistant, or nurse's aide; a full examination is not required. If high blood pressure is found, a doctor should confirm it, and you should carefully attend to the measures needed to keep it under control.

• If you are a woman over twenty-five, you should have a "Pap smear" taken every year or so. Some authorities now recommend beginning Pap smear testing at the age of beginning sexual activity, decreasing frequency to every three to five years after the first three are negative, and again increasing the frequency to every one or two years after age forty. This test detects cancer of the womb (cervix), and in early stages this cancer is almost always curable. See "For Women Only" (p. 319) for more information on Pap smears and instructions on breast self-examination.

• Women over age twenty-five should practice breast self-examination monthly. Any suspicious changes should be checked out with a physician; the great majority of breast cancers are first detected as suspicious lumps by the patient. Women with large breasts cannot practice self-examination with as much reliability as other women and may wish to discuss other screening procedures with their doctor. In general, we do not like to recommend mammography as a screening procedure for women below the age of fifty, but there are exceptions, such as women who have already had a breast tumor or women with a strong history of breast cancer in their family.

• A test for glaucoma (a treatable disease that can cause blindness) should be done every few years after age forty if there is a family history of glaucoma. Most cases of this disease are discovered during eye examinations, so it is generally advisable that such examinations include a routine check for glaucoma.

• Tuberculosis skin tests (PPD or Tine Test) or periodic chest X rays are indicated if there has been any possibility of exposure to this disease. If the skin test was negative and becomes positive, check with your doctor.

• Dental checks can save teeth, and regular dental examinations are recommended. The primary purpose of an annual dental examination is to find and fill cavities; the benefits of other aspects of the examination ritual are less well established.

• Screening tests of urine, tests for blood in the stool after age thirty, and regular sigmoidoscopy after age fifty are of more dubious value. Some doctors feel that these are worthwhile, and others do not.

The importance of these few examinations is underscored by their availability as a public service, free of charge, at many city and county clinics. These are the crucial elements of periodic checks; others are optional and controversial.

Congratulations: You just saved an executive examination costing $400.

Are "complete" checkups ever worthwhile? Yes. The first examination by a new physician allows you to establish a relationship with the doctor. Increasingly, the periodic checkup is being used not as much for the detection of disease as for the opportunity to counsel the patient about the health habits described in Chapter 1, so that patients can do a better job of taking care of themselves.

MULTIPHASIC SCREENING

The term "multiphasic" simply means that many laboratory tests are performed in an attempt to find abnormalities that are not readily apparent. Some multiphasic screening programs involve fifty or more tests, including blood studies, urinalysis, X rays, electrocardiograms, and other procedures. With automation, these tests can be performed quickly and economically.

Experience with these screening systems over the years has shown that many laboratory abnormalities are detected but surprisingly few major problems that need attention are found. No laboratory test is perfectly accurate, and each test has a certain number of "false positives" associated with it. There is danger that the doctor may feel obligated to follow up the "false positive" test with additional tests, thereby unnecessarily increasing both the patient's cost and worries.

Because of these problems, we do not routinely recommend multiphasic screening except as part of a total health care program, such as the Kaiser-Permanente Health Plans. In such programs, multiphasic screening has allowed more effective use of nurse practitioners and has encouraged more efficient health care delivery systems. Some physicians also feel that multiphasic screening is an effective way to reassure the "worried well." That is, a negative multiphasic screening examination may help people who are overly concerned about their health to accept the fact that medical treatment is not likely to help them with their problems. Thus, like the complete physical examination, multiphasic screening may be of value not so much for the detection of disease as for providing a good opportunity for reassurance and counsel.

Screening for disease detection is justified only for those individual tests that can detect important and treatable problems. For many people, the blood pressure measurement is by far the most important test.

EARLY TREATMENT

An effective health maintenance strategy includes seeking medical care promptly whenever an important new problem or finding appears. If you have a lump in your breast, unexplained weight loss, a fever for more than a week, or if you have begun to cough up blood, you should seek medical attention without delay. These may not represent true emergencies, but they do indicate that professional attention should be sought within a few days. Most times, nothing will be seriously wrong; on other occasions, however, an early cancer, tuberculosis, or other treatable disease will be found.

The guidelines of Part 2 of this book can help you select those instances in which you should seek medical care. In many cases, you can take care of yourself with home treatment. However, you must respond appropriately when professional care is needed.

To ensure timely treatment you need to have a plan. Think things through ahead of time. Do you have a doctor? If you need emergency care, where will you go? To an emergency hospital? To the emergency room of a general hospital? To the on-call physician of a local medical group? If you are not sure what to do after consulting this book, who can you call for further advice? Have you written down the phone numbers you need?

Only rarely will you need emergency services. But the time that you need them is not the time to begin wondering what to do. If you have a routine problem that requires medical care, where will you go? Is there a nearby doctor? Who has your medical records? Chapter 3, "Finding the Right Physician," and Chapter 7, "Choosing the Right Medical Facility," will help you answer these questions. But plan ahead.

IMMUNIZATIONS

Immunizations have had far greater positive impact upon health in the developed nations than all of the other health services provided by physicians. Only a few years ago, smallpox, cholera, paralytic polio, diphtheria, whooping cough, and tetanus killed large numbers of people. These diseases are now effectively controlled by immunization in the United States and in most other developed nations. Smallpox has been eradicated from the entire world, and there is no longer any need for smallpox immunization. An incredible success story!

Frequent immunization is not needed now because these diseases occur less often and because we know that the immunizations provide protection for a long time. Thus, tetanus boosters are not required more often than every ten years for adults who have had the basic series of tetanus injections. As these conditions become rare, the problems of side effects from the inoculations are in some instances as great as the risk of the illness.

Keep a careful record of your immunizations in the back of this book. Do not allow yourself to be reinoculated just because you have lost records of previous immunizations. If you haven't had a tetanus shot for ten years or so, ask for a booster shot while visiting the doctor for another reason. You can save future trips to the doctor by being protected for the next ten years. In general, do not seek out the optional immunizations. Flu shots, for example, are only partially effective and often cause a degree of illness themselves; they are recommended only for the elderly and for those with severe lung diseases.

TABLE 2–1	Age	Immunization
Recommended Immunization Schedule	2 months	DPT (diphtheria, pertussis, tetanus), and Oral Polio
	4 months	DPT and Oral Polio
	6 months	DPT and Oral Polio
	15 months	Measles
	18 months	DPT and Oral Polio
	5 years	DPT and Oral Polio
	12 years	Rubella (only for females with a rubella hemagglutination test that is negative or less than 1:16)
	Every 10 years	T(d) (adult tetanus, diphtheria)

We recommend that the optional immunizations (including mumps, hepatitis, pneumovac, and flu) be taken only upon the recommendation of your doctor, and then only after careful discussion. In general, do not initiate requests for these inoculations. They have a definite role for some people, but not for all.

Finally, here is a summary of what you need to remember about preventive medicine:

• You don't need frequent checkups if you feel well, except for a few specific tests. Blood pressure, Pap smears, breast examination, tuberculosis screening, glaucoma testing, and dental checks are the most important; most people will not even need all of these. Most of these procedures can be obtained through public health departments at city or county expense. Take your doctor's advice concerning the need for a urinalysis, urine culture, tests of the stool for blood, rectal examination, or sigmoidoscopy.

• Elaborate physical examinations or multiphasic screening may detect trivial abnormalities and thus worry you unnecessarily.

• Complete physical examinations should include counseling on health habits.

• You should have a plan for obtaining medical care before the need arises.

• You should be immunized according to recommended schedules, but you need "boosters" only occasionally in adult life.

If you follow these general principles and if you moderate your habits as discussed in the first chapter, you are well on the way toward taking care of yourself.

3 Finding the Right Physician

Who is the right doctor for you? There are all kinds of physicians, and the distinctions among them can be confusing. This chapter is designed to help you understand the different types of doctors and how they conduct their medical practices. This chapter contains some guidelines to help you choose the right doctor for you and your family.

THE FAMILY DOCTOR

The primary care physician, who used to be termed a "GP" or "General Practitioner," is now commonly called a "Family Practitioner." The family practitioner is a specialist too and has had several years of advanced training in family practice. A specialist in internal medicine or pediatrics often serves as a primary care physician.

Primary care physicians represent the initial contact between the patient and the medical establishment. They accept responsibility for the continued care of a patient or a family and perform a wide variety of services. Usually, they have had some training in internal medicine, pediatrics, and gynecology. In the past, primary care physicians performed both major and minor surgery; but in recent years this practice has become much less common, and the family doctor will usually refer major surgical problems to surgeons. Obstetrics and gynecology, the female specialties, are not always handled by primary care physicians.

Family practitioners serve as the quarterbacks of the medical system and may direct and coordinate the activities they do not perform personally. Other than the patient, the primary care physician makes the most important decisions in medicine by determining the nature and severity of the problem as well as recommending approaches to its solution.

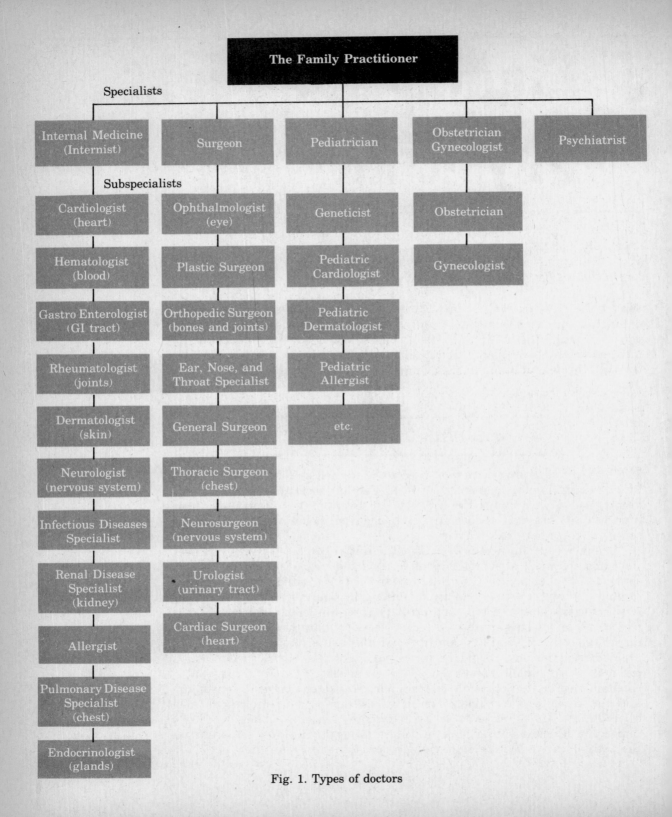

Fig. 1. Types of doctors

THE SPECIALISTS

The five major clinical specialties are internal medicine, surgery, pediatrics, obstetrics and gynecology, and psychiatry. There are other specialties such as radiology, clinical pathology, and anesthesiology, but they are not included in our chart because the patient seldom goes directly to such physicians. The largest specialty is internal medicine. Physicians may refer to this specialty as "medicine" and to its practitioner as an "internist." The internist is sometimes confused with the "intern." An intern is a recent medical school graduate who is undergoing hospital apprenticeship in any specialty; an internist is a specialist in internal medicine and has usually completed three or more years of training after graduation from medical school. Each of the other specialties and family practice has a similar length of training. As noted, family practice is now a specialty as well, although often not referred to as such.

THE SUBSPECIALISTS

Subspecialties have developed within the major specialty areas; some are listed in Fig. 1. In internal medicine, there is a specialist for nearly every organ system. Thus, cardiologists specialize in the heart; dermatologists, the skin; neurologists, the nervous system; renal disease specialists, the kidneys; and so forth. Within surgery, different types of operations have defined the specialties of particular surgeons. The ophthalmologist performs surgery on the eyes; the ear, nose, throat (ENT) specialist on those areas; the thoracic surgeon in the chest; and the cardiac surgeon on the heart. The general surgeon operates in the abdominal cavity as well as other areas.

Within childhood medicine, or pediatrics, specialties have developed similar to those within adult internal medicine. In addition, since certain problems, particularly genetic and developmental ones, are more common in children, subspecialties unique to pediatrics have developed.

Increasingly, the specialty "obstetrics and gynecology" has been divided and is practiced by the obstetrician who delivers babies and the gynecologist who deals with diseases of the female organs.

Psychiatry does not have formal subspecialties, but a variety of schools of psychotherapy exist, such as Freudian and Jungian. Recently, obesity, alcoholism, and other specific problems have become subjects for separate disciplines within psychiatry.

There are other specialties and other names for doctors, and the full classification is more complicated than that which we show in Fig. 1. For example, where does the podiatrist fit? The physiatrist? The chiropractor? But for most purposes you will find that Fig. 1 is a good guide.

The different kinds of doctors provide their services under various arrangements: sometimes they practice alone, sometimes in groups, often under different financial conditions. You should know the strengths ⹁nd weaknesses of each. By combining the right doctor with your medical and financial needs, you have a better chance of good medical care.

TYPES OF PRACTICE ARRANGEMENTS

Solo Practice

The solo practitioner is a physician without partners or organizational affiliation and may be a family practitioner, a specialist, or a subspecialist in any of the medical disciplines. The solo practitioner generally works from an office which may or may not be near a hospital. With a solo practitioner, each time you are sick you will probably be seen by the same person. In small communities and rural areas, a solo practitioner may be the only source of medical care.

In recent years, busy solo practitioners have sometimes employed "nurse practitioners" or "physician's assistants" to enable them to care for a larger number of patients. Experience to date indicates that these health professionals, who are not doctors, provide excellent care in many areas of medicine.

It is rumored that in the old days a doctor was always available. One doubts that this was ever true, at any rate, it is not true now. The typical solo practitioner spends several weeks of the year on vacation or attending medical meetings. The doctor goes to concerts and parties like everybody else and may spend a weekend at a cabin in the mountains. Such diversions are important for the mental health of the physician. On the other hand, this means that you will not always see the same physician, even if your doctor is a solo practitioner; your doctor's answering service may refer you to another physician who is "on call."

Group Practice

The medical group or "group practice" came into being some years ago as an answer to some of the problems of single practice. The sharing of night and weekend coverage, the lowering of office costs by shared expense, the availability of consultation, and a more medically stimulating environment for the physician all contributed to the increase in group practices. Group practices come in all sizes and varieties. The smallest group practice is the partnership; there may be two partners or more. The partners may be incorporated into a "medical corporation."

Fee-for-Service

The quality of medical care is not determined by the method of payment; nevertheless, there are psychological factors in payment arrangements which everyone should understand.

"Fee-for-service" is an awkward term that describes the traditional method of paying the doctor in the United States. A service is performed and payment is given for that service. The more services provided, the higher the patient's bill and the higher the physician's income. Nearly everyone else in the United States is paid by salary, and piecework payment for physician services has been severely criticized by some.

When payment is determined by the number of services, there is a financial incentive to increase the number of services. On the other hand, "customer satisfaction" becomes important to the physician. A good "bedside manner" may be developed and extra services may be provided in response to special problems. Since considerable effort is expended in maintaining the relationship with the patient, respect of physicians by patients tends to be greatest in areas where physicians are paid for each service.

On the other hand, problems have been attributed to this payment system. It has been charged that patients have been seen too frequently, given too many medications and too many shots, had too many diagnostic procedures performed, and undergone too much surgery as a result of this financial incentive. Studies have suggested that the physician in the fee-for-service setting provides many more services than physicians paid by salary. Controversy remains as to whether these additional services represent better care or simply greater expense.

Prepaid Practice

In prepaid practice, a group of physicians offers a plan which looks like an insurance policy but actually represents a rearrangement of the traditional incentives. The patient knows in advance the medical expenses for the year. A set monthly amount is paid regardless of whether the medical facility is used frequently or not at all. When the patient needs a doctor, little or no additional expense is involved. The physician is now given an incentive to minimize the number of services provided, since the amount of money to be earned is already determined.

Advocates of prepayment have argued that the physician now has an incentive toward "preventive medicine" and is more likely to treat conditions early rather than letting them get out of control. Some observers doubt that this is true. It is evident in many prepaid group practices that little attention is given to preventive medicine; indeed, sometimes the very opposite has been observed. However, prepaid group practices do decrease the overall cost of medical care, usually at a savings of approximately 20 percent; this is achieved by a lower use of expensive hospital care. Studies that compare the quality of medical care under the different payment conditions have not shown a difference. Thus the average patient in the prepaid plan saves money and avoids the nuisance of excessive medical procedures, with no apparent decrease in the quality of the care.

On the negative side, many patients are not happy with prepaid group practices. The most common complaints are that lines are too long, the physicians are too impersonal, and that the patients "feel like a number." Prepaid systems have been burdened by the few patients that overuse the system; in many plans, 25 percent of the patients use 75 percent of the services. The excessive services received by these few people increase the payments for the rest. The prepaid group practice has a less direct stake in patient satisfaction than the fee-for-service physician. The physician is now given the incentive to minimize the number of services provided since the amount of money is already determined. The dedication of most physicians works to counteract these financial forces. Still, as a patient, you should be aware of the potential problems with the system you choose.

WHICH DOCTOR IS RIGHT FOR YOU?

Given the choice of many kinds of physicians, medical practices, and payment schedules, which doctor is right for you? Medically, seeing a different physician each time seems to work about as well as seeing the same physician consistently, if your medical record is good or if the problem is a new one. However, many patients and physicians feel that the depth of the relationship is impaired when frequent doctor changes are made.

Here are some things to remember when choosing a physician:

The type of physician is usually not as important as the individual physician. You can go to a family practitioner, a pediatrician, an internist, or a subspecialty internist for your primary care. Women sometimes use a gynecologist as their primary physician and have a Pap smear, breast examination, and blood pressure check during routine visits.

If you have a defined special problem, a subspecialist may be the best physician for you. The majority of your care can be provided by one physician and referral to other doctors can be arranged when needed.

You may want everyone in your family to see the same physician. This avoids the inconvenience of having several different doctors. More important, the physician who sees the entire family is better able to understand individual problems.

Rely upon your friends' experiences with their doctors. Question them closely about office practices.

If you know a doctor or nurse personally, ask them for a recommendation or call the head nurse at your local hospital. In most communities there are a few doctors to whom all the doctors and nurses go. These are always good doctors, but it is sometimes difficult to find out who they are. When you need the name of a physician and cannot obtain reliable information elsewhere, call your county medical society. They will have a list of physicians in the area who will accept new patients. Note that the medical society is providing information, not making recommendations; any member of the local society who is available may be given to you as a name. If you live near a medical school, you can obtain the names of their clinical faculty.

When choosing a doctor, do not place much emphasis on the social status of the office address, the depth of the carpet, the clothing of the staff, or the hairstyle of the physician. Also, don't worry about the length of the wait. The practice of good medicine means that the physician's working day will be busy, some problems will require more time than anticipated, and emergencies may arise in the middle of the day. Delays occur in the best organized practices, particularly with the most conscientious physicians. Take something useful to do in the waiting room; don't depend on the office magazines. The central question is this: Is this physician acting in the best interests of each patient? You may be waiting now, but you may need this same special attention later.

HOW TO DETECT POOR MEDICAL SERVICE

There are some tip-offs to poor medical practices. If you are taking three or more different medicines daily, you are probably receiving poor advice, unless you have a serious medical problem. If nearly every visit to the physician results in an injection or a new prescription, there may be a problem. Be wary if the physician recommends a costly service when you are not aware of any problem. Ask about any tests you do not understand. If your questions remain unanswered or if the physician fails to perform any physical examination at all, it's time to worry.

Under each of the medical problems in Section II, we give you an idea of what to expect at the doctor's office. If the physician does not perform these actions, there is cause for some questioning. Expectations noted in this book are conservative and should be met in large part by most good physicians.

Free choice of physicians is available in the United States. For the "free market" to work effectively, you must be willing to "vote with your feet." In other words, if you cannot communicate effectively with your physician, seek another physician. If your questions are not adequately answered, go somewhere else. If practice does not live up to your expectations and to the guidelines of this book, select another physician.

But remember that your physician is human too. The physician is faced with a continual barrage of complaints from patients which cannot

Finding the Right Physician

be solved coming from patients who demand solutions. Don't use the physician for trivial problems. Don't erode medical ethics by requests for misleading insurance claims, exaggerated disability statements, or repeated prescriptions for pain medication. The high ethical standards of the medical profession continue to impress us; still, human is human, and sometimes problems begin with unconscious manipulation by the patient.

Support good medical practices and become a committed medical consumer. If you believe that women should be in medicine, don't avoid female physicians when you seek your own personal care. If you would like to see more family physicians in this country, don't seek a specialist to direct your own care. If you like house-calls, respect the physician who will make them. If you want physicians to settle in your geographical area, patronize the physician closest to your home. If cost is important to you, compare the charges of several physicians.

"Doctor-shopping"—going from physician to another to find one who will give you the treatment you want even if it is not warranted—will almost certainly result in poor care. Find a physician who suits you, even if you must change doctors several times. But when you find a satisfactory situation, stay with it. Change early but not often.

Using the guidelines of this chapter, you can arrange for the physician and payment system that will best fit your medical needs.

4 Aging and Vitality

New understanding of the aging process has been achieved over the past several years, and the implications are startling. Aging, like health, is now known to be under personal control to a much greater extent than previously thought. To a considerable degree, you can decide not to age. This chapter reviews this new information, which gives yet another meaning to the phrase "take care of yourself."

THE BAD NEWS: YOU CAN'T LIVE FOREVER

Humans are mortal. Like dogs, hamsters, horses, and other animals, humans have a fixed average life span for their species. If you do not die of illness or accident, you will die a natural death when you reach the end of your life span. There are no exceptions to the biological rules that determine the length of life. This is the "bad news."

The human life span appears to be fixed at an average of about 85 years of age, with an absolute maximum life duration of about 115 years. Studies of ancient humans suggest that this maximum duration of life has been constant for some 100,000 years. Intuitively, most of us recognize that eventually the function of our vital organs, which become less efficient with increasing age, will no longer support life, and that at this time we will die a natural death, of "old age." As disease is prevented by the patient or successfully treated by the doctor, "life expectancy" can be increased. By following good health habits as outlined in this book and preventing your own premature death, you can increase your "life expectancy" but not your maximum life span.

Often these simple facts have not been directly faced, and thus for a long time research in human aging was a quest for the secrets of longevity and even immortality. Predictions that we would soon live to be 200 years old because of vitamin C, vitamin E, Gerovital, or some other magical elixir have obscured a more reasonable quest—increased vitality in old age.

Four popular myths have increased the confusion. The "myth of the super-centenarian" states that there are some people who live to be more than 120 years old. Scientists have sought individuals claiming great age, but in every instance the claims could not be verified. The oldest person, a Japanese, has attained a verified age of 115 years. In the United States no one has yet reached the age of 114. The reasons for the false claims are varied—ignorance, avoidance of military service, prestige, and others—but now there is no question that this myth is false.

The "myth of Shangri-la" claims that there are distant mountain regions, perhaps in Peru, Tibet, or Soviet Georgia, where people have found the secret of long life. Recently, careful studies of these proposed regions have exploded this myth. There is systematic age exaggeration in these locations, due principally to ignorance but more recently influenced by the tourist attraction provided by the claims.

The "myth of Methuselah" holds that persons lived to great ages, but only in the past. The 969 years of Methuselah remains the record claim of all time, and Adam is said to have lived well over 900 years. Acceptance of these ages hinges upon the question of literal interpretation of the Book of Genesis, since there are no other supporting documents. At any rate, the duration of life of the Biblical patriarchs has little apparent relevance to our present day.

The "myth of the Fountain" had its clearest expression in the search of Ponce de León for the legendary Fountain of Youth, said to be somewhere near the present location of Disney World. The "fountain" theme is present in the histories of nearly every culture and has its counterpart in rejuvenating elixirs that are promoted even at this time. Suffice it to say that these claims remain as false and diverting as they have been in the past. Indeed, as we shall see, there are ways to slow the aging process, but they have nothing to do with magic potions.

If all disease and accidents are eliminated, the natural human life span centers at an average of approximately 85 years, with 95 percent of the population dying between the ages of 73 and 97. The life span of our modern society, for the first time in history, is beginning to approach these average figures, as deaths due to diseases have been greatly reduced. Many major diseases of previous years, such as smallpox, polio, tuberculosis, diphtheria, tetanus, and rheumatic fever have been nearly eliminated as threats to life. In 1900, the average person died of illness or accident at 47 years of age. Now, the average is 72 years and is still rising. The natural life span has not changed, but the average life expectancy is now much greater.

As illness is cured or prevented, it is more common for us to live into "old age," and to almost the very end of our natural life span. Obviously, the closer we get to the ideal, the harder it is to make further progress. If the life span will not be extended in our lifetimes (and almost all scientists agree), we must focus our efforts elsewhere. We must be concerned with the quality of life rather than its duration. We must put the myths behind us and look instead to what might be done to increase vigor and vitality in old age. And here the news is much better.

THE GOOD NEWS: YOU CAN STAY YOUNG

You can slow down your own aging. Almost every important aspect of aging can be modified, by you. The difference between biological age and chronological age can be as much as thirty years.

What is aging anyway? Is it birthdays? White hair? Wrinkled skin? The problem with any definition of growing old is that aging is not one thing but many. Scientists have worked with many different markers of aging, including blood pressure, skin elasticity, grey hair, cholesterol, reaction time, and lung capacity. None of these describe aging very well, and with all of them some people seem to age much more rapidly than others.

In approaching old age, most people fear the loss of the ability to get around easily, loss of intellect and memory, and development of some lingering and painful disease. In sum, most people think of old age as dependence upon others, inability to take care of themselves, and increasing loneliness and isolation. Old age thus has little to do with the number of birthdays, the color of hair, or spots on the skin.

Scientists have now begun to study the differences between individuals. Why do some people age more rapidly in particular ways than others? Can we identify the good factors in the "slow agers" and apply them to others? This is the source of the good news: the factors can be identified, and they can be modified.

Consider a simple example of the beginning jogger. Scientists know that our ability to run a given distance at maximum speed decreases by about one to two percent for every year of life over age thirty. This is the aging process, and similar declines in function occur in every body organ and function. As you grow older, your maximum ability decreases, very slowly but very steadily.

But beginning runners improve steadily even as they grow older. Year after year they can improve running times and become more fit and physically stronger. Loss of mobility is one of the three great fears of growing old. Yet in this case mobility improves with age, and the same thing happens regardless of the age at which the activity is started—this is a paradox, representing in an important way a reversal of what we think of as growing old.

How can we improve with age when our maximum ability is decreasing by perhaps two percent each year? The answer: we were not previously operating at our maximum ability. Few of us are working at our limit in any area; if we are not, then we can improve despite increasing age.

How can we improve? The answer is again obvious: practice. If we wish to maintain or improve a skill or function, we must use that skill or function. If we don't use it, we will lose it. If we do not train and work at a function, that function ages more rapidly.

Can we slow the progression of all aging markers? Probably not. At this time, it appears that some features of increasing age cannot be altered. Some of these are listed in Table 4–1. These features relate, for the most part, to fibrosis—the accumulation of fibrous scar tissue in our tissues. This fibrosis is not reversible, and its accumulation may represent the biological imperative that ultimately limits our life span.

The list given in Table 4–2 represents the good news. There are far more aspects of aging that can be modified than cannot, and the modifiable features are the ones that most of us think of as the most important.

TABLE 4–1 **Unavoidable Aspects of Aging**	Greying of Hair Loss of Skin Elasticity Development of Cataracts Fibrosis of Arteries

TABLE 4–2 **Modifiable Aspects of Aging**	Feature	Modifying Factors
	Physical fitness	Exercise, weight control, nonsmoking
	Heart reserve	Aerobic exercises
	Mobility	Stretching exercises
	Blood pressure	Exercise
	Intelligence	Practice
	Memory	Practice
	Reaction time	Exercise
	Isolation	Socialization

Studies have now shown that training and use can improve scores on intelligence tests, even in individuals over the age of seventy; that the loss of short-term memory often associated with aging can be improved by practice in related areas; and that reaction times in active people of ages sixty and seventy can be as quick as those of typical sedentary twenty-year-olds. Change has been scientifically demonstrated for each of the important features listed. The crucial aspects of aging, like health, are under individual control, within broad limits.

Our society has not encouraged the avoidance of aging, and this has resulted in an apparent aging rate that is unnecessarily rapid. We have expected the older individual to be less active, perhaps as a reward for a long period of hard work. We have tried too often to take care of our senior citizens rather than trying to help our elders take care of themselves. We have not fully respected the value of accumulated wisdom and have almost forced people to retire at the early age of sixty-five. We have failed to recognize that by so doing we increase financial dependence, remove the individual from the stimulation of new inputs, decrease social interactions which prevent isolation, and reduce the sense of contribution which affects the feeling of self-worth.

The study of the modifiable aspects of aging has just begun, and it represents a new scientific frontier. In most areas we do not yet know how much change is possible, nor do we know the best way to accomplish it. The following principles are speculative in part and general in nature. But as we move from our preoccupations with disease and longevity, these principles represent an approach to the maintenance of a full and vigorous life.

PRINCIPAL PRINCIPLES

The avoidance of aging requires a strategy, and a general strategy of six interrelated principles is outlined below.

1. Maintain Independence

Personal autonomy and confidence appear to be the underlying requirements for preservation of vitality. Psychologists have developed at least two theories to explain these observations. First, health and avoidance of depression have been linked to the prevention of "helplessness," a feeling that there are no options, nothing is worthwhile, and that there is no way to avoid the situation. Second, a related theory uses the awkward term "locus of control" to differentiate those people who act as though they are in control of their environment (internal control) and those who act as though they are controlled by their environment (external locus of control). Either way, personal autonomy, plans for the future, looking forward, and taking care of yourself are critically important.

2. Moderate Your Habits

This subject is discussed in Chapter 1 as a means to good health. It is even more important as a means of slowing the aging process. The cigarette smoker, heavy drinker, or fat person ages faster than their more moderate counterparts. And the avoidance of chronic diseases such as emphysema, cancer, and arteriolosclerosis makes it much easier to maintain vigor in later life.

3. Keep Active

Exercise regularly and pleasurably, at least four days a week for at least fifteen minutes a day. Use your muscles, and build up your heart reserve. Your cells will become more efficient in the use of oxygen, and you will increase your stamina through the rest of the day. Stretching exercises will give you flexibility and help avoid muscle strain. Walk, jog, bicycle, or swim regularly. Play tennis or some other sport for fun. If you have a medical problem or if you are starting out in poor shape, take it slow and easy at first. There is no hurry, and you can take a year or more to get back into shape. But develop a lifelong habit and maintain it.

4. Be Enthusiastic

The enthusiasm of youth is always tempered by the wisdom of increasing years, and this is undoubtedly good in part. But it seems that our society sometimes places a value on indifference and grudging acceptance. To stay young you need to act young in some sense, and this means that enthusiasm is perfectly permissible. What do you really want to do? Work, travel, sport, hobby? Do it. Plan ahead and savor the anticipation. Do new things, change hobbies, develop new skills. And enjoy them. You are not old as long as you look forward with real pleasure to anticipated events in the future.

5. Have Pride

Psychologists use the term "self-image" in order to avoid some of the negative associations of the term "pride," but this is really what it is. "Pride" is a vice, but having a good "self-image" is a virtue. You must think well of yourself. Individuals with low self-image are sick more often, become depressed, and appear to age more rapidly. Pride can take almost any form, such as in personal appearance, household maintenance, family, friends, work, hobby, play. There are things that you do well. Be proud of what you do.

6. Be An Individual

As you grow older, you are more and more unique. There is no one else with your particular set of life experiences, insights, and beliefs. These are your strengths, and they make you interesting to others. Cultivate this individuality. As you actively grow and change, your personal uniqueness increases. Your individuality is not set early in life but develops as you develop. Avoid conformity for its own sake, both with your peer group or your own earlier behaviors and beliefs.

A frequent problem of increasing age is a monotony of inputs: the same newspaper, television programs, magazines, and set of acquaintances with pretty much the same opinions about everything. You need to vary your ingrained habits so that you are exposed to uncomfortable opinions, challenges to your established thinking, and new political inputs, so that your unique synthesis of the conflicting threads of our complex society can grow. This may entail new classes, seminars, hobbies, interest groups, or whatever. Don't let yourself become predictable. You are unique.

Perhaps you see a paradox in that you cannot outlive the life span of our species but can modify the rate at which you age. How can this be?

Oliver Wendell Holmes, Sr., once wrote whimsically about the wonderful "one-hoss shay": A deacon, perhaps dismayed by the constant breakdowns of current products, built his own horseless carriage to exacting specifications. Everything was so well made that it could not break down. The one-hoss shay performed marvelously and was used for generations. Its parts were so perfectly matched that none could be the first to fail. But after exactly one hundred years of perfect performance, it suddenly collapsed into a pile of dust. It had aged, and finally all the parts failed simultaneously in an almost triumphant terminal collapse.

There are limitations to the avoidance of aging. A decline in maximal performance of about 1 to 2 percent per year after age thirty is not avoidable. But there are many examples of what can be achieved and what cannot. Churchill, Mao, Tito, Picasso, Grandma Moses, Bertrand Russell, George Bernard Shaw, Mary Baker Eddy, Albert Schweitzer, Michelangelo, Pablo Casals, and many others have shown creativity and leadership after the age of eighty-five and often into their tenth decade. None had discovered the elusive Fountain of Youth. All exemplified the principles of the preceding section. None eluded the statistical boundaries that define our mortality. But all showed the potential for vital life until its very end, as expressed by the allegory of the "wonderful one-hoss shay."

The paradox is resolved if we consider the consequences of an unchangeable life span and a changeable rate for aging. Our period of vigorous and vital life can be prolonged, and our final period of infirmity can be shortened. Fears of dependence and lingering illness can be reduced. Taking care of yourself does not result in a longer old age. To the contrary, what we usually think of as old age is compressed into a shorter period, since the period of adult vigor is prolonged.

In many ways these implications represent a celebration of life. Psychologists have shown that death is feared less than depression, isolation, infirmity, sickness, and increasing pain in the final days of life. Yet these are the very factors that can be modified and avoided through personal action.

The life course we suggest here, with careful personal attention to the determinants of poor health such as smoking, drinking to excess, inactivity, and overweight, is no longer in dispute. But psychologists who have studied the reasons people change habits have pointed out that a promise of longer life has very little "incentive value." Life changes that must be undertaken in youth are unlikely if the reward is additional months or years of dependent living many years in the future.

Taking care of yourself, in all of the senses of this book, has much more relevant dividends. The rewards of the avoidance of aging are immediate, at any age. They include more vigor, more stamina, fewer sick days, and they range from greater intellectual exhilaration to a more active sex life. The additional months and years of vigor replace those that otherwise might have represented dependence and depression.

The new challenges to society must be faced. Soon over 90 percent of the population will live to be over seventy years of age. The vitality of our increasingly elderly population will depend upon the independence of these individuals. Presently our society does not encourage independence in the elderly. We must abandon the concepts that turn people "out to pasture" and the programs that forsake autonomy for regimented total care. The future is bright, if we attend to it.

5 Special Problems of the Senior Citizen

Medical problems are different for the older patient for various reasons: the way that the body reacts to illness or medication, the difficulties that are likely to be present at the same time, the special illnesses that occur only in the elderly, and because our society has not yet learned the lessons of the previous chapter. A detailed treatment of the new subject area known as geriatric medicine would require several volumes; here we briefly describe a few of the most important considerations.

SOME QUESTIONS OF MEDICATION

As we grow older, above the age of thirty, we begin to lose a part of our "organ reserve." In youth, our hearts can pump ten times the amount of blood required to sustain life, our kidneys can excrete six times the waste products that we produce in our bodies each day, and every other organ has similar reserve powers which fortunately are very seldom required. After age thirty, we begin to lose this reserve at a rate of one or two percent each year. We don't even notice the loss, unless we are in a situation in which we really need it. Loss of reserve power means that it is more difficult to restore the equilibrium of the body after a severe insult to a body function.

As we age, our bodies detoxify drugs at a slower rate. In medical terms, the drug is metabolized more slowly. A little goes a long way. In essence, we can get the same effect for a lower dosage; the regular dose of a drug can become an overdose. The first rule that a good physician observes with an older patient is to keep the dose low.

Side effects of medications can simulate disease, and unwary physicians and patients often mistake a drug reaction for an underlying medical problem. A small dose of codeine may cause severe fatigue and sleepiness, a little digitalis may cause profound nausea and vomiting, a diuretic to remove fluid from the ankles may cause dizziness and kidney problems. The second rule that a good physician observes is to suspect that the whole problem might be a minor drug reaction, cured simply by removing the offending drug.

Entirely new side effects can appear in the elderly. A sleeping pill may keep the patient awake. A tranquilizer may excite the patient or cause severe depression. These paradoxical reactions are not fully understood, but they are very common. Again, the good physician and the thoughtful patient or relative will suspect the drug first.

THE PROBLEM OF THE MULTIPLE PROBLEM

Most of the major diseases of our time are more common in the older patient. Diabetes, atherosclerosis, osteoarthritis, cancer, and the other major problems are more common with increasing age. And the older patient, with less organ reserve, may have several problems at once, thus creating special difficulties.

In Section II we have provided decision charts for dealing with the common problems that come up. The charts work almost all of the time for the young patient, but not as often for the patient who has more than one problem. If you already have one significant medical problem, a second one is more serious than if it occurred when you were in good health. Because the simple rules do not apply as well in this situation, you have to use more judgment. In general, a combination of problems is more serious than the sum of the problems dealt with by themselves.

One problem can easily complicate another. High blood pressure can increase kidney failure which can increase blood pressure. A problem of breathlessness caused by the heart can complicate breathlessness caused by lung disease. Arthritis can increase inactivity which leads to blood clots in the legs. Your approach to these problems must be a compromise in which all aspects of the situation are considered. You need a doctor to help you in these decisions much more often than in the uncomplicated, isolated illnesses of relative youth.

THE PROBLEM OF MULTIPLE MEDICATIONS

In medical slang, using too many medications is termed "polypharmacy." A patient may be taking a diuretic (water pill), a uricosuric to help eliminate the uric acid caused by the water pill, a tranquilizer for anxiety, a sedative to sleep, an antacid to settle the stomach, a hormone to replace lost glandular functions, a pain medication for arthritis, an antiinflammatory agent for muscle aches, a laxative to help elimination, miscellaneous vitamins and minerals "just in case," iron for the blood, and additional medicines whenever a new problem comes up. This is polypharmacy, and it is usually a prelude to disaster. It happens most often in an older patient, and usually the use of all the drugs has built up over a long time. Often the physician prescribing a new agent is not even aware of the long list of drugs already being taken.

The side effects of these many medications add up and may cause illness. Even more importantly, the drugs may interact. Sedatives can dangerously slow the metabolism of coumadin, a blood thinning drug. The action of the uric acid drug may be blocked by aspirin. Antacids can destroy the effectiveness of antibiotics. Antiinflammatory drugs can cause retention of fluid which requires a water pill or diuretic for relief. As we indicated, drug interactions are so complicated that no physician or scientist fully understands them.

Use as few drugs as possible. No drug interactions can occur if only a single drug is taken. This is not possible for all patients at all times, but if your drug intake is minimal, your doctor can usually find combinations that are known to work well together.

These are our three general principles:

(1) Avoid tranquilizers (nerve pills), sedatives (sleeping pills), and analgesics (pain pills) whenever possible. These drugs have many bad effects and often do not solve the basis of the problems.

(2) Use lifestyle change instead of medication whenever possible. Avoiding salt in your diet is better than taking a "water pill," exercise programs can reduce the need for blood pressure medications, and weight reduction will usually work better than pills for diabetes. There are many other examples listed throughout this book.

(3) Get rid of the optional medications. Crucial drugs make up less than 10 percent of all prescriptions in the United States. Over 1.5 billion prescriptions are written each year in our country; this represents 8 prescriptions for every man, woman, and child. And the figure is much higher for the elderly.

In addition to tranquilizers, sedatives, and minor pain medications, optional drugs include allopurinol (Zyloprim) given for uric acid elevation without gout, diuretics (water pills) given for "fluid retention" in the absence of an actual disease, hormonal supplements that are not related to a disease, and the pills (oral hypoglycemics) given for adult diabetes. There are many others. This is not to say that these drugs are not beneficial on occasion, but more often they are not necessary. The decision to use them must be made with caution.

DIABESITY

There is no such disease as diabesity, and yet it is one of the most common problems encountered in the older patient. Diabesity is the combination of diabetes and obesity, and the two go together much like Tweedledum and Tweedledee (who probably had diabesity themselves).

If you are overweight, you are much more likely to have elevated blood sugar in your urine (diabetes), and if you have diabetes, you are very likely to be overweight. The combination is called diabesity.

The terminology of diabetes is confusing. Older people with diabetes almost always have the mild form, variously called adult-onset diabetes, Type II diabetes, noninsulin dependent diabetes mellitus, or NIDDM. This is a very different condition than the juvenile (Type I) diabetes that begins early in life and often has serious complications. The childhood diabetic may go into diabetic coma and almost always requires insulin as a treatment. The older diabetic usually does not require any medication.

Only a few years ago, it was felt that all diabetics should be on medication to control their blood sugar, and drugs that could be taken by mouth were developed (Orinase, Diabinase, DBI) for this purpose. Studies, some of them still controversial, began to show serious side effects from these drugs and/or failure to improve the problem with the diabetes. Sometimes patients who received the drugs fared worse than those who received nothing at all. Gradually, these medications are being given to fewer and fewer patients. They do have a place, but only in special situations.

At the same time, it was increasingly recognized that the blood sugar level would improve with weight loss and exercise. Indeed, the majority of "diabetic" obese older individuals who are successful in reducing to a normal body weight and developing a regular exercise program lose all signs of this major disease. Thus we have a problem in terminology. Is a condition that is remedied with diet and exercise a disease? Or just a bad habit?

Not all people with diabesity will totally improve with weight reduction and exercise; some also need to pay special attention to their diet. Your physician can advise you about the specifics of the diet that you need; the principles are to avoid getting too much carbohydrate (sugars and starches) at one time, and to spread your calorie intake out over the day so that you don't get too many calories at any one time. A few people may still require drugs if these measures do not suffice.

Diabesity is a sign of accelerating aging in your body, and should be taken as a major signal to revitalize. You need to be taking better care of yourself.

DEPRESSION

Down in the dumps. Hopeless and helpless. All of your best days behind you. No one really cares. And you keep growing older.

Depression represents one of our great fears of aging. Ever[y]
these feelings to some extent. There is no need to be ashamed
feelings; they are justified and normal, and they are nearly un[...]

The depth and duration of depression vary greatly among
A severe depression may cause weight loss, sleeplessness, slow[...]
ment and speech, and may be complicated by fear that a canc[...]
In a severe depression, suicide may be contemplated. Severe [...]
quires professional help. It can be alleviated, but sometimes i[...]
a while to improve.

Most depression in older individuals is much more easily
often the depressive symptoms are not even recognized as de[...]
depressed patient may complain of fatigue, insomnia, constip[...]
in the muscles and joints. Once the problem is recognized a[...]
origins in depression, recovery is likely.

If you think you may be depressed, check the drugs you are taking.
The easiest way to cure depression is to stop taking a drug that is causing
it. "Downers," which are frequently used as tranquilizers, can cause
depression and have very little use in the care of the older person. Codeine
and other painkillers, as well as antihistamines, can also cause or aggravate depression. Even sleeping pills, because of the unnatural type of sleep
they induce, can contribute to depression. Some arthritis medicines, notably prednisone and indomethacin, can cause depressive reactions.

The principles of the previous chapter will help you to alleviate depression. Increase your activity and exercise. Change your pace. Visit friends.
Go on a vacation. Start new hobbies. Do some things you've always wanted
to do but kept postponing. Project and anticipate future events. Make long-
range plans. Set intermediate goals. Work at living. Plan an exciting future event and begin saving and planning for it.

Know your limits. Get help if you can't alleviate your depression, when
it is very severe, or involves thoughts of suicide. Most depressions ease and
disappear if you work at life, but some need some special care.

VITAMINS

Unless you have an unusual medical condition or eat an incredibly unbal-
anced diet, you do not require vitamin supplements. If you have pernicious
anemia, you may need vitamin B_{12} shots; vitamin D is sometimes prescribed for severe osteoporosis, iron and other minerals may be needed on
occasion; and folic acid is needed once in a while for another kind of
anemia.

Having made the above statement, we must confess that we don't
think vitamin supplements or even "megavitamin" programs do much
harm. As a rule, only vitamins A and D are likely to be toxic in large
doses. There is more emotionalism about vitamins than about almost any
subject, and if someone tells us that they are benefiting from a particular

...min program, we encourage them to continue it. Generally, the potential harm of these programs involves their cost and the possibility that needed medical care may not be undertaken because of the assumption that the vitamins are enough.

We feel very differently about the systematic hoaxes that use vitamins as a gimmick. In these promotions the "secret tonic" may be vitamins, minerals, gerovital, or snake oil, but the sales pitch is the same: you need the secret tonic and must buy it from the promoter (who makes a large profit from the transaction).

Laetrile is not actually a vitamin but is promoted as one. Often but not always it is offered as part of an exploitation scheme. While medical authorities have raised alarms over the small amount of cyanide contained in Laetrile, its real harm comes from the theft of dignity. It is difficult enough to treat cancer without spending the last few days of your life realizing that you were deluded by a monumental swindle. Scientific evidence that this agent is not effective in treatment of any form of cancer is now accumulating and is now conclusive.

The megavitamin situation is more whimsical, and aside from a few prominent book authors no one is making very much money from these proffered solutions to the difficulties of life. Vitamin C has been most imaginatively promoted. As evidence mounted that it did not help the common cold it was advocated for cancer treatment. As evidence grew that it didn't work there it was touted as an arthritis cure. We have studied its effects in arthritis and can't find any. We suspect that next it will be suggested that it helps stop hardening of the arteries.

Common sense is your best guide to vitamin use. Consider it carefully.

PREVENTING ARTHRITIS

To an extent, we all experience some degree of osteoarthritis as we get older and our joint cartilage wears down. But, some people have a lot of osteoarthritis at a relatively early age and others have very little at an advanced age. The goal with arthritis, as with other aspects of aging described in the previous chapter, is to slow its development. This is best begun early in life, but the lifestyles that postpone arthritis help at any age; they also help the heart and blood vessels. The following three principles may sound familiar, for they are echoed in many other parts of this book.

First, KEEP FIT. Exercise increases the strength of the bones and the stability of the supporting ligaments and tendons. Exercise nourishes the joint cartilage by bringing nutrients to the cartilage and removing waste products. Regular, gently graded, permanent exercise programs are required.

Second, CONTROL YOUR WEIGHT. Being overweight places unnecessary stress on joints by changing the angles at which the ligaments attach to the bone as well as by the additional impact on the feet, ankles, knees, hips, and lower back.

Third, PROTECT YOUR JOINTS. Listen to the pain messages that your body sends, and perform activities in the least stressful way. Joints, ligaments, and tendons can be damaged by misuse of a part that is already injured. If you are suffering with discomfort from an activity, do not take a pain pill so that you can continue the activity. Listen to the pain message and change the activity appropriately.

The postponement or management of arthritis is a large and complex subject. We have written extensively about these problems in *Arthritis: A Comprehensive Guide*, and about what you can do to help yourself in *The Arthritis Helpbook*. (See the reference section at the end of this book.)

OSTEOPOROSIS

Sometimes it seems as though almost everyone is "suffering from osteoporosis," yet osteoporosis is really not even a disease. In this condition, the bones gradually lose much of their calcium and become weaker and more brittle. But they do not hurt! You can't "suffer" from osteoporosis; indeed, you can't even tell that you have it.

There is a tendency for all of us to lose calcium from our bones as we get older, particularly if we are not active. Exercise, particularly weight-bearing exercise like walking, acts to keep the bones strong. Hormones, such as cortisone or prednisone, can cause a much more rapid loss of calcium. Women tend to lose calcium, particularly after menopause, when loss is rapid. Some diseases also cause loss of calcium.

While osteoporosis is not a disease, it can lead to serious problems with broken bones. The vertebrae in the back can collapse and cause much discomfort. A fall can result in a fracture that would not have occurred if the bones were of normal strength. A fracture of the hip is particularly serious, but almost any bone can break.

Medical treatment can help somewhat. You need enough calcium in your diet, but excessive amounts are not absorbed by the body. Vitamin D and similar compounds may help some people. Hormone (estrogen) treatment is occasionally undertaken and can slow the process, but it carries significant risks.

Prevention is important, and you should start early. It is useful to maintain some calcium in your diet, perhaps by drinking a glass of milk a day. Osteoporosis is a very gradual process, occurring over many years, and prevention must continue similarly. Exercise and activity are the most important features of your prevention program. Avoid drugs such as prednisone whenever possible. If you have had a fracture, find out what your doctor thinks about vitamin D treatment, calcium supplements, or hormone treatments.

THE ACTIVATED ELDER

This is the bottom line. The special problems of the senior citizen are not so different, but they are more difficult. Even more than young people, elders need to take care of themselves. We do not mean to imply that these problems are easy or that they can be entirely resolved. They are very complex, and your solutions, as you grow older, are more likely to be partial solutions rather than total cures. But the solutions are largely in your own hands, and as you increasingly take charge of the management of your own health, you grow more confident and more independent. "Do not go gentle into that good night," said Dylan Thomas.

6 The Office Visit

A visit to the doctor's office can be a mysterious undertaking. This chapter will help you understand the procedures a physician follows when you come to the office with a medical problem. It will stress the importance of your active participation in these procedures and the advantages of strictly following your doctor's instructions.

THE MEDICAL HISTORY: TELLING IT LIKE IT IS

The medical history is the most important communication between the patient and the physician. Your ability to give a concise, organized description of your illness is essential. The patient who rambles on about irrelevant details and doesn't mention real fears and problems is his or her own worst enemy. An inability to give a good medical history is expensive in terms of your health and your dollars.

Most people do not realize that every physician uses a similar process to learn a patient's medical history. Obviously, the physician must organize information to be able to remember it accurately and to reason correctly. Knowledge of the organization can help you give accurate information to your doctor. The physician organizes information under five headings: the chief complaint, the present illness, the past medical history, the review of systems, and the social history. Physicians will not always request information in the same order, but the following descriptions will help you understand the purposes of the medical interview in which you are participating.

The Chief Complaint

Following the initial greeting, the "chief complaint" is usually the first information sought by the physician. This question may take several forms: "What bothers you the most?" "What brings you here today?" What's the trouble?" or "What is your biggest problem?" The purpose of such questions is to establish the priorities for the rest of the medical history process. Be sure you express your problem clearly. Know in advance how to state your chief complaint: "I have a sore throat." "I have a pain in my lower right side." Any of the problems listed in the second section of this book may be your chief complaint, and there are hundreds of less common problems.

Think of the "chief complaint" as the title for the story you are about to tell the doctor. Do not give the details of your illness at this time, Instead, title your illness appropriately and provide the doctor with a heading under which to understand your problem.

Sometimes you may go to the physician with more than one problem, and you may not know if the problems are related. Identify this situation for the doctor. "I seem to have three problems: sore throat, skin rash, and cloudy urine." The physician can then investigate each of these areas.

Tell it like it is. If you have a sexual problem, do not say that your chief complaint is that you're "tired and run down." If you are afraid that you have cancer, do not say that you came for a "checkup." If you mislead the physician because of embarrassment, the real reason for your visit may never be determined. You will compromise the physician's ability to be of assistance. An honest description is your best guarantee that your problems will be attended to correctly.

The Present Illness

Next, your physician will want to hear the story behind your chief complaint. This section of the interview will be introduced by a question such as: "When did this problem begin?" "When were you last entirely well?" or "How long has this been going on?" The first fact the physician wants to establish is how long you have had the problem. Be sure that you know the answer to this question in advance: "Yesterday." "On June 4th." "About the middle of May." If you are uncertain as to the date the problem began, state the uncertainty and tell what you can. "I am not sure when these problems began. I began to feel tired in the middle of February, but the pain in the joints did not begin until the end of April." The physician can then determine the starting point for the illness.

After you define the starting point for the problem, the doctor will want to establish the sequence of events from that time until the present. Tell the story in the order it occurred. Do not use "flashbacks"; you will only confuse yourself and your physician. Do not attempt to tell everything you can remember about the illness, but highlight those events which seem most important to you. Use short, clear sentences. Do not include irrelevant occurrences in your family or social situation. Your cause is not aided by reference to the relatives who were visiting you at the time, the purchases you made at the shopping center, or the state of international affairs. If you confuse your story, the chances for a successful solution to your problems are decreased.

As you recount the sequence of the problem, sketch the highlights as you perceive them.

I was well until I developed a sore throat four weeks ago. I had a fever and some swollen glands in my neck. This lasted about a week, and then I felt better although still tired. One week ago the fever returned. I began to have pains in my joints, beginning with the right knee. The joint pain moved around from one joint to another, and I had pain in the shoulders, elbows, knees, and ankles. Over the last three days I have had a red rash over much of my body. I have not taken any medications except aspirin, which helps a little.

The physician may interrupt the story to ask specific questions. At the end of the story, questions may be asked about problems that you have not mentioned. By making your account well organized and then allowing the physician to ask additional questions, you provide information in the most effective way.

If you have several problems to recount, the history of each may be told separately, or they may be intertwined in a single story. The physician can help you choose the most appropriate procedure.

Supporting information can be extremely important. Know which medications you have taken before and during the course of the present illness. Bring the medication bottles to the physician. If you are pregnant or could be pregnant, tell the physician. If X rays or laboratory tests have been performed during the course of the illness, attempt to make these materials or a report of the results available to the physician. Mention any allergic reactions that you have to drugs. If other physicians have been consulted, bring those medical records with you. Attempt to be a careful observer of your own illness. Your observations, if carefully made and recounted, are more valuable than any other source of information.

The Past Medical History

After hearing your chief complaint and a history of your medical problem, your physician will want more background information about your general health. At this point, information that did not appear important earlier may be relevant. The physician will ask specific questions and will be assisted by direct, reasonably brief answers. You will be asked about your general health, hospitalizations, operative procedures, allergies, and medications. The physician may be interested in childhood illnesses as well as those occurring during adult life. (Record this information in Section III so it will be readily available.)

The subjects most frequently misreported are allergies and medications. If you report a drug "allergy," describe the specific reaction you experienced. Many drug side effects (such as nausea, vomiting, or ringing in the ears) are *not* allergic reactions. Physicians are rightfully wary of prescribing drugs to which an allergy has been reported. If you report an allergy to a drug to which you are not allergic, you may deprive yourself of a useful method of treatment. Be thorough when reporting medications. Birth control pills, vitamins, aspirin, and laxatives are medications that are frequently not reported. On occasion, each of these may be important in diagnosis or treatment of your medical problem.

The Review Of Systems

Next, your physician will usually review symptoms related to the different body systems; there are standard questions for each system. Your physician may begin with questions about the skin, then ask about the head, eyes, ears, nose, and throat, and then begin to move down the body. Questions about the lymph glands, the lungs, and the heart are followed by questions about the stomach, intestines, and urinary system. Finally there will be questions about muscles, bones, and the nervous system. In this questioning, the physician is looking for information that may have been missed previously and for additional factors that may influence the choice of therapy. A very detailed "review of systems" will only be taken when you are having a complete health examination.

The Social History

Finally, questions relating to your "social history" are addressed. Here, the physician may wish to know about your job, family, and interpersonal stresses. Questions may concern smoking, drinking, use of drugs, and sexual activity. Knowledge of exposures to chemical or toxic substances may be sought. Questions are sometimes intensely personal. However, the answers can be of the utmost importance in determining your illness and how it can be best treated. A detailed social history should be expected only in a complete health examination.

THE MEDICAL HISTORY AS AN INFORMATION SOURCE

The physician has three major sources of information: the medical history, the physical examination, and laboratory tests. Depending on the illness, any one of the three may be the most important. The medical history is the only source of information that is directly controlled by the patient. It is frequently termed "subjective" by physicians because the information cannot be directly verified. To the extent that you provide your physician with clear, accurate data, you increase the probability of an accurate diagnosis and successful treatment of your problem.

LEARN TO OBSERVE YOURSELF

The careful physical examination requires skill and experience. Some important observations can be made at home, and if you can report accurate information on these points, you can further help your doctor.

Temperature: Don't say "fever" or "running a temperature" or "burning up." Buy a thermometer, read the instructions, practice shaking the thermometer down, and be able to report the exact temperature. If you have a small child, buy a rectal thermometer and learn how to use it.

Pulse: If the problem involves a rapid or forceful heartbeat, know exactly how fast it is beating. Feel a pulse in the arm or throat, or put an ear to the chest. Count the exact number of beats occurring in one minute, or have someone do this for you. If you think that there is a problem with the pulse, determine whether the beat is regular or irregular. Is the heart "skipping a beat," "turning flip-flops," "missing every other beat," or is it completely irregular? A pulse irregularity is often gone by the time you reach the doctor. If you can describe it accurately, your doctor may be able to understand what happened. For more information, refer to Problem 76: Palpitations.

Breast: The mammary tissue is normally a bit lumpy. Adult women should carefully examine their breasts every month in order to detect changes. Press the breast tissue against the chest wall, not between the fingers. Try several positions— lying down, sitting, and with the arm on the side being examined raised over the head. Look particularly for differences between the two breasts. If you note a suspicious lump, see the doctor immediately. Many women delay out of fear. Please don't. Very few lumps are cancerous, but if the lump is malignant, it is important that it be removed early. Often the patient can feel a lump that the doctor misses; help the doctor locate the problem area. Detailed instructions for a self-examination can be found in "For Women Only" in Section II.

Weight: Changes in weight are frequently very important. Know what your normal weight is. If your weight changes, know by how much and over what period it changed.

Other Findings: Know your body. When something changes, report it accurately. A change in skin color, a lymph gland on the back of the neck, an increase in swelling in the legs, and many other new events are easily observed. Just as important, knowledge of your body will help you to avoid reporting silly things. The "Adam's apple" is not a tumor, "knobs" on the lower ribs or pelvis are usually normal, the vertebra at the lower neck normally sticks out, and there is a normal bump at the back of the head— the "knowledge bump." We have known patients to report each of these as emergencies.

ASK AND LISTEN: GET GOOD ADVICE THEN FOLLOW THROUGH

If you are a typical patient, you carry out less than one-half of the instructions given to you by your physician. Think back to your last encounter with your physician. After you started to feel better, did you discontinue the medication prematurely? Do you have pills left over from your last prescription? Did you honestly adhere to diet recommendations? Did you restrict or increase your activity as instructed? Did you take medication irregularly or exactly as prescribed? When a new illness occurred in your family, did you use "leftover" medication? If you did none of these things, you are a remarkable patient. We suspect that many patients don't understand their doctor's advice in the first place, so not following it is hardly surprising.

Let's look at the consequences of not following instructions:

First, there is the obvious waste of your time and money. You have sought expensive advice. As indicated in this book, there are many occasions when you do not require such advice. The advice will not always help, and sometimes it will be wrong. However, after you seek advice, it is foolish not to understand it clearly and then follow it. After you have arranged transportation to your doctor's office, waited until you could be seen, spent time with a trained professional, proceeded to a pharmacy, purchased medication, and finally returned home, you have invested a considerable amount of time and effort. Don't waste it by not getting your questions answered, accepting advice you don't understand or know you won't follow, or failing to follow through.

Second, there can be serious medical consequences if you don't follow instructions. The disease may persist; it may come back; you may have complications, side effects, or drug interactions. The most frequent consequence is that your problem may persist. For example, if you have an ulcer, the pain will usually respond to appropriate treatment within a few days. However, the ulcer crater, often large enough to stick your thumb into, has barely begun to heal. If treatment is not continued throughout a period of about six weeks, complete healing of the ulcer crater may not occur, and the symptoms of the persisting condition may recur as soon as treatment is discontinued.

With urinary tract infection, the symptoms of urinary burning, lower abdominal pain, and frequent urination usually disappear in the first forty-eight hours of treatment. However, the bacteria that are responsible for the condition may not be totally destroyed for several more days. If antibiotic treatment is not continued until the condition is under control, the infection may come back, necessitating repeated medical attention. As another example, when you go to the physician for a sore throat, your physician is treating you mainly to prevent complications. Serious complications of strep throat include damage to the heart (acute rheumatic fever) and to the kidneys. These complications are unusual if ten days of antibiotic therapy is taken. However, you will feel well after forty-eight hours and may neglect further therapy. This is a major reason that long-acting penicillin shots may be prescribed for strep throat, since the physician is certain by giving you an injection that you will receive all the medication. In every scientific study, the shots have proved superior to medication taken by mouth in preventing complications. Oral medication is not inferior, but patients are not always reliable in taking it.

Sometimes patients take too much medication. Many operate on the theory that if a little bit is good, a lot is better. All drugs are alien to the body and basically must be considered to be "poisons." When used in excess of recommended dosage, you may encounter increased side effects, dependence, addiction, or even death. You are gambling with your life when you increase the dosage without knowing if it is safe to do so.

Finally, drug interactions may occur. If a patient fails to report that other medication is being taken, the physician may prescribe a new drug that has unfortunate interactions with the original medication. This represents a breakdown in your communication with your physician.

Most important, the patient who accepts and then disregards instructions contributes to the dissipation of trust between patient and physician. Frequently, the patient who most strongly maintains that the physician "never explains things" is the same patient who disregards instructions. Not following "doctor's orders" can add a fundamental dishonesty into the patient-physician relationship. Future events cannot be correctly interpreted by the physician without accurate historical information. As a result, you receive more shots and fewer oral medications, and frequent visits are necessary so that the physician can check up on you. More blood tests are ordered to measure the actual blood levels of drugs you are supposed to be taking. Directness and honesty in the communication between doctor and patient can help avoid these problems. In this book we are often critical of medical practices. Here, we suggest that when communication is poor the blame must be shared.

UNDERSTAND AND ADHERE
TO YOUR PROGRAM

First, insist on understanding the importance of the medication and the instructions. Second, consider whether following the instructions poses any special problems. Third, adhere to the agreed program. Fourth, if medication is left over after the course of therapy, destroy it.

You must understand the instructions given to you. If you are confused, ask questions: "Could you go over that again?" "I don't understand what this medication is for." "Do I really have to be treated in the hospital?" "How much will this cost?" "Are there any risks to this drug?" Ask your doctor to write out the instructions. Understand the importance of each drug or treatment. In some instances it does not matter if you take the medicine regularly; in these circumstances the drug gives only symptomatic relief and should be discontinued as soon as possible. Be sure that you understand whether or not it is necessary to continue the medication after you feel well.

Consider the entire prescribed program. You may have difficulties not known to your physician. Perhaps you have trouble taking a medication at work, or you anticipate trouble with a prescribed diet. Perhaps reasons unknown to your physician prevent you from undertaking the recommended activity. If more than one medication has been prescribed initially, it may be more desirable for you to take them all at once. When such questions arise, ask in advance. Frequently, if you raise these questions with your physician, your treatment program can be modified so that you feel more comfortable. The keynote is honesty. Don't say that you will do something that you know you will not do. Express your worries.

After an agreed program has been developed, follow it closely. If you notice side effects from the program, call the physician and inquire. If the side effects are serious, return for an examination. Make a chart of the days of the week and the times when medications are to be taken. Note on the chart when you take the medicines. This is not an insult to your intelligence; this practice is universally used in hospitals by trained personnel to insure that medication schedules are maintained accurately. At home, you and your family are the custodians of your health. Do not view this task more lightly than it is viewed by professionals.

When pills remain at the end of a course of therapy, flush them down the toilet. A medicine chest containing old prescription medicines presents multiple hazards. Every year, children and adults die from taking leftover drugs. Children take birth control pills, adults brush their teeth with steroid creams, and the wrong medication is taken because one bottle was mistaken for another. If you give your leftover tetracycline to your children with their next cold, you may cause mottling of their teeth. If tetracycline becomes outdated and is subsequently used, dangerous liver damage may result. When a new illness occurs, the situation is confused if you have already taken leftover medications. Sometimes it will be impossible to make an accurate identification of a bacterium by culture, or the clinical picture of the disease may be distorted.

The doctor-patient encounter is the most reliable protection against serious illness. Value the opportunity for such attention, utilize it selectively, and follow the program you and your doctor develop to the maximum extent possible.

7 Choosing the Right Medical Facility

A wide variety of medical facilities are available to prospective patients—hospitals, emergency rooms, convalescent homes, and clinics. There are sufficient choices to satisfy most individual preferences. It's important to know the facilities in your area and to make your choices before you need the services.

To select the best facilities, you will need to understand the terms "primary," "secondary," and "tertiary" care. Primary medical care is provided by a physician at the office or at an emergency room or clinic. This care may be obtained by a patient without the referral of another physician. It is often called "ambulatory care" or "outpatient care." Secondary care is that provided by the typical community hospital, and the physicians involved may be specialists or subspecialists. As a rule, access to this care requires the referral of a physician. Much secondary care is "inpatient" or hospital care. Tertiary care includes special and extraordinary procedures such as kidney dialysis, open-heart surgery, and sophisticated treatment of rare diseases. This type of care is found at university-affiliated hospitals and regional referral centers.

When you select a medical facility, you want close primary care with good access to secondary care. Tertiary care is often a great distance from your home and may not be needed during your entire lifetime.

HOSPITALS

Private or community hospitals are the most common hospital facilities in the United States. These hospitals are usually nonprofit and contain from 50 to 400 beds. Sometimes they have been financed with funds from doctors practicing in the area. More frequently, nonprofit organizations aided by government funds for hospital construction, have financed the facility.

The quality of care in these institutions is largely dependent upon the physician in charge of your case. Relatively few physician actions come under serious review. A physician is not always present in the hospital at all times. Nevertheless, private hospitals usually give personalized care of high quality. The hospital is quiet and orderly. In the great majority of cases, facilities are adequate for the care required.

Public hospitals include city, county, public health service, military, and Veterans Administration hospitals. These hospitals are generally large, with from 500 to 1000 beds. They have permanent full-time staff, and physicians are present in the hospital at all times. Usually they have a "house staff," with interns and resident physicians always available. As befits their larger size, they offer more services and frequently have associated rehabilitation units or nursing homes. Activities in the public hospital are more visible, and the efforts of each physician are scrutinized by others. The quality of care you receive depends upon the overall quality of the institution. The presence of interns and residents may pose some minor inconveniences to you as a patient, but their presence is an excellent guarantee of good care. The physician-in-training has hospital patient care as his or her primary responsibility and is not greatly involved with office practice and administrative tasks.

Many public hospitals have the reputation for providing service to the poorer economic classes. Within the community, they are often perceived as offering substandard service. These accusations are usually grossly unfair. While not always quiet and orderly, and often not physically attractive, these hospitals give dependable and excellent care. When available, they should be seriously considered by individuals of all economic classes.

The teaching hospital is one associated with a medical school. Teaching hospitals are large and have from 300 to 2000 beds. These hospitals always have interns and residents as well as medical students on the hospital wards. They have superb technical resources, and it is here that the most extraordinary events of medicine take place. Open-heart surgery, transplantation of kidneys, elaborate nurseries for the newborn, support for management and rare blood diseases, and other marvels are all available here. Dozens of people may be concerned with the well-being of a particular patient. Crucial medical decisions are thoroughly discussed, presented at conferences, and reviewed by many personnel.

On the other hand, the quality of personal relationships at teaching hospitals is variable. Many patients feel that they are treated in an impersonal way, and that their laboratory tests receive more attention than their human and social problems. Since these institutions are on the frontier of medicine, there is a tendency to emphasize the new and elaborate procedures, when older and more modest ones might have served as well. With the inexperience of some members of the care team, there is a tendency to order more laboratory tests than would have been considered necessary for the same condition in a private hospital. The sick patient is sometimes confused by having to relate to a large number of doctors and students. Medical educators are concerned with such criticisms and have moved to correct some of the problems. However, excesses of technological medicine still occur in these institutions.

KNOW WHEN TO USE THE HOSPITAL

The hospital is expensive. It is not home or hotel. Lives are saved and lost. The hospital must be used and it must be avoided. To manage these contradictions, the need for hospitalization for you or a member of your family must be carefully considered in each instance.

Don't use the hospital if services can be performed elsewhere. The acute (short-term) general hospital provides acute general medicine; it does not perform other functions well.

Don't use the hospital for a rest; it is not a good place to go for rest. It is busy, noisy, unfamiliar, and populated with unfamiliar roommates. Its nights are punctuated with interruptions, and it has an unusual time schedule. It has many employees, a few of whom will be less thoughtful than others.

Don't use the hospital for the "convenience" of having a number of tests done in a few days. It does not provide tests in the most efficient manner; indeed, most laboratories and X-ray facilities are not open on the weekend, and special procedures may require several days just to be scheduled.

Many people have urged that we establish a system of "hoptels," which would provide lodging at minimal cost, allow for efficient test performance, and are appropriate for periods of rest and minimal activity. A number of experiments along these lines are under way. Until more appropriate facilities are available, however, use the acute hospital with great reluctance.

Over a century ago, the Hungarian physician Inaz Philipp Semmelweiss (1818–65) noted that mothers giving birth at home and their infants fared better than those in the hospital, and that the existence of the often fatal "childbed fever" was one of the risks of the hospital. This problem, due to poor hygiene in the delivery rooms, has long since been corrected. But in our present age, new evidence suggests that for many conditions home treatment may work better than treatment in the hospital. For example, home treatment for minor heart attacks has been reported as possibly better than hospital treatment. It is apparent to most hospital visitors that the crisis atmosphere of the short-term acute hospital does not promote the calmest state of mind for the patient. Many therapeutic features of the home cannot be duplicated in the hospital.

The hospice movement attempts to provide humane, caring, medically sound treatment with a minimum of the technological trappings of the hospital. Hospice and home care programs are growing rapidly and are very worthwhile.

EMERGENCY ROOMS

The emergency room has become the "physician" for many patients. Patients who cannot find a physician at night, or who don't know where else to go, are increasingly coming to emergency rooms. Thus, the typical emergency room is now filled with nonemergency cases. The various problems are all mixed together: trivial illnesses which could have been treated with the aid of this book, routine problems more easily and economically handled in a physician's office, specialized problems which should have been dealt with at a time when the hospital facilities were fully available, and true emergencies. Even though the emergency room is not designed for the purpose it now serves, it does a surprisingly good job of delivering adequate care.

However, there are major disadvantages to using an emergency room as your sole medical contact. Emergency rooms make little or no provision for continued care. In the emergency room you will usually be seen by a different physician each time. The emergency room physician will attend to the chief problem reported by the patient but seldom has sufficient time to complete a full examination or to deal with underlying problems. While simple X-ray facilities are available, procedures such as gallbladder studies and upper G.I. series are arranged with difficulty. Thus evaluation of a complicated problem is not handled well by emergency room facilities. When a true emergency occurs, patients with less urgent problems are shunted aside. You cannot estimate with any certainty how long you will have to wait for treatment in an emergency room. Emergency room fees, because they support equipment required to handle true emergencies, are higher than those of standard office visits. Emergency room services are not always covered by medical insurance, even when the policy states that the costs of emergency care are included. With many policies, the nature of the illness determines whether or not it is covered. You may end up paying a large bill if you go to the emergency room with a sore throat.

The smoothly functioning emergency room is a dramatic place and provides one of the finest examples of a service profession at work. Using the procedures outlined in this book, you can use this valuable resource appropriately.

SHORT-TERM SURGERY
CENTERS

Recently, a number of facilities specially designed for short-term surgery (requiring only a short stay; overnight at the most) have appeared. Obviously such surgery is minor, and the patient must basically be in good health. Since such centers are able to avoid some of the overhead of a hospital, they often charge less for the use of their facilities. But since they do not have the capability to handle difficult cases or complications, you should use them only for minor procedures.

CONVALESCENT FACILITIES

Nursing homes and various types of rehabilitation facilities provide for the patient who does not require more expensive care but cannot be adequately managed at home. The quality of these facilities ranges from abysmal to superb. In the best circumstances, with dedicated nursing and regular physician attendance, a comfortable and homelike situation for the patient can accelerate the healing process. In other cases, disinterest, inadequate facilities, and minimal care are the rule. Before suggesting or accepting referral to a nursing home facility, visit the facility or have a friend or relative visit it for you. In the convalescent setting, your comfort with the arrangements is essential. The same checkout practice should be used for a hospice; most are good, but some are not.

FREE CLINICS

"Free clinics" have developed in many areas of the country. In some cases, they have appeared because the general medical care in the community has been poor. In others, clinics have developed to deal with undesired pregnancies, drug use, or venereal disease. These clinics are high in idealism and often short of money. Sympathetic care from sensitive individuals is the rule. Facilities will be limited, but considerable thought will have been given to those services provided, so that relatively little is lost.

These clinics provide care for many who would not find it available elsewhere. However, the financial instability and political ferment of many free clinics make their continued existence uncertain; these clinics come into and go out of existence with regularity. Free clinics do not present challenge to organized medicine but serve to remind it of its inequities. In most cases, they deserve broader community support than they receive.

It will be worth your time to investigate the various medical facilities in your area. If you can, visit them and ask questions. "Is there emergency care?" "Is there always a doctor on duty?" "What are your payment arrangements?" Then choose the facility that best meets your needs.

8 Reducing Your Medication Costs

Legal drugs are a multibillion dollar industry. Your contribution to this windfall is largely voluntary. The size of the contribution is determined by your physician, your pharmacy, and yourself.

Drugs are life-saving, dangerous, curative, painful, pain-relieving, and easy to misuse. Most are basically poisons, as they act to block one or more of the natural body defense mechanisms, such as pain, cough, inflammation, or diarrhea. Drugs interact with other drugs, causing hazardous chemical reactions. They have direct toxic reactions on the stomach lining and elsewhere in the body. They cause allergic rashes and shock. They are foreign chemicals and have severe toxic effects when taken in excess. Under some circumstances they probably cause cancers, and some drugs decrease the ability of the body to fight infections.

If you do *not* receive a prescription or a sample package of medication from your physician, consider this good news rather than rejection or disinterest. Take the fewest possible drugs for the shortest possible time. When drugs are prescribed, take them regularly and as directed, but expect that your medication program will be thoroughly reviewed every time you see your doctor.

Most drugs are given as "symptomatic medications," that is, they do not cure your problem but perhaps only given some relief for the symptoms of the problem. If you report a new minor symptom every time you see your physician and urgently request relief from the symptom, you will probably be given additional medications. You are unlikely to feel much better as the result of the extra medications, and you are nearly certain to function at a lower level as a human being. Unless you have a serious illness, you will seldom need to take more than one or two medications at a time. Many perceptive observers have argued that the present practice of using drugs to control symptoms is only a temporary phase in the history of medicine.

YOUR PHYSICIAN CAN SAVE YOU MONEY ON DRUGS

Your physician plays a major role in the cost of drugs by choosing the drugs to be prescribed. For example, if you have an infection due to bacteria, you may be given tetracycline or erythromycin. Tetracycline costs about three cents a capsule, while erythromycin costs about twenty-five cents. At the physician's option, a steroid prescription for asthma may be prednisone at two cents per tablet or methylprednisolone at twenty cents per tablet. Medically, such drug choices are between agents of similar effectiveness. If your physician prescribes a drug by its trade name, in most states the pharmacist must fill the prescription with that particular brand-name product. The brand-name product frequently costs many times more than its "generic" equivalent. Does your physician know the relative cost of alternative drugs? Many doctors do not.

The drug-prescribing habits of different physicians can be divided into two groups: the "additive" and the "substitutive." With each visit to an "additive" physician, you receive a medication in addition to those you already have. With a "substitutive" physician, the medication you were previously taking is discontinued and a new medicine is substituted. Usually the "substitutive" practice is advantageous to your health as well as your pocketbook.

Most of the time, medication can be taken by mouth. The common reason for requiring medication by injection is the physician's uncertainty that you will take the medication as prescribed; by injecting it, there is no question that the medication has been taken. However, as a thoughtful and reliable patient, you can assure your physician that you will comply with an oral regimen. Taking medication orally is less painful, less likely to result in an allergic reaction, and far less expensive. There are exceptions, but whenever possible you should take medication by mouth rather than by injection.

If it is clear that you must take a medication for a prolonged period, ask the physician to allow refills on the prescription. With many drugs it is not necessary to incur the expense of an additional physician visit just to get a prescription written. However, under some circumstances, the physician may prefer to examine you before deciding whether the drug can be safely continued or is still required. Ask your physician if refills on the prescription are permitted.

The careful physician will ensure that you fully understand each drug that you are taking, the reasons you are taking it, the side effects that may arise, and the expected length of time that you will be taking the medication. A daily medication schedule will be arranged so that it is convenient as well as medically effective. If the program is confusing, ask for written instructions. It is crucial that you understand the why and how of your drug therapy. Do not leave the physician's office for the pharmacy without understanding your medications.

REDUCING COSTS AT THE PHARMACY

Studies indicate that the pharmacy is the single most important factor in drug costs. For the most part, the pharmacist no longer weighs and measures individual chemical formulations. Much of the activity in the pharmacy consists of relabeling and dispensing manufactured medication. Medication is thus usually identical at different pharmacies; you should choose the least expensive and the most convenient place. Comparison shop. Discount stores often sell the same medication at significantly lower prices. If a considerable sum of money is involved, you should compare prices by telephone before purchasing the medication. Don't buy from a pharmacy that won't give you price information over the phone.

Unfortunately, even though your physician writes a prescription by "generic" name rather than brand name, the pharmacist is not required to give you the cheapest of the equivalent alternatives. The pharmacy often stocks only one manufacturer's formulation of each drug. Thus, even though your physician has been careful to prescribe a less expensive preparation, the pharmacist may substitute the more expensive alternative that is in stock. There is no way to detect this problem except to get direct price quotes from different pharmacies.

The majority of pharmacies charge a percentage markup. Their pricing is determined by the wholesale price, which is multiplied by a fixed profit figure. A sliding scale may be used, but profit is largest on the largest sales. Other pharmacies work on a specific charge per prescription. These pharmacies add a constant fee to the wholesale price. With a small drug bill, you will be better off with the percentage markup formulas. If you are buying a significant quantity of expensive medication, application of the one-time fixed charge may be less costly. Knowledge of these practices and aggressive comparison shopping is essential for you to control costs.

ULTIMATELY, YOU CONTROL YOUR DRUG COSTS

You are the ultimate determinant of your own drug costs. In this age, visits to the physician frequently are requests for medication. If your satisfaction with the physician depends on whether or not you are given medication, you are working against your own best interest. If you go to a physician because of a cold and request a "shot of penicillin," you are asking for poor medical practice. Penicillin should only infrequently be given by injection, and it should not be given for uncomplicated colds. Your physician knows this but may give in to your pressure.

Reducing Your Medication Costs

The most frequently prescribed medications in the United States, making up the bulk of drug costs, are tranquilizers, minor pain relievers, and sedatives. These are not scientifically important medications. This prescription pattern arose, at least in part, because of ill-advised consumer demand. You can decrease the cost of medications by using some of the techniques discussed previously; you can eliminate them almost completely by decreasing your pressure to receive and utilize medications that you do not require.

9 The Home Pharmacy

To effectively treat the minor illnesses that appear from time to time in your family, you need to have some medications on hand and know where to obtain others as you need them. Your stock should include only the most inexpensive and frequently needed medications. They will deteriorate with time and should be replaced at least every three years.

Table 9-1 lists the essential products for a home medical shelf; Table 9-2 gives a more complete list of agents that may sometimes be needed. The guidelines for common medical problems in Section II indicate when and why to use each medication. In this chapter we provide commentary on drug dosage and side effects; since these are subject to changes, you should carefully read the instructions that come with the medication. Our discussion will add some perspective to the manufacturer's statements.

TABLE 9–1 **Your Home Pharmacy**	Aspirin	For fever, headache, minor pain
	Antacid	For stomach upset
	Adhesive tape and bandages	For minor wounds
	Hydrogen peroxide	For cleansing wounds
	Sodium bicarbonate	For soaking and soothing
	Liquid acetaminophen	For pain and fever
	Syrup of ipecac	To induce vomiting

Note that only five items appear in Table 9-1 for the adult patient, and only one of these (aspirin) is a drug that is taken internally. You do not need most of the items that are currently in your medicine cabinet. It is best to dispose of them.

Reading the labels of compounds available at the supermarket can be a little frightening. It is in the manufacturer's interest to extol the product's benefits while including strong warnings, in small print, concerning its possible side effects. Surprisingly, it is also in the manufacturer's interest to recommend the smallest dosage that is likely to have any effect. In short, you are exhorted to buy the drug but not to cause any trouble, especially legal trouble due to side effects. Be this as it may, you must accept certain truths about drugs:

The Home Pharmacy

• Used in effective dosages, all drugs have the potential for side effects. Many common drugs have some side effects, such as drowsiness, that are impossible to avoid at effective dosages.

• Misuse of over-the-counter drugs can have serious consequences. Do not assume that a product is automatically safe because it does not require a prescription.

TABLE 9–2

Medications For Sometime Use

This expanded list contains medicines that not all people will need. Nearly all of the home treatment recommended in this book may be carried out with the use of these agents.

Ailment or Need	Medication
Allergy	Antihistamines
	Nose drops and sprays
Antiseptic	Hydrogen peroxide, iodine
Colds and coughs	Cold tablets, cough syrups
Constipation	Milk of magnesia, bulk laxatives
Dental problems (preventive)	Sodium fluoride
Diarrhea	Kaopectate, Parepectolin
Eye irritations	Eye drops and artificial tears
Fungus	Antifungal preparations
Hemorrhoids	Hemorrhoid preparations
Pain and fever	Aspirin, acetaminophen
in children:	Liquid acetaminophen, rectal suppositories of aspirin
Poisoning (to induce vomiting)	Syrup of Ipecac
Skin rashes	Hydrocortisone cream
(soaking and soothing)	Sodium bicarbonate (baking soda)
Sprains	Elastic bandages
Stomach, upset	Antacid (nonabsorbable)
Sunburn (preventive)	Sunscreen agents
Wounds (minor)	Adhesive tape, bandages

The rational approach to this dilemma is for you to learn something about the drugs that may be useful to you. This is the reason for this chapter.

There are hundreds of over-the-counter medicines available at your supermarket or drugstore. For most purposes there are several medicines that are almost identical. This has posed a problem for us in the organization of this chapter; if we discuss drugs by chemical name, the terms are long and confusing, while if we use the brand name, we may appear to favor the product of a particular manufacturer when there are equally satisfactory alternatives. We have decided, instead, to give some clues to reading the list of ingredients on the package so that you can figure out what the drug is likely to do. We do not include all available drugs, but we do mention some representative alternatives. The brand names listed in this chapter are vigorously marketed and should be available almost everywhere. They are *not* necessarily superior to alternatives that are not listed, which contain similar formulas.

ALLERGY

Antihistamine Decongestant Compounds: Allerest, Sinarest, Sinutab, Dristan

The many over-the-counter drugs designed for treatment of minor allergic symptoms are similar to the cold compounds described below, but they less frequently contain pain and fever agents like aspirin or acetaminophen. Usually these drug compounds contain an antihistamine and a decongestant agent, which can be identified from the label. If you tolerate one of these drugs well and get good relief, it may be continued for several weeks (for example, through a hay fever season) without seeing a physician. The same sort of drug taken as nose drops or nasal spray should be used more sparingly and only for short periods, as detailed below in "Nose Drops and Sprays." You can purchase the ingredients of the compound separately, and we advise you to do so.

Reading the labels: The decongestant is often phenylephrine, ephedrine, or phenylpropanolamine. If the compound name is not familiar, the suffix "-ephrine" or "-edrine" will usually identify this component of the compound. The antihistamine is often chlorpheniramine (Chlor-trimeton) or pyrilamine. If not, the antihistamine is sometimes (but not always) identifiable on the label by the suffix "-amine."

Dosage: As per product directions. Reduce dose if side effects are noted, or try another compound.

Side effects: These are usually minor and disappear after the drug is stopped or decreased in dose. Agitation and insomnia usually indicate too much of the decongestant component. Drowsiness usually indicates too much antihistamine. If you can avoid the substance to which you are allergic, it is far superior to taking drugs which, to a certain degree, inevitably impair your functioning.

Nose Drops and Sprays: Afrin, Neo-Synephrine, Dristan, Sinarest, Contac

A runny nose is often the worst symptom of a cold or allergy. Because this complaint is so common, remedies are big business, and there are many advertised that claim to decrease nasal secretions. Many of these preparations are "topical," as with nose drops and sprays, and act directly on the inflamed tissue. There are some problems associated with the use of these compounds.

The active ingredient in these compounds is a decongestant drug—ephredrine or phenylephrine. When applied, you can feel the membranes shrinking down and "drawing," and you will note a decrease in the amount of secretion. In other words, the medication is effective and can relieve symptoms.

The major drawback is that the relief is temporary. Usually the symptoms return in a couple of hours, and you need to repeat the dose. This is fine for a while. But these drugs work by causing the muscle in the walls of the blood vessels to constrict, decreasing blood flow. After many applications, these small muscles become fatigued and fail to respond. Finally, they are so fatigued that they relax entirely and the situation becomes worse than it was in the beginning. This is medically termed "rebound vasodilatation" and can occur if you use these drugs steadily for three days or more. Many patients interpret these increased symptoms as a need for more medication. Taking more only makes the problem increasingly worse. Therefore, use nose drops or sprays only for a few days at a time. After several days rest, they may be used again for a few days.

Dosage: These drugs are almost always used in the wrong way. If you can taste the drug, you have applied it to the wrong area. If you don't bathe the swollen membranes on the side surface of the inner nose, you won't get the desired effect. Apply small amounts to one nostril while lying down on that side for a few minutes so that the medicine will bathe the membranes. Then apply the agent to the other side while lying on that side. Treat four times a day if needed, but do not continue for more than three days without interrupting the therapy.

Side effects: Rebound vasodilatation from prolonged use is the most common problem. If you apply these agents incorrectly and swallow a large amount of the drug, you may experience a rapid heart rate and an uneasy, agitated feeling. The drying effect of the drug can result in nosebleeds. Try to avoid the substances to which you are allergic rather than treating the consequences of exposure. Often simple measures like changing a furnace filter or using an air conditioner to filter the air will improve symptoms.

COLDS AND COUGHS

Cold Tablets: Coricidin, Dristan, Contac

Dozens of products are widely advertised as being effective against the common cold, and the choice is confusing. Surprisingly, many give satisfactory symptomatic relief. While we do not feel that these compounds add much to standard treatment with aspirin and fluids, many patients feel otherwise, and we do not discourage their use for short periods.

These compounds usually have three basic ingredients. The most important is aspirin (or acetaminophen), which acts to reduce fever and pain. In addition, there is a decongestant drug, which acts to shrink the swollen membranes and the small blood vessels, and an antihistamine which acts to block any allergy and dry the mucus.

Reading the labels: The decongestant is often phenylephrine, ephedrine, or phenylpropanolamine. If the compound name is not familiar, the suffix "-ephrine" or "-edrine" will usually identify this component of the compound. The antihistamine is often chlorpheniramine (Chlor-trimeton) or pyrilamine. If not, the antihistamine is usually (but not always) identifiable on the label by the suffix "-amine."

Occasionally, a "belladonna alkaloid" is added to these compounds to enhance other actions and reduce stomach spasms. In the small doses used there is little effect from these drugs, which are listed as "scopolamine," "belladonna," or something similar. Other ingredients that may be listed contribute little. Do not use products with caffeine if you have heart trouble or difficulty sleeping. Do not use products with phenacetin over a long period because kidney damage has been reported.

These products, then, contain the much promoted "combination of ingredients" approach. As a general rule, single drugs are far preferable to combinations of drugs; they allow you to be more selective in treatment of symptoms, and consequently you take fewer drugs. The ingredients in combination products are available alone and should be considered as alternatives. The major ingredient, aspirin, is discussed below. Pseudoephedrine is an excellent decongestant and is available without prescription in 30-mg and 60-mg tablets. Chlorpheniramine, a strong antihistamine, is now available without prescription in the standard 4-mg size. When possible, consider applying medicine directly to the affected area, as with nose drops or sprays for a runny nose.

Finally, note that the commonly prescribed cold medicines (Sudafed, Actifed,Dimetapp) are really just more concentrated and expensive formulations of the same type of drugs that are available over the counter. Is it worth a trip to the doctor just for that?

Dosage: Try the recommended dosage. If no effect is noted, you may increase the dosage by one-half. Do not exceed twice the recommended dosage. Remember that you are trying to find a compromise between desired effects and side effects. Increasing the dosage gives some chance of increased beneficial effects, but it guarantees a greater probability of side effects.

Side effects: Drugs that put one person to sleep will keep another awake. The most frequent side effects of cold tablets are drowsiness and agitation. The drowsiness is usually casued by the antihistamine component, and the insomnia or agitation results from the decongestant component. You can try another compound that has less or none of the offending chemical, or

65

you can reduce the dose. There are no frequent serious side effects; the most dangerous is drowsiness if you intend to drive or operate machinery. Rarely, the "belladonna" component will cause dryness of mouth, blurring of vision, or inability to urinate. Aspirin's usual side effects—upset stomach or ringing in the ears—may also be experienced.

COUGH SYRUPS

This is a confusing area, with many products. To simplify, consider only two major categories of cough medication: "expectorants" and "cough suppressants." The expectorants are usually preferable, since they liquefy the secretions and allow the body's defenses to get rid of the material. Cough suppressants should be avoided if the cough is bringing up any material or if there is a lot of mucus. In the late stages of a cough, when it is dry and hacking, compounds containing a suppressant may be useful. We prefer compounds that do not contain an antihistamine since the drying effect on the mucus can harm as much as help.

Reading the labels: Glyceryl guaiacolate, potassium iodide, and several other frequently used chemicals cause an expectorant action. Cough suppressant action comes principally from narcotics, such as codeine. Over-the-counter cough suppressants cannot contain codeine. They often contain dextromethorphan hydrobromide, which is not a narcotic but is a close chemical relative. Many commercial mixtures contain a little of everything and may have some of the ingredients of the cold compounds as well. We will discuss only glyceryl guaiacolate (Robitussin, 2/G) and dextromethorphan (Romilar) specifically; follow the label instructions for other agents.

Glyceryl Guaiacolate: Robitussin, 2/G

This cough medicine acts to draw more liquid into the mucus that triggers a cough and thus to liquefy these mucus secretions so that they may be coughed free. The resulting cough is easier and less irritating. For a dry hacking cough remaining after a cold, the lubrication alone often soothes the inflamed area. The basic component in these medications, glyceryl guaiacolate, does not suppress the cough reflex but encourages the natural defense mechanisms of the body. There is controversy over its effectiveness, but it appears to be safe. It is not as powerful as the codeine-containing preparations, but for routine use we prefer it to prescription drugs. The two common brand-name products (Robitussin and 2/G) are medically equivalent but have a slightly different taste. Pepper and garlic, usually not thought of as medicines, have a similar effect.

Reading the labels: These drugs are also available in combination with decongestants and cough suppressants; the decongestants may carry a "-PE" suffix for "phenylephrine" and the cough suppressants a "-DM" for "dextromethorphan."

Dosage: One or two teaspoonfuls, three or four times daily for adults; one-half teaspoon for children of ages six to twelve; one-fourth teaspoon for children between the ages of one and six. Call your physician if you have a sick and coughing child less than a year old.

Side Effects: No significant problems have been reported. If preparations containing other drugs are used, side effects from the other components of the combination may occur.

Dextromethorphan: Romilar

This drug "calms the cough center," which is to say that it makes the areas of the brain that control coughs less sensitive to the stimuli that trigger coughs. No matter how much is used, it will seldom decrease a cough by more than 50 percent. Thus you cannot totally suppress a cough; this is actually beneficial because the cough is a protective reflex. This drug may be used with dry hacking coughs that are preventing sleep or work.

Dosage: Adults often require up to twice the recommended dosage to obtain any effect, but do not exceed this amount. A higher dose may produce problems, not further benefit.

Side effects: Drowsiness is the only side effect that has been reliably reported.

CONSTIPATION

We prefer a natural diet, with natural vegetable fiber residue, to the use of any laxative. But if you must use a laxative, the most attractive alternatives are psyllium as a bulk laxative or milk of magnesia to hold water in the bowel and soften the stool.

Bulk (psyllium-containing) Laxatives: Metamucil, Effersylium

These substances—refined from the psyllium seed—can help both diarrhea and constipation. It draws water into the stool, forms a gel or thick solu-

67

tion, and thus provides bulk. It is not absorbed by the digestive tract but only passes through; thus it is a natural product and essentially has no contraindications or side effects. However, it doesn't always work; a similar effect can probably be obtained by eating enough celery. It has been recommended as a weight reduction aid when taken before meals because it induces a feeling of fullness which may reduce appetite; however, it doesn't seem very effective in this role.

Dosage: One teaspoonful, stirred in a glass of water, taken twice daily is a typical dose. A second glass of water or juice should also be taken. Psyllium is also available in more expensive, individual-dose packets, for times when you don't have a teaspoon. The effervescent versions mix a bit more rapidly and taste better to some people.

Side effects: If the bulk laxative is taken without sufficient water, the gel that is formed could conceivably lodge in the esophagus (the tube that leads from the mouth to the stomach). Sufficient liquid will prevent this problem.

Milk of Magnesia

This home remedy has been on most bathroom shelves since the days of our grandparents. Milk of magnesia has two actions: as a laxative it causes fluid to be retained within the bowel and in the feces; as an antacid it neutralizes the acid in the stomach. It is an effective antacid, but unfortunately, when taken in a sufficient dose to help an ulcer patient (see "Antacids"), it causes quite severe diarrhea. A single dose is relatively well tolerated, so a mild upset stomach may be treated with milk of magnesia.

Magnesium is the active ingredient in milk of magnesia. While milk of magnesia cannot be termed a "natural" laxative, it is mild and less subject to abuse than many alternatives.

Dosage: For the adult, 30 cc (two tablespoons) liquid may be taken at bedtime as a laxative or up to once daily, as required, to quiet stomach upset. It produces its laxative effect in approximately eight hours. If the stomach is not soothed, use another antacid more frequently. Give one-half dose to children of ages six to twelve; one-fourth dose to children of ages three to six. As with other antacids, two tablets are roughly equal in chemical content to two tablespoons liquid. However, the liquid is more effective as an antacid.

Side Effects: Milk of magnesia is more difficult to misuse because it causes diarrhea before any more serious effects. Too much magnesium is harmful to the body, but you won't ingest that much unless you use a bottle a day. There is some salt present, so be careful if you are on a low-salt diet. Milk of magnesia is a "nonabsorbable" antacid, so it does not greatly affect the acidity of the body. However, it should never be used by people who have kidney disease.

DENTAL CARE

Take care of your teeth; they help you chew. There is good evidence that preventive measures can save teeth. Brush your teeth as recommended, and use dental floss to clean the difficult areas between the teeth. Many doctors feel that flossing is the most important preventive for adult tooth decay. The use of water jets (such as Waterpic) to remove food products from between the teeth and to prevent the buildup of tartar remains controversial. We believe that such devices, used regularly, are helpful, but the evidence for their effectiveness is incomplete.

Sodium Fluoride

If your water supply is fluoridated, your fluoride intake is adequate and you do not need to supplement your diet. The ground water in many areas is naturally fluoridated. Find out if your water is fluoridated or not, whether naturally or by chemical treatment; your local health department usually has the answer. If it is not fluoridated, it is important for you to supplement your children's diet with fluoride. There remains argument as to whether fluoride continues to be required after the teeth have been formed, but all authorities agree that fluoride is needed through age ten. To be certain, you may wish to continue fluoride supplements for several years longer, until all the molars are in. Adults probably do not require dietary fluoride, although the painting of teeth with fluoride paste by the dentist is still felt to be helpful, as is stannous fluoride toothpaste.

Dosage: Fortunately, it is relatively easy to supplement with fluoride when the water supply is not treated. Buy a large bottle of fluoride tablets in a soluble form. Most tablets are 2.2 mg and contain 2 mm of fluoride; the rest is a soluble sugar. A child under the age of three needs approximately 0.5 mg per day, and a child between the ages of three and ten needs 1 mg, or one-half tablet. The tablets may be chewed or swallowed. They may also be taken in milk; they do not alter the taste. In states where fluoride is available only by prescription, request a prescription from your doctor or dentist on a routine visit.

Side Effects: Too much fluoride will mottle the teeth and will not give additional strength, so do not exceed the recommended dosage. At recommended dosage, there are no known side effects; fluoride is a natural mineral present in many natural water supplies.

DIARRHEA

For occasional loose stools, no medication is required. A clear liquid diet (for example, water or ginger ale) is the first thing to do for any diarrhea.

When diarrhea is severe, Kaopectate is the first medicine to try at home. When it does not control the diarrhea, stronger agents containing substances such as paregoric may be needed. Protracted diarrhea may require the help of a physician.

Kaopectate

Kaopectate is a combination of a claylike substance (Kaolin) and pectin, a substance found in apples. The different ingredients have a gelling effect which helps to form a solid stool.

Dosage: For adults, four to eight tablespoons after each bowel movement; for children of ages three to twelve, one to four tablespoons; for children below age three, call the doctor. With this dosage schedule, more severe diarrhea is treated more vigorously, and minor problems require little medicine.

Side effects: None have been reported.

Paregoric-Containing Preparations: Parepectolin, Parelixir

In addition to a gelling substance, these compounds contain a narcotic (paregoric) which acts to decrease the activity of the digestive tract and thus to slow down the diarrhea. These drugs should be used only when a clear liquid diet and Kaopectate have failed to control frequent diarrhea (one or more watery stools per hour).

Dosage: The amount indicated in the table below is given after each loose bowel movement. No more than four doses should be given in an eight-hour period without the approval of your physician.

Age	Dose
1 to 3 years	1/2 to 1-1/2 teaspoons
3 to 6 years	1-1/2 to 2 teaspoons
6 to 12 years	2 to 3 teaspoons
over 12 years	1 to 2 tablespoons

Side effects: A narcotic overdose with paregoric is extremely rare. Drowsiness or nausea occur occasionally and are indications that the drug should be withdrawn. "Overshoot" can occur, in which the diarrhea is controlled so completely that bowel movements don't occur for a week, so be careful.

Psyllium Hydrophilic Mucilloid: Metamucil, Effersyllium

This substance—refined from the psyllium seed—can help both diarrhea and constipation. It draws water into the stool, forms a gel or thick solution, and thus provides bulk. Their use is discussed on page 67.

EYE IRRITATIONS

The tear mechanism normally soothes, cleans, and lubricates the eye. Occasionally, the environment can overwhelm this mechanism, or the tear flow may be insufficient. In these cases the eye becomes "tired," feels dry or gritty, and may itch. A number of compounds that may aid this problem are available.

Murine, Visine

There are two general types of eye preparations. One class contains compounds intended to soothe the eye (Murine). Added to the compounds may be substances that shrink blood vessels and thus "get the red out" (Visine); these substances are decongestants. Their capacity to soothe is debatable. The use of decongestants to get rid of a bloodshot appearance is totally cosmetic. It is possible that such preparations can actually interfere with the normal healing process, although this is probably unusual.

Methylcellulose Eyedrops

The second group of preparations makes no claims of special soothing effects and contains no decongestants. They are solutions with concentrations like those of the body so that no irritation occurs. Their purpose is to lubricate the eye, to be "artificial tears." These are the preparations preferred by ophthalmologists for minor eye irritation. Methylcellulose eyedrops are an example of this type.

Prefrin

Prefrin is a substance that lies somewhere between the two types of eye preparations discussed above; it contains both substances that effectively soothe and lubricate the eye, and a decongestant.

Dosage: Use as frequently as neeeded in the quantity required. You can't use too much, although usually a few drops give just as much relief as a bottleful. If your problem of dry eyes is constant, you should check it out with the doctor, since an underlying problem could be present. Usually the symptom of dry eyes lasts only a few hours and is readily relieved. Too much sun, wind, or dust usually causes the minor irritation.

Side effects: No serious side effects have been reported. Visine and other drugs containing decongestants tend to sting a bit.

None of these drugs treat eye infections or injuries or remove foreign bodies from the eye. In Section II, we give instructions for more severe eye complaints. Refer to: Problem 77, Foreign Body in Eye; Problem 78, Eye Pain; Problem 79, Decreased Vision; Problem 80, Eye Burning, Itching, and Discharge.

Zinc Oxide Powders and Creams

These agents aren't magic, but they are good for ordinary problems. The creams soothe the irritated area while the body heals the inflamed vein. They also help toughen the skin over the hemorrhoids so that they are less easily irritated. Don't trap bacteria beneath the creams; apply them after a bath when the area has been carefully cleaned and dried.

Reading the labels: We do not advocate the use of creams that contain ingredients identified by the suffix "-caine," because repeated use of these local anesthetics can cause further irritation. The other heavily advertised products, in our opinion, offer no advantages over zinc oxide.

Dosage: Apply as needed, following label directions.

Side effects: Essentially none.

PAIN AND FEVER

Aspirin

Aspirin is the superdrug. It controls fevers, helps pain, and reduces inflammation. It is the only significant active ingredient in many nonprescription cold and pain remedies and is the unnamed "ingredient doctors recommend most." Although great quantities of it have been consumed, it nevertheless has an enviable safety record. You can kill yourself with an overdose of aspirin, but it is extremely difficult for an adult to do so.

Aspirin is somewhat of an anachronism at the drug counter. If it were developed as a new drug today, it would be available only by prescription. It can be purchased over the counter because it was in wide use before the present regulations were in force. Paradoxically, this familiarity with aspirin makes it difficult for the physician. Often, a patient does not accept a suggestion for the use of aspirin, because aspirin is equated with disinterest or neglect on the part of the physician. The patient may also reject it because of a sensationalistic article that describes severe side effects and implies that aspirin is the cause of much human illness.

The truth in medicine is seldom sensational and is usually consistent with common sense. All drugs are hazardous; aspirin can cause serious problems on occasion, but this is rare if the drug is used properly. Usually a drug alternative to aspirin is more dangerous, has not been studied as completely, and is much more expensive. In addition, the alternative is often not as effective. Prescription pain relievers such as Darvon or codeine

(1/2 grain) are approximately as strong as aspirin but often do not result in real improvement.

The claims for excessive purity of expensive preparations of aspirin aren't of much medical relevance. For ourselves, we buy a big jar of the cheapest U.S.P. aspirin at the cut-rate drugstore. If the bottle contains a vinegary odor when opened, the aspirin has begun to deteriorate and should be discarded. Aspirin usually has a shelf life of about three years, although shorter periods are sometimes quoted. (Note: U.S.P. stands for "United States Pharmacopeia." While not an absolute guarantee that the drug is the best, it does mean that the drug has met certain standards in composition and physical characteristics. The same is true of the designation N.F., which stands for "National Formulary.")

Dosage: In adults, the standard dose for pain relief is two tablets taken every three to four hours as required. The maximum effect occurs in about two hours. Each standard tablet is 5 grains (300 mg or 0.3 g). If you use a nonstandard concoction, you will have to do the arithmetic to calculate equivalent doses. The terms "extra-strength," "arthritis pain formula," and the like merely indicate a greater amount of aspirin per tablet. This is medically trivial. You can take more tablets of the cheaper aspirin and still save money. When you read that a product "contains more of the ingredient that doctors recommend most," you may be sure that the product contains a little bit more aspirin per tablet; perhaps 325 to 400 mg instead of 300.

Here are some hints for good aspirin usage. Aspirin treats symptoms; it does not cure problems. Thus, for symptoms such as headache or muscle pain or menstrual cramps, don't take it unless you hurt. On the other hand, for control of fever, you will be more comfortable if you repeat the dose every three to four hours during the day, since this prevents the fever from moving up and down. The afternoon and evening are the worst, so try not to miss a dose during these hours. If you need aspirin for relief from some symptom over a prolonged period, check the symptom with your doctor. Relief from pain or fever is not very different if you increase the dose, and you are more likely to irritate your stomach, so take the standard dose even if you still have some discomfort.

For control of inflammation, as in serious arthritis, the dose of aspirin must be high, often sixteen to twenty tablets daily, and must be continued over a prolonged period. A physician should monitor such treatment; it is relatively safe but problems sometimes occur.

In children, a dose of about 1 grain (60 mg) for each year of age is appropriate, with an adult dose for children over ten years old. Children's aspirin comes in 1.25-grain (75 mg) tablets which taste good; please do not allow them to be taken as candy by a small child.

Aspirin can be given as a rectal suppository if vomiting prevents taking medication by mouth; the dosage is the same. Five-grain and 10-grain suppositories may be cut to prepare smaller doses for smaller people. Suppositories will irritate the rectum if used repeatedly, so try to limit their use to two or three doses. These suppositories require a prescription.

Side effects: Aspirin frequently upsets the stomach or causes ringing in the ears. If the stomach is upset, try taking the aspirin a half-hour after meals, when the food in the stomach will act as a buffer. Coated aspirin (such as Ecotrin or A.S.A. Enseal) will almost totally protect the stomach. However, some people do not digest the coated aspirin and so receive no benefit. Buffering is sometimes added to aspirin to protect the stomach and may help a little. If you take a lot of aspirin and desire a buffered preparation, we recommend a combination made with a nonabsorbable antacid (as in Ascriptin or Bufferin) rather than an absorbable antacid, as in some buffered aspirins. Nonabsorbable antacids are much easier on your system. Over the short-term, the buffering makes little difference and there is controversy as to whether it works anyway. If your ears ring, reduce the dose—you are taking too much.

Asthma, nasal polyps, deafness, serious bleeding from the digestive tract, ulcers, and other major problems have been associated with aspirin. However, such problems are unusual and almost always disappear after the aspirin is stopped. Conversely, some studies suggest that aspirin might be good treatment for hardening of the arteries; but this has by no means been proven.

Aspirin comes in combination with many other remedies not described in this book, most frequently caffeine and phenacetin ("APC Tabs"). Some scientists think these agents increase the painkilling effects; others dispute this. They do increase the side effects, and we find little use for them. Do not use products with caffeine if you have heart trouble or difficulty in sleeping; do not use products with phenacetin over a long period because kidney damage has been reported.

Acetaminophen: Tylenol, Datril, Liquiprin, Tempra

Aspirin is the drug of first choice for treatment of minor pains and fever. Acetaminophen, available in several brand-name preparations, is the second choice. It is slightly less predictable than aspirin, somewhat less powerful, and does not have the antiinflammatory action that makes aspirin so valuable in treatment of arthritis and some other diseases. On the other hand, it does not cause ringing in the ears or upset the stomach—common side effects with aspirin. Most pediatricians feel that acetaminophen is preferable for use by children for these reasons. In the British Commonwealth, this drug is known as paracetamol.

Dosage: Acetaminophen is used in doses identical to those of aspirin. For adults, two 5-grain tablets every three to four hours is the standard dose. In children, 1 grain per year of age every four hours is satisfactory. There is never a reason to exceed these doses, since there is no additional benefit in taking higher amounts. Acetaminophen is available in liquid preparations that are palatable for small children. These are usually administered by a dropper, and the package insert gives the amount for each age range.

Side effects: These are seldom experienced. If you suspect a side effect, call your physician. A variety of rare toxic effects have been reported, but

none are definitely related to the use of this drug. Like aspirin, acetaminophen comes in multiple combination products which offer little advantage.

PAIN AND FEVER: CHILDHOOD

The principles and drugs used to control minor pain and fever in the child
are the same as in the adult, but there are differences in the importance of
treatment and in the method of administration. In the child, fever comes
on more rapidly and may rise much higher, even with a minor virus. The
fever must be controlled; high fever can lead to a frightening temporary
epilepsy, with seizures or "fits." Thus, while control of the fever in an
adult is principally for the comfort of the patient, fever control in the child
actually prevents serious complications. It can be difficult to get a sick
small child to take medication, thus different methods of administration
are sometimes needed.

If the child has a rash, a stiff neck, difficulty in breathing, is lethargic,
or looks very ill, call or visit the doctor. Be particularly careful with children under one year of age. Phone advice is graciously available in most
areas; don't hesitaste to call if you have a question. Many times, despite a
high fever, the child will look fine and not even be very irritable. In such
cases, treatment and observation at home are adequate. Physicians frequently prefer a phone call to a visit, because if the visit can be avoided,
other children in the waiting room or office are not exposed to the virus.

Liquid Acetaminophen or Aspirin

Most pediatricians prefer acetaminophen or sodium salicylate to aspirin for
the small child, principally because these agents have less chance of causing stomach upset. The liquid preparations are easier to administer and
are better tolerated by the stomach. (If vomiting makes it impossible to
keep even these liquid medicines down, the use of rectal suppositories of
aspirin can be very helpful.)

Dosage: For liquid acetaminophen or aspirin preparations, follow the label
advice. Administer every four hours. During the period from noon to midnight, awaken the child if necessary. After midnight, the fever will usually
break by itself and become less of a problem, so if you miss a dose it is
less important. But check the child's temperature at least once during the
night to make sure. Remember, these drugs only last about four hours in
the body, and you must keep repeating the dose or you will lose the effect.
Some pediatricians recommend alternating aspirin and acetaminophen at
two-hour intervals for high fevers.

Aspirin Rectal Suppositories

Aspirin rectal suppositories are available only by prescription in most localities. The dose is the same as by mouth; 1 grain (60 mg) for each year

of age per four hours; after age ten, use the adult dose. One-grain supposi-tories are manufactured but are sometimes difficult to find. If necessary, cut the larger 5-grain suppositories to make an approximate equivalent to the dose needed. Use a warm knife and cut them lengthwise. Ask your physician for a prescription for aspirin rectal suppositories on a routine visit if you can't get them over the counter. Keep them in stock at home. Use them only when vomiting prevents retention of any oral intake, and do not exceed three doses for any one illness without contacting your physician.

Use of suppositories confuses many parents. The idea is to allow the medicine to be absorbed through the mucus membranes of the rectum. Re-move the wrapper before use! When inserting the suppository, firm but gentle pressure will cause the muscles to relax around the rectum. Be pa-tient. In small children, the buttocks may need to be held or taped to-gether to prevent expulsion of the suppository.

Side effects: Rectal aspirin can irritate the rectum and cause local bleed-ing; therefore it should only be used if the ordinary routes of administra-tion are impossible—even then, if more than two or three doses seem to be required, call your physician for advice.

Other Measures

Cool or lukewarm baths are also useful in keeping a fever down. During the bath, wet the hair as well. Keep the patient in a cool room, wearing little or no clothing.

POISONING

To Induce Vomiting: Syrup of Ipecac

Keep this traditional remedy handy if you have small children. With most poisonings, promptly induced vomiting will empty the stomach of any poi-son that has not already been absorbed. Do *not* use any agent to cause vomiting if the poison swallowed is a petroleum-based compound or a strong acid or alkali (see Section 2, Problem 1, Oral Poisoning). Vomiting should be induced immediately when poisoning is due to a plant or a drug.

It is far better to keep toxic chemicals out of a child's reach than to have to use ipecac. When you buy ipecac, use the purchase as a reminder to check the house for toxic chemicals that a child might reach and move them to a safer place. If your child does swallow something, the sooner the stomach is emptied the milder the problem will be, with the exceptions listed above. There is no time to buy ipecac after your child has swallowed poison; therefore you should have it on hand—just in case it's ever needed.

Dosage: One tablespoon of ipecac may suffice for a small child; two table-spoons are necessary for older children and adults. Follow the dose with as much warm water as can be given, until vomiting occurs. Repeat the dose in fifteen minutes if you haven't had any results.

Side effects: This is an uncomfortable medication, but it is not hazardous unless vomiting causes vomited material to be thrown down the windpipe into the lungs. This can cause pneumonia, so do not induce vomiting in a patient who is unconscious or nearly unconscious, and do not cause vomiting of flammable materials which can be inhaled into the lung and cause damage. Call the local poison control center in any potentially severe poisoning. In this setting, giving ipecac on the way to the hospital may be helpful and even can be lifesaving, but the experts at the poison control center can tell you for sure. Poisoning from medicine or a poisonous plant should be treated with ipecac.

SKIN DRYNESS

Moisturizing Creams and Lotions: Lubriderm, Vaseline, Corn Huskers, Nivea

There is little to be said about the various kinds of artificial materials that human beings apply to their skin in the attempt to temporarily improve its appearance or retard its aging. The various claims are not scientifically based, and long-term benefits have not been demonstrated. In some areas, it has been postulated that they are harmful rather than beneficial.

Sometimes, dry skin can actually cause symptoms, thus becoming a medical problem. Then something that is safe, nontoxic, nonallergenic, and that provides relief is needed. Of the products available over the counter, Lubriderm, Vaseline, or Corn Huskers lotion are as good as any. Nivea is effective, but a few people are sensitive to the lanolin it contains. Remember that bathing or exposure to detergents may contribute to the drying of skin. Decreasing the frequency of baths or showers, wearing gloves when working with cleansing agents, and other similar measures are more important than using any lotion or cream.

Dosage: Per product label.

Side effects: Essentially none except for the rare lanolin sensitivity mentioned above.

SKIN RASHES

Hydrocortisone Creams: Cortaid, Dermolate, Lanacort, Caldecort

For temporary relief of skin itching and rashes such as poison ivy and poison oak, hydrocortisone cream (0.5%) has recently become available over the counter. This is a strong, local antiinflammatory preparation; in general, it is as effective as anything that your doctor can prescribe. Used for a short period of time, these creams are safe and almost totally nontoxic. They will clear up many minor rashes, but they "suppress" a condition rather than "cure" it.

Dosage: Rub a very small amount into the rash. If you can see any cream remaining on the skin, you have used too much. Repeat frequently as needed, which often is every two to four hours.

Side effects: Over the long-term, these creams can cause skin atrophy and wasting, so limit their use to a two-week period. Beyond this time, check with your doctor. Theoretically, these creams can make an infection worse, so be careful about using them if the "rash" seems as though it might be infected. Don't use these creams around the eyes, and do not take them by mouth.

SKIN FUNGUS

Antifungal Preparations: Tinactin, Selsun, Desenex

Fungal infections of the skin are not serious, so treatment is not urgent. In general, the fungus needs moist undisturbed areas to grow and will often disappear with regular cleansing, drying, and application of a powder to keep the area dry. Cleansing should be performed twice daily.

If you need a medication, there are effective nontoxic agents available. For athlete's foot, use one of the zinc undecylenate creams or powders, such as Desenex. In difficult cases, tolnaftate (Tinactin) is very effective. This agent is useful for almost all skin fungus problems, but is is more expensive. For superficial fungus infection, particularly those causing patchy loss of skin color, selenium sulfide (Selsun Blue) is often quickly effective. It is sold as a shampoo, but you can use it as a medicinal cream.

Dosage: For athlete's foot, use as directed on the label. For other skin problems, selenium sulfide is available by prescription in a 2.5% solution. Over the counter, a 1% solution is available as Selsun Blue shampoo. Use the shampoo as a cream and let it dry on the lesions; repeat several times a day to compensate for the weaker strength.

Side effects: There are very few. Selenium sulfide can burn the skin if used to excess, so decrease application if you notice any irritation. Selenium may discolor hair and will stain clothes. Be very careful when applying any of these products around the eyes. And don't take them by mouth.

SUNBURN PREVENTION

Sunscreen Products: Pre-Sun, Block-Out, Paba-Film, Pabonal

Dermatologists continually remind us that sun is bad for the skin. Exposure to the sun accelerates the skin aging process and increases the chance of skin cancer. Advertisements, on the other hand, continually extol the virtues of a suntan, and as a nation we spend much of our youth trying to achieve a pleasing skin tone, with disregard for the later consequences of solar radiation. The sunscreen agents can be used to prevent burning but allow you to be in the sun. If the skin is unusually sensitive to the sun's effects, a more complete block of the rays is best. Partial blocking of the sun's rays is provided by Block-Out and Paba-Film, while Pabonal and Pre-Sun block out virtually all rays. Suntan lotions that are not sunscreen agents block relatively little solar radiation.

Dosage: Apply evenly to exposed areas of skin as directed on the label.

Side effects: Very rare skin irritation or allergy.

SPRAINS

Elastic Bandages

Elastic (Ace) bandages are periodically used by any family. You will probably need both a narrow and a broader width. If problems are recurrent, the one-piece devices designed specifically for knee and ankle are sometimes more convenient. All of these bandages primarily provide gentle support, but they also act to reduce swelling. Elastic bandages should be used if they make the injured part feel better. The support given is minimal and reinjury is possible, despite the bandage. Thus it is not a substitute for a splint, a cast, or a proper adhesive-type dressing when these are needed. Perhaps the most important function of these bandages is as a reminder to you that you have a problem so that you are less likely to reinjure the part.

Dosage: Support should be continued well past the time of active discomfort to allow complete healing and to help prevent reinjury; this usually requires about six weeks. During the latter part of this period, use of the bandages may be discontinued except during activities that will likely stress the injured part. Remember that reinjury is still possible while these bandages are being used.

Side effects: The simple elastic bandage can cause trouble when not properly applied. Problems arise because the bandage is applied too tightly, and circulation in the limb beyond the bandage is impaired. The bandage should be firm but not tight. The limb should not swell, hurt, or be cooler beyond the bandage. There should not be any blueness or purple color to the limb. When wrapping the bandage, start at the most distant area to be bandaged and work toward the trunk of the body, making each loop a little looser than the one before. Thus a knee bandage should be tighter below the knee than above, and an ankle bandage should be tighter on the foot than on the lower leg. Many people think that because a bandage is elastic it must be stretched. This is not the case. The stretching is for when you move. Simply wrap the bandage as you would a roll of gauze.

UPSET STOMACH

Absorbable Antacids: Baking Soda, Alka-Seltzer Gold, Tums

The main ingredient in these products is sodium bicarbonate, which neutralizes acid, at least in a test tube. In the human stomach, its action is not so clear. For one thing, it may be absorbed through the walls of the stomach, thus not helping with the acid problem there, and in large doses it may upset the body's own chemistry. More important, there may be "rebound" after taking sodium bicarbonate; that is, the stomach may be stimulated to secrete more acid. This, of course, only adds to the problem and may be one reason that any relief that is provided is short-term. For these reasons, we prefer the nonabsorbable antacids.

Nonabsorbable Antacids: Maalox, Gelusil, Mylanta, Alugel, Wingel, Riopan

The nonabsorbable antacids are an important part of the home pharmacy. They help neutralize stomach acid and thus decrease heartburn, ulcer pain, gas pains, and stomach upset. Since they are not absorbed by the body, they usually do not upset the acid-base balance of the body and are quite safe.

Almost all of these antacids are available in both liquid and tablet form. For most purposes, the liquid form is superior. It coats more of the surface area of the gullet and stomach than the tablets do. Indeed, if not well chewed, the tablets may be almost worthless. Still, during work or play a bottle can be cumbersome, and a few tablets in a shirt pocket or handbag may help out with midday doses.

Reading the labels: Nonabsorbable antacids contain magnesium or aluminum, or both. As a general rule, magnesium causes diarrhea and aluminum causes constipation. Different brands are slightly different mixtures of the salts of these two metals, designed to avoid both diarrhea and constipation. A few brands also contain calcium, which is mildly constipating; in general the calcium-containing preparations should be avoided.

Different products differ in taste. While there are some differences in potency, most people will ultimately select the particular antacid that has a taste they can tolerate and that doesn't upset their bowels. Keep trying different brands until you are satisfied.

Dosage: Two tablespoons (30 cc) or two tablets, well-chewed, is the standard adult dose. Use one-half the adult dose for children of ages six to twelve, and one-quarter the adult dose for children of ages three to six. The frequency of the dose depends upon the severity of the problem. For stomach upset or heartburn, one or two doses may often suffice. For gastritis, several doses a day for several days may be needed. For ulcers, six weeks or more may be needed, with the medication taken as frequently as every hour or so; this type of program should be supervised by a physician.

Side effects: In general, the only problem is the effect on the bowel movements. Maalox tends to loosen the stools slightly, Mylanta and Gelusil are about average, and Alugel and Aludrox (with more aluminum) tend to be more constipating. Adjust the dose and change brands as needed. Check with your doctor before using these compounds if you have kidney disease, heart disease, or high blood pressure. Some brands contain significant quantities of salt and should be avoided by people on a low-salt diet. Riopan has the lowest salt content of the popular brands.

WARTS

Wart Removers: Compound W, Vergo

Warts are a curious little problem. The capricious way in which they form and disappear has led to countless myths and home therapies. They can be surgically removed, burned off, or frozen off, but they also will go away by themselves or after treatment by hypnosis. Warts are caused by a virus and are a reaction to a minor local viral infection. If you get one, you are likely to get more. When one disappears, the others often follow. The exception is plantar warts, on the sole of the foot, which will not go away by themselves and not always with home treatment; the physician may be needed.

Over-the-counter chemicals for treatment of warts are moderately effective. They contain a mild skin irritant. By repeated application, the top layers of the wart are slowly burned off, and eventually the virus is destroyed.

Dosage: Apply repeatedly, as directed on the product label. Persistence is necessary.

81

Side effects: These products are effective because they are caustic to the skin, therefore be careful to apply them only to the wart, and be very careful around the eyes or mouth.

WOUNDS (Minor)

Adhesive Tape, Bandages

Bandages really don't "make it better." Sometimes leaving a minor wound open to the air is preferable to covering it. Still, a home medical shelf wouldn't be complete without a tin of assorted adhesive bandages. In order to fashion larger bandages, you also need adhesive tape and gauze. Bandages are useful for covering tender blisters, keeping dirt out of wounds, and keeping the edges of a cut together. They have some value in keeping the wound out of sight and thus are of cosmetic importance.

Dosage: For smaller cuts and sores, use a bandage from the tin. Usually, leaving the bandage on for a day or so is long enough; change the bandage if you wish to use it longer. For cuts, apply the bandage perpendicular to the cut, and draw the skin toward the cut from both sides to relax skin tension before applying the bandage. The bandage should then act to keep the edges together during healing. For larger injuries, make a bandage from a roll of sterile gauze or from sterile 2 x 2″ or 4 x 4″ gauze pads, and firmly tape it in place with adhesive tape. Change the bandage daily. If you see white fat protruding from the cut, see the doctor.

Side effects: If the wound isn't clean when you cover it with a bandage, you may hide a developing infection from early discovery. Clean the wound and keep it clean. The bandage should be changed if it becomes wet. Some people are allergic to adhesive tape; they should use one of the paper tapes which are nonallergenic. If adhesive tape is left on for a week or so it will irritate almost anyone's skin, so give the skin a rest. Some patients leave a bandage on too long because they are afraid of the pain as they remove the bandage—particularly if there is hair caught in the tape. For painless removal, soak the adhesive tape in nail-polish remover (applied from the back) for five minutes. This will dissolve the adhesive and release both the skin and hair.

Antiseptics and Cleansers: Hydrogen Peroxide, Iodine

A dirty wound often becomes infected; if dirt or foreign bodies are trapped beneath the skin, they can fester and delay wound healing. Only a few germs are introduced at the time of a wound, but they may multiply to a very large number over several days. The purposes of an antiseptic are to remove the dirt and kill the germs. Most of the time, the cleansing action is the more important because many antiseptic solutions, such as hydrogen peroxide, Merthiolate, Zephiran, or Mercurochrome, really aren't very good at killing germs. Antibiotic creams (such as Bacitracin and Neosporin) are expensive, usually not necessary, and of questionable effectiveness. Hydrogen peroxide, which foams and cleans as you work it in the wound, is a good cleansing agent, and iodine is a reasonably good agent with which to kill germs. Scrupulous attention to the initial cleaning of a wound and the scrubbing out of any imbedded dirt particles are crucial to good healing. Do this even though it hurts and bleeds. For small, clean cuts use soap and water followed by iodine and then soap and water again. For larger wounds use hydrogen peroxide with vigorous scrubbing. Betadine is a nonstinging iodine preparation. First-aid sprays are a waste of money.

Dosage: Do not use hydrogen peroxide that is at a strength of more than 3%, such as that used for bleaching hair. Most hydrogen peroxide is sold at the 3% strength and may be used at full strength. Pour it on and scrub with a rough cloth. Wash it off and repeat. Continue until there is no dirt visible beneath the level of the skin. If you can't get it clean, go to the doctor.

Iodine is painted or wiped onto the wound and the surrounding area. Wash it off within a few minutes, leaving a trace of the iodine color on the skin.

Side effects: Iodine will burn the skin if left on full strength, so be careful. Iodine is poisonous if swallowed; keep it away from children. Hydrogen peroxide is safe to the skin but can bleach hair and clothing, so try not to spill it. Some people are allergic to iodine; discontinue use if you get a rash.

Soaking Agent: Sodium Bicarbonate (Baking Soda)

Sodium bicarbonate (baking soda, $NaHCO_3$) is a very useful household chemical. It has three principal medical uses: As a strong solution, it will draw fluid and swelling out of a wound, and will act to soak and clean the wound at the same time. As a weaker solution, it acts to soothe the skin and reduce itching; thus it is helpful in conditions ranging from sunburn to poison oak to chicken pox. If taken by mouth, it serves as an antacid and may help heartburn or stomach upset.

Dosage: (1) For soaking a wound: one tablespoon to a cup of warm water. If a finger or toe is injured, it may be placed in the cup; for other wounds a wash cloth should be saturated with the solution and placed over the wound as a compress. Generally, a wound should be soaked for five to ten minutes at a time, three times a day. If the skin is puckered and "waterlogged" after the soak, it has been soaked too long. A cellophane or plastic wrap may be placed over the cloth compress to retain heat and moisture longer. (2) For soothing the skin: from two tablespoons to a half-cup in a bath of warm water; blot gently after the bath and allow to dry on the skin; repeat as often as necessary. (3) As an antacid: one teaspoonful in a glass of water, every four hours as needed—but only occasionally (see Antacids).

Side effects: There are none as long as the baking soda is only applied to the skin. Be careful if you take it by mouth: First, there is a lot of sodium in it, and if you have heart trouble, high blood pressure, or are on a low-salt diet, you can get into a lot of trouble. Second, if you take it for many months on a regular basis, there is some evidence that it may result in calcium deposits in the kidneys, and thus in kidney damage. As an antacid it is "absorbable" and is thus more dangerous than antacids that are not absorbed by the intestine.

VITAMIN DEFICIENCY

Vitamin Preparations

Americans are said to have the most expensive urine in the world. Much of its added worth comes from unneeded vitamins which are excreted unchanged in the urine and cannot aid the body. Most vitamins are chemically known as coenzymes. They are essential to normal function but are required in only very small amounts. With an ordinary diet, many times the required amounts of vitamins are provided. Vitamin supplementation is needed only by severe alcoholics or by people with unusually limited diets.

Megavitamin doses, providing many times the known requirements for vitamin C, vitamin E, and other vitamins, have been advocated by a few people. Considering the biological role of vitamins in enzyme systems, the available vitamin supply to primitive societies, and the forces of evolution, we find it difficult to conceive of a role for such extra vitamin therapy. Extra vitamins have not been shown to decrease common colds, improve sex life, restore lost energy, or to cure or prevent cancer or arthritis. Doctors, who can get vitamins free, almost never take them. Nor do we, the authors, take vitamins or give vitamins to our families.

Unless a physician documents a vitamin deficiency and recommends a supplement, use of vitamins is entirely optional. It's your money. If you want to buy vitamins, select the cheaper "house" brands which are not advertised heavily.

Dosage: As specified by a physician for the individual's use.

Side effects: Vitamin A, vitamin D, and vitamin B6 (Pyridoxine) can cause severe problems when excessively large doses are taken. Vitamin C is theoretically toxic when taken in large doses but has not yet proved to be much of a practical problem. Other vitamins have not been as well studied, but no serious side effects are known.

10 Avoiding Medical Fraud

At least $3 billion yearly are spent on frauds, hoaxes, and false cures. You probably contribute to this windfall. When you buy worthless drugs as a result of television advertisements, take massive amounts of the vitamin-of-the-month, or send away for "cures" advertised in the back of magazines, you are paying part of this bill. You are being hustled.

You can recognize a hustle. There are four questions, one or more of which will usually identify the dishonest marketer. The questions are: What is the motive? What are the claims? Do experts in the field use the service? Does the service make sense? Let's examine these questions.

What Is the Motive of the Marketer?

Make some rough estimates of the proposed service as a business. Is it a revolving-door operation, where people walk in one door with their money and soon thereafter leave without it? What is the average fee paid by the customer? How many patients are seen each hour? The product of these two numbers represents the hourly income of the operation. If this gross amount exceeds one hundred dollars per professional employee, watch out. Many patients have paid hundreds of dollars to have their arthritis "treated" with ordinary "flu shots" which should represent a trivial charge. Medicines may be repackaged and marked up and misrepresented. The hustler is doing it for the money. Don't be misled by a "loss leader" that is an apparent bargain. Look at the total cost over the long term.

What Are the Promises and Claims Made?

Are they vague? Misleading? A typical advertisement urges purchase of a product "containing an ingredient recommended by doctors." This is clearly intended to deceive; the advertiser knows that if the ingredient were named, you would recognize it to be relatively ineffective for the problem or readily available at less expense.

Beware of testimonials, coupons, and guarantees. If a product or service is advertised by testimonial, it is probably of marginal value or lower. A testimonial may consist of "before and after" pictures. It may be a story told by a presumed patient relating success with the treatment. On occasion, testimonials will be totally fabricated. However, even if the testimonial is accurate, it provides no reliable information. Your interest is not whether the proposed service has *ever* helped anyone but whether it is likely to help you. There is an important difference in these statements.

Coupons are another clue to bad services. Worthwhile treatments are not marketed through magazine and newspaper coupons. "Guarantees" in medicine are almost a guarantee that the product or service is worthless. In medicine, a guarantee is not possible. There are always exceptions, as well as the possibility of unfortunate results. No worthwhile medical service is accompanied by a money-back guarantee. Thus it isn't that the guarantee will not be honored (which is probably also the case) but that the offer itself strongly suggests a suspicious product.

Do Experts In the Field Use the Service?

Does your doctor take the vitamin you are considering? Does the doctor's family? Do arthritis doctors who have arthritis wear copper bracelets? Do cancer doctors use laetrile when they or their spouses have cancer? Doctors (and their families) get cancer and other diseases just as frequently as anybody else. If any treatment had the remotest chance of benefiting one of these serious conditions, the physician would use that product. In point of fact, physicians do not use these marginal services. Instead, doctors have decreased their cigarette smoking. They have taken up jogging and other regular forms of exercise. They have not endorsed megavitamin therapy, diet fads, and other popular fancies by their own use, except in unusual instances.

Who, if anyone, endorses the service? Is it endorsed by a national professional organization? Or by a national consumer organization? Direct product endorsement by such organizations is rare but of great value if given. Endorsement of toothpaste containing stannous fluoride by the American Dental Association is an example. Consumers Union and its magazine *Consumer Reports* may be relied upon for thoughtful discussions of the medical issues of the day. Another excellent source is the newsletter of the Center for Consumer Health Education, 380 West Maple Avenue, Vienna, Virginia 22180.

Does the Proposed Service Make Sense?

This is the final test. Frequently, frauds and promotion of false cures are successful because no one really asks whether it makes common sense. Do you really think that creams will improve your bust line? Or that you can lose weight only in the hips? Or that a vitamin will help your sex life? Or that a lamb's embryo will keep you young? By definition, a false cure has a false rationale. This rationale is often weak and easily identified as such.

Three Examples

Three of the oldest and largest medical rackets victimize people who have the problems of obesity, arthritis, or cancer.

Overweight people appear to be particularly willing victims for the fringe health entrepreneur. As we noted in Chapter 1, successful weight control is achieved gradually, through moderate programs, and must be sustained for a lifetime. A weight-loss program has merit when it projects its program for a prolonged period. There is negligible medical benefit (and quite possibly harm) in weight loss that occurs abruptly and lasts only a few weeks or months. Individuals with a significant weight problem face a very difficult task requiring intense commitment, long-term discipline, and considerable emotional distress. We applaud the courage of those who undertake such a program and the fortitude of those able to maintain an important but difficult task.

The fraudulent approach is to promise a shortcut. A gadget of some type, massage, a miracle diet, an appetite suppressant, a food supplement, or some other mechanism is promoted as a way to "lose weight fast and easy." "Fast" and "easy" do not describe safe and effective weight loss programs.

The facts are relatively straightforward. Most overweight people do not succeed in both losing weight and maintaining a steady desirable level under any program. The best results have been obtained under medically supervised programs, and with reputable, long-term programs such as "Weight Watchers." Spot-reducing (reduction of fat at one particular point in the body such as the hips or legs) does not work. Massage is not an effective way to lose weight. Appetite suppressants have not been successful over the long term. A brief period of weight loss frequently occurs with any technique promoted. Almost any program has an occasional success, but it is the individual and not the fad that is responsible for this improvement.

Arthritis is another ideal subject for exploitation. Arthritis problems are often chronic and discouraging. A widespread myth exists that arthritis cannot be treated by traditional medicine. But the tragedy of false fads in arthritis is aggravated by this myth, because good treatment is available for almost all patients. Patients are often unnecessarily crippled because they avoided sound, established medical approaches. The fourth test for recognizing a hustle in the area of arthritis is that of use: Does it make sense? Diet for arthritis? You can understand a diet for losing weight, but what does it have to do with pain in the joints? Vinegar and honey for arthritis? Copper bracelets?

A legend persists that other countries have better drugs for arthritis than the United States. It is true that the Food and Drug Administration has rather carefully limited approval of new therapies for arthritis. There have been, at most points in recent years, several drugs available in Mexico, Canada, and Europe which are not yet licensed in the United States. However, none of these drugs is a major addition to existing therapy. The position of the Food and Drug Administration has been to insure as carefully as possible the safety of new medications before allowing them to enter the market. There are no magical new drugs.

The legend of dramatic new treatments has led to fraudulent medical operations just over the Mexican border. (Such operations should not be confused with the very fine medicine available at many locations in Mexico.) These "arthritis mills" attract patients who come long distances to be seen briefly and then return to the United States with bags and boxes full of medications. Patients are told a variety of things about these medications, but it is usually suggested that they are being given drugs not available in the United States. We have had occasion to analyze the contents of such medications, and the active ingredient has uniformly been a drug related to cortisone; a drug called phenylbutazone is often present in combination with it. Both are available and frequently prescribed in the United States, but they are hazardous and have resulted in fatalities. Ill-conceived therapies with such drugs often make patients feel better over the first few days and weeks; such short-term improvement is what keeps the waiting rooms full. Over the longer term, increased disability and even death can result. Common sense suggests that the best medical care in the world is unlikely to be found in Mexican border towns. When you suspend common sense, you can lose more than money.

Acupuncture has received great publicity and is under intensive evaluation as a treatment for arthritis. The early studies suggest a minor effect in pain relief, less strong than the effect of aspirin. However, final information is not yet available. Other fad cures, such as cocaine or flu shots or bee venom have already been definitely discredited.

DMSO is a special case. This drug was removed from medical testing programs because of fears of toxicity but now is back as a legal remedy in some states, with limited distribution. We have studied it, and as a liniment, it is good. But it is not an active medication against arthritis. It will not help rheumatoid arthritis or osteoarthritis. Crazy things are being said about this drug, which is an industrial solvent. Don't believe everything that you hear.

Cancer is the area of the cruelest hoaxes. In some cases, when cancer has already spread throughout the body, orthodox medicine cannot help the patient very much. In this setting, the vultures move in. "What have you got to lose?" is their call. The answer is that you may lose courage, dignity, and money. The tragedy of quack cancer treatments is that you have nothing to gain.

Cancer is not one but many diseases, requiring many different approaches to treatment. Very effective treatment is available for some cancers, and new techniques are being applied as fast as they can be proven effective. The great majority of cancer patients can be helped by present medical treatment. Many agencies and patients are working very hard to contribute to knowledge in cancer. This is a sophisticated field, with many minds working toward solutions. It is highly unlikely that significant discoveries will come in the form of apricot pits or horse serum. In our own experience, we have seen hundreds of patients take dozens of different "cures"; not a single one has received benefit.

You are hustled because you want to believe. Your wish that the claims might be true does not make them become so.

Section II THE PATIENT AND THE COMMON COMPLAINT

A How to Use This Section

In this section, you will find general information and decision charts for nearly one hundred common medical problems. The *general information* on the left-hand page will give you background on a specific medical problem and will help you interpret the decision chart. It will also provide instructions for home treatment, as well as what to expect at the doctor's office, if you go. The *decision chart* on the right-hand page will help you decide whether to use home treatment or consult a physician. To gain the most benefit from this part of the book, use these simple guidelines:

Emergencies. Before dealing with any medical problem at home, the first question to ask is whether or not emergency action is necesary. Often the answer is obvious. The great majority of complaints are quickly recognized as minor. The true emergency is hard to ignore. The information in part B, Emergencies, presents a commonsense approach to several problems that require immediate action. All decision charts assume that emergency symptoms have been considered first.

Finding the right chart for your medical problem. Determine your "chief complaint" or symptom—for instance, a cough, an earache, or chest pains—look it up in the Table of Contents, or in the Index, and then turn to the appropriate pages.

Multiple problems. If you have more than one problem, you may have to use more than one decision chart. For example, if you have abdominal pain, nausea, and diarrhea, look up your most serious complaint first, then the next most serious, and so on. You may notice some duplication of questions in the decision charts, especially when the symptoms are closely related. If you use more than one chart, take the most "conservative" advice; if one chart recommends home treatment and another advises a call to the physician, then call the doctor.

Using the charts. First, read all of the general information under your particular problem, then go to the decision chart. Start at the top and follow the arrows. Skipping around may result in errors. Each question assumes that all previous questions have been answered. The general information under the medical problem will help you understand the questions in the chart. If this general material is ignored, a question may be misinterpreted and the wrong course of action selected.

If the chart indicates home treatment. Don't assume that an instruction to use home treatment guarantees that the problem is trivial and may be ignored. Home therapy must be approached conscientiously if it is to work. If over-the-counter medicines are suggested, look them up in the Index and read about dosage and side effects in Chapter 9 before you use them.

There are times when home treatment is not effective despite conscientious application, and in these cases, a physician should be consulted. The length of time you should wait before consulting a doctor is indicated in the general information for each problem. The home treatment we include in these pages is what most physicians recommend as a first approach to these problems. If it doesn't work, think the problem through again. If you are seriously worried about your condition, call the doctor.

If the chart indicates that you should consult a physician. This does not necessarily mean that the illness is serious or dangerous. Often you are directed to the doctor because a physical examination needs to be performed or because certain facilities of the physician's office are needed. The chart will refer you to a physician with different levels of urgency. "See physician now" means right away. "See physician today" indicates that the visit should be the same day. "Make appointment with physician" means a less urgent situation; the visit should be scheduled but may take place any time during the next few days. We try to give you the medical terminology related to each specific problem. With this information, you will be able to "translate" the terms your doctor may use during your visit or telephone call.

In this revised edition we are encouraging use of the telephone by instructing you to "call physician now" or "call physician today." Often a phone call will enable you and your physician or nurse to make decisions that will avoid unnecessary visits and to use medical care more wisely. Remember that most physicians do not charge for telephone advice but regard it as part of their service for regular patients. Don't abuse this in an attempt to avoid paying for necessary medical care. At the same time, if every call results in a routine recommendation for a visit, then you are probably not getting useful information from the call.

With these guidelines, you will be able to use the decision charts to quickly locate the information you need, while not burdening yourself with information that you do not require. Examine some of the charts now; you will quickly learn how to find the answers you need.

B Emergencies

Emergencies require prompt action, not panic. What action you should take depends on the facilities available and the nature of the problem. If there are massive injuries or if the patient is unconscious, you must get help immediately. Go to the emergency room if it is close. If it isn't, you can often obtain help over the phone by calling an emergency room or the rescue squad. This is especially important if you think that someone has swallowed poison.

The most important thing is to *be prepared*. Record the phone numbers of the nearest emergency facility, poison control center, and rescue squad in the front of this book. Know the best way to reach the emergency room by car. Develop these procedures *before* an actual emergency arises.

When to call an ambulance. Usually the slowest way to reach a medical facility is by ambulance. It must travel both ways and often is not twice as fast as a private car. If the patient can readily move or be moved, and a private car is available, use the car and have someone call ahead. The ambulance is expensive and may be needed more urgently at another location, so engage it with care.

The ambulance brings with it a trained crew, who know how to lift a patient to minimize chance of further injury. Oxygen is usually available; splints and bandages are carried; and in some instances, life-saving resuscitation may be employed en route to the hospital. Thus the patient who is gravely ill, has a back or head injury, or is severely short of breath may benefit from care afforded by the ambulance attendants.

In our experience, ambulances are too often used as expensive taxis. The type of accident or illness, the facilities available, and the distance involved are all important factors in deciding whether an ambulance should be used.

The instruction charts in the rest of this book assume that no emergency signs are present. These signs "overrule" the charts and dictate that medical help be sought immediately. Be familiar with the following emergency signs:

Major injury. Common sense tells us that the patient with a broken leg or large chest wound deserves immediate attention. Emergency facilities exist to take care of major injuries. They should be used promptly.

Unconsciousness. The patient who is unconscious needs emergency care immediately.

Active bleeding. Most cuts will stop bleeding if pressure is applied to the wound. Unless the bleeding is obviously minor, a wound that continues to bleed despite the application of pressure requires attention in order to prevent unnecessary loss of blood. The average adult can tolerate the loss of several cups of blood with little ill effect, but children can tolerate only smaller amounts, proportional to their body size. Remember that active and vigorous bleeding can almost always be controlled by the application of pressure directly to the wound and that this is the most important part of first aid for such wounds.

Stupor or drowsiness. A decreased level of mental activity, short of unconsciousness, is termed "stupor." A practical way of determining if the severity of stupor or drowsiness warrants urgent treatment is to note the patient's ability to answer questions. If the patient is not sufficiently awake to answer questions concerning what has happened, then urgent action is necessary. Children are difficult to judge, but the child who cannot be aroused needs immediate attention.

Disorientation. In medicine, disorientation is described in terms of time, place, and person. This simply means that a patient cannot tell the date, the location, or who he or she is. The person who does not know his or her own identity is in a more difficult state than the person who cannot give the correct date. Disorientation may be part of a variety of illnesses and is especially common when a high fever is present. The patient who previously has been alert and then becomes disoriented and confused deserves immediate medical attention.

Shortness of breath. Shortness of breath is described more extensively in Problem 75. As a general rule, immediate attention is needed if the patient is short of breath even though resting. However, in young adults the most frequent cause of shortness of breath at rest is the hyperventilation syndrome, Problem 69, which is not a serious concern. Nevertheless, if it cannot be confidently determined that shortness of breath is due to the hyperventilation syndrome, then the only reasonable course of action is to seek immediate aid.

Cold sweats. Sweating is the normal response to elevated temperature. It is also the natural response to stress, either psychological or physical. Most people have experienced sweaty palms when "put on the spot" or stressed psychologically. As an indication of physical stress, "cold sweat" is helpful in determining the urgency of a problem. Cold sweat is a common effect of severe pain or serious illness. Sweating without other complaints is unusual; as an isolated symptom it is not likely to be serious. In contrast, a cold sweat in a patient complaining of chest pain, abdominal pain, or lightheadedness indicates a need for immediate attention. Remember, however, that aspirin often causes sweating in lowering a fever; sweating associated with the breaking of a fever is not the "cold sweat" referred to here.

Severe pain. Surprisingly enough, severe pain is rarely the symptom that determines if a problem is serious and urgent. Most often it is associated with other symptoms that indicate the nature of the condition; the most obvious example is pain associated with major injury—like a broken leg— which itself clearly requires urgent care. The severity of pain is subjective and depends upon the particular patient; often the magnitude of the pain has been altered by emotional and psychological factors. Nevertheless, severe pain demands urgent medical attention, if for no other reason than to relieve the pain.

Much of the art and science of medicine is directed at the relief of pain, and the use of emergency procedures to secure this relief are justified even if the cause of the pain eventually proves to be inconsequential. However, the patient who frequently complains of severe pain from minor causes is in much the same situation as the boy who cried "wolf"; calls for help will inevitably be taken less and less seriously by the doctor. This situation is a dangerous one, for the patient may have more difficulty in obtaining help when it is most needed.

Work out a procedure for medical emergencies. Develop and test it before an actual emergency arises. If you plan emergency action ahead of time, you will decrease the likelihood of panic and increase the probability of providing the proper care quickly.

We have not attempted to teach complex first-aid procedures such as cardiopulmonary resuscitation (CPR) or the abdominal-thrust (Heimlich) maneuver. To use these procedures correctly you need intensive instruction and an opportunity to practice these skills. Providing these is beyond the capability of the printed word. Community organizations such as the American Red Cross and the American Heart Association offer training in these procedures.

C Poisons

1 Oral Poisoning

Although poisons may be inhaled or absorbed through the skin, for the most part they are swallowed. The term *ingestion* refers to oral poisoning.

Most poisoning can be prevented. Children almost always swallow poison accidentally. Keep harmful substances, such as medications, insecticides, caustic cleansers, and organic solvents like kerosene, gasoline, or furniture polish, out of the reach of children. The most damaging are strong alkali solutions such as drain cleaners (Drano and others), which will destroy any tissue with which they come in contact.

Treatment must be prompt to be effective, but accurate identification of the substance is as important as speed. *Don't panic.* Call the doctor or poison control center immediately and get advice on what to do. Attempt to identify the substance without causing undue delay. Always bring the container with you to the emergency room. Life-support measures take precedence in the case of the unconscious victim, but the ingested substance must be identified before proper therapy can be instituted.

Suicide attempts cause many significant medication overdoses. Any suicide attempt is an indication that help is needed. Such help is not optional, even if the patient has "recovered" and is in no immediate danger. Most successful suicides are preceded by unsuccessful attempts.

Home Treatment

All cases of poisoning require professional help. Someone should call for help immediately. If the patient is conscious and alert and the ingredients swallowed are known, there are two types of treatment: those in which vomiting should be induced, and those in which it should not. Vomiting can be very dangerous if the poison contains strong acids, alkalis, or petroleum products. These substances can destroy the esophagus or damage the lungs as they are vomited. Neutralize them with milk while contacting the physician. If you don't have milk, use water or milk of magnesia.

Vomiting is a safe way to remove medications and suspicious plants. It is more effective and safer than using a stomach pump and does not require the doctor's help. Vomiting can sometimes be achieved immediately by stimulating the back of the throat with a finger (don't be squeamish!), or by giving two to four teaspoons of *syrup* (*not* extract) of ipecac, followed by as much liquid as the patient can drink. Vomiting follows usually within twenty minutes, but since time is important, using your finger to induce vomiting is sometimes quicker. Or you can try both methods. Mustard mixed with warm water also works. If there is no vomiting in twenty-five minutes, repeat the dose of syrup of ipecac. Collect the vomitus so that it can be examined by the physician.

Before, after, or during first aid, contact a physician. Many communities have established poison control centers to identify poisons and give advice. These are often located in emergency rooms. Find out if such a center exists in your community, and if so, record the telephone number both on the accompanying decision chart and in the front of this book. Quick first aid and fast professional advice are your best chance to avoid a tragedy.

If an accidental poisoning has occurred, make sure that it doesn't happen again. Put poisons where children cannot reach them. Flush old medications down the toilet.

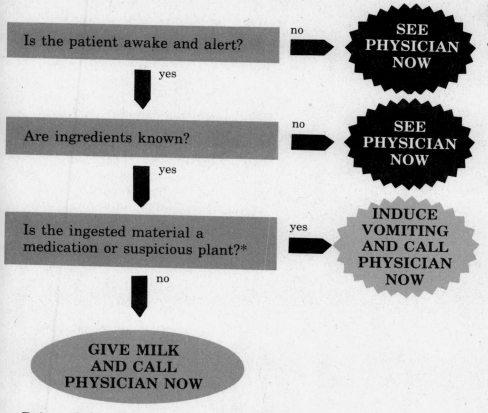

Is the patient awake and alert? — no → **SEE PHYSICIAN NOW**

yes ↓

Are ingredients known? — no → **SEE PHYSICIAN NOW**

yes ↓

Is the ingested material a medication or suspicious plant?* — yes → **INDUCE VOMITING AND CALL PHYSICIAN NOW**

no ↓

GIVE MILK AND CALL PHYSICIAN NOW

Poison Control Center Telephone Number _____

Emergency Room Telephone Number _____

* Do not induce vomiting if the patient has swallowed any of the following:

Acids: battery acid, sulfuric acid, hydrochloric acid, bleach, hair straightener, etc.

Alkalis: Drano, drain cleaners, oven cleaners, etc.

Petroleum Products: Gasoline, furniture polish, kerosene, oil, lighter fluid, etc.

What to Expect at the Doctor's Office

Significant poisoning is best managed at the emergency room. Treatment of the conscious patient depends on the particular poison and whether vomiting has been achieved successfully. If indicated, the stomach will be evacuated by vomiting or by the use of a stomach pump. Patients who are unconscious or have swallowed a strong acid or alkali will require admission to the hospital. Observation at home is important for those who are not admitted to the hospital.

D Common Injuries

2 Cuts (Lacerations)

Most cuts affect only the skin and the fatty tissue beneath it. Usually they heal without permanent damage. However, injury to internal structures such as muscles, tendons, blood vessels, ligaments, or nerves presents the possibility of permanent damage. Your physician can decrease this likelihood.

It may be difficult for you to determine whether major blood vessels, nerves, or tendons have been damaged. Bleeding that cannot be controlled with pressure, numbness or weakness in the limb beyond the wound, or inability to move fingers or toes normally call for examination by a physician.

Signs of infection—such as pus oozing from the wound, fever, extensive redness and swelling—will not appear for at least twenty-four hours. Bacteria need time to grow and multiply. If these signs do appear, a physician must be consulted.

Stitching (suturing) a laceration is a ritual in our society. The only purpose in suturing a wound is to pull the edges together to hasten healing and minimize scarring. Stitches are not recommended if the wound can be held closed without them, since they injure tissue to some extent.

See the doctor if the edges of the wound cannot be kept together, if signs of infection are present, or if the cut is not healing well within two weeks. Stitching must be done within eight hours of the injury, because germs begin to grow in the wound and can be trapped under the skin, causing it to fester.

A cut on the face, chest, abdomen, or back is potentially more serious than one on the legs or arms (extremities). Cuts on the trunk or face should be examined by a physician unless the injury is very small or shallow. A call to the doctor's office will help you decide if the doctor's help is needed.

Facial wounds in a young child who drools are often too wet to treat with bandages, so the doctor's help is usually needed. Because of potential disfigurement, all but minor facial wounds should be treated professionally. Stitching is often required in young children who are apt to pull off bandages, or in areas that are subject to a great deal of motion, such as the fingers or joints. Cuts in the palm that become infected can be difficult to treat, so do not attempt home treatment unless the cut is shallow.

Home Treatment

Cleanse the wound. Soap and water will do, but be vigorous. Hydrogen peroxide (3%) may also be used. Make sure that no dirt, glass, or other foreign material remains in the wound. Antiseptics such as Mercurochrome and Merthiolate are unlikely to help, and some are painful. Iodine will kill germs, but it is not really needed and is also painful. (Betadine is a modified iodine preparation that is painless but costly).

The edges of a clean, minor cut can usually be held together by "butterfly" bandages or, preferably, "steristrips"—strips of sterile paper tape. Apply either of these bandages so that the edges of the wound join without "rolling under."

See the doctor if the edges of the wound cannot be kept together, if signs of infection appear (pus, fever, extensive redness and swelling), or if the cut is not healing well within two weeks.

Removing Stitches

Your doctor will tell you when the stiches are to be removed. Unless there

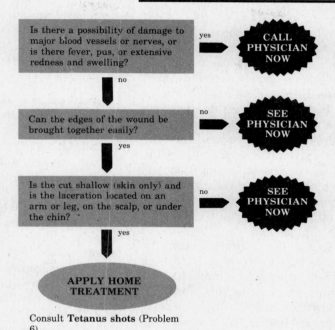

Is there a possibility of damage to major blood vessels or nerves, or is there fever, pus, or extensive redness and swelling? — yes → **CALL PHYSICIAN NOW**

no ↓

Can the edges of the wound be brought together easily? — no → **SEE PHYSICIAN NOW**

yes ↓

Is the cut shallow (skin only) and is the laceration located on an arm or leg, on the scalp, or under the chin? — no → **SEE PHYSICIAN NOW**

yes ↓

APPLY HOME TREATMENT

Consult **Tetanus shots** (Problem 6).

is some other reason to return to the doctor, you can perform this simple procedure. First, gently lift the stitch away from the skin by grasping a loose end of the knot; tweezers help. Sometimes in order to accomplish this, a scab must be removed by soaking. Next, cut the stitch at the end as close to the skin as possible and pull it out. A pair of small, sharp scissors or a fingernail clipper works well. It is important to get close to the skin so that a minimum amount of the stitch that was outside the skin is pulled through. This reduces the chance of contamination and infection.

What to Expect at the Doctor's Office

The wound will be thoroughly cleansed and explored to be sure that no foreign particles are left and that blood vessels, nerves, and tendons are undamaged. The physician may use an anesthetic to deaden the area. Be aware of any allergy to lidocaine (Xylocaine) or other local anesthetics; report any possible allergy to the physician. The physician will determine the need, if any, for a tetanus shot and decide whether antibiotics are needed (they usually are not). Lacerations that may require a surgical specialist include those with injury to tendons or major vessels, especially when this damage has occurred in the hand. Facial cuts may also require a surgical specialist if a good cosmetic result appears difficult to obtain.

3 Puncture Wounds

Puncture wounds are those caused by nails, pins, tacks, and other sharp objects. The most important question is whether a tetanus shot is needed. Consult **Tetanus Shots** (Problem 6) to determine this. Puncture wounds do occasionally require further medical attention.

Most minor puncture wounds are located in the extremities, particularly in the feet. If the puncture wound is located on the head, abdomen, or chest, a hidden internal injury may have occurred. Unless a wound in these areas is obviously shallow see a physician.

Injury to a tendon, nerve, or major blood vessel is rare but can be serious. Injury to an artery may be indicated by blood pumping vigorously from the wound; injury to a nerve usually causes numbness or tingling in the wounded limb, beyond the site of the wound; injury to a tendon causes difficulty in moving the limb (usually fingers or toes) beyond the wound. Major injuries such as these occur more often from a nail, ice pick, or large instrument than with a narrow implement such as a needle.

To avoid infection, be absolutely sure that nothing has been left in the wound. Sometimes, for example, part of a needle will break off and remain in the foot. If there is any question of a foreign body remaining, the wound should be examined by the physician.

Signs of infection do not occur immediately at the time of injury; they usually take at least twenty-four hours to develop. The formation of pus, a fever, or severe redness and swelling are indications that the wound should be seen by a physician.

Many physicians feel that puncture wounds of the hand, if not very minor, should be treated with antibiotics. Once started, infections deep in the hand are difficult to treat and may lead to loss of function. Call the physician for advice if a puncture wound of the hand has occurred.

Home Treatment

Clean the wound to prevent infection. Let it bleed as much as possible to carry foreign material to the outside, since you cannot scrub the inside of a puncture wound. Do not apply pressure to stop the bleeding unless there is a large amount of blood loss and a "pumping," squirting kind of bleeding. The wound should be washed thoroughly with soap and warm water and checked as thoroughly as possible for remaining foreign objects. Hydrogen peroxide (3%) can also be used to cleanse the wound.

Soak the wound in warm water several times a day for four to five days. The object of the soaking is to keep the skin puncture open as long as possible, so that any germs or foreign debris can drain from the open wound. If the wound is allowed to close, an infection may form beneath the skin but not become apparent for several days. Consult **Tetanus Shots** (Problem 6).

See the physician if there are signs of infection or if the wound is not healed within two weeks.

What to Expect at the Doctor's Office

The physician will answer the questions on the opposite chart by history and examination. The wound will be surgically explored if necessary. More frequently, it will be observed for a reaction to a foreign body over the next few days. If a metallic foreign body is suspected, X-rays may be taken. Be prepared to tell the physician the date of the last tetanus

Is the wound located in an extremity?

no → **SEE PHYSICIAN NOW**

yes ↓

Are any of the following present?
(a) Injury to a major nerve or blood vessel
(b) Any foreign material in the wound
(c) Fever, pus, or extensive redness and swelling.

yes → **SEE PHYSICIAN NOW**

no ↓

Is this a puncture wound of the hand?

yes → **CALL PHYSICIAN TODAY**

no ↓

APPLY HOME TREATMENT

Consult **Tetanus Shots** (Problem 6).

shot. Most physicians will recommend home treatment. Antibiotics will only rarely be suggested. In puncture wounds caused by bird shot, the shot may be left in the skin. Occasionally glass or wood may be left in for a period of time to give the body time to push it to the surface.

4 Animal Bites

The question or rabies is of uppermost concern following an animal bite. The main carriers of rabies are wild animals, especially skunks, foxes, bats, raccoons, and opossums. Rabies is also carried, though rarely, by cattle, dogs, and cats, and it is extremely rare in squirrels, chipmunks, rats, and mice. Although 3000 to 4000 animals with rabies are found each year, only one or two humans annually contract the disease in the United States. Rabid animals act strangely, attack without provocation, and may foam at the mouth. Be concerned if the attacking animal has any of these characteristics.

Any bite by an animal other than a pet dog or cat requires consultation with the physician as to whether or not the use of antirabies vacine will be required. If the bite is by a dog or a cat, the animal is being reliably observed for sickness by its owner, and its immunizations are up to date, then consultation with the physician is not required. If the bite has left a wound that might require stitching or other treatment, consult **Cuts** (Problem 2) or **Puncture Wounds** (Problem 3). You should also check **Tetanus Shots** (Problem 6).

Home Treatment

An animal whose immunizations are up to date is, of course, unlikely to have rabies. However, arrange for the animal to be observed for the next fifteen days to make sure that it does not develop rabies. Most often, the owners of the animal can be relied on to observe it. If the owners cannot be trusted, then the animal must be kept for observation by the local public agency charged with that responsibility. Many localities require that animal bites be reported to the health department. If the animal should develop rabies during this time, a serious situation exists and treatment by a physician must be started immediately.

For the wound itself, use soap and water. Treat bites as you would treat cuts or puncture wounds, depending on its appearance.

What to Expect at the Doctor's Office

The physician must balance the usually remote possibility of exposure to rabies against the hazards of rabies vaccine or antirabies serum. An unprovoked attack by a wild animal or a bite from an animal that appears to have rabies may require both the rabies vaccine and the antirabies serum. The extent and location of the wounds also play a part in this decision; severe wounds of the head are the most dangerous.

A bite caused by an animal that has then escaped will often require the use of at least the rabies vaccine. This is one of the most difficult decisons in medicine. Rabies vaccine is administered in fourteen to twenty-one daily injections, which are followed by booster injections ten to twenty days after the initial series. The vaccine will often cause local skin reactions as well as fever, chills, aches, and pain. Severe reactions to the vaccine are rare. The antirabies serum, unfortunately, has a high risk of serious reactions. The serum is given both directly into the wound and by intramuscular injections.

Many physicians give a tetanus shot if the patient is not "up to date" because tetanus bacteria can (rarely) be introduced by an animal bite. Be sure you know when the last tetanus shot was received.

Is this a bite by a dog or cat whose rabies immunizations are current and who is presently being observed?

no →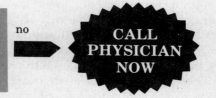

CALL
PHYSICIAN
NOW

yes ↓

Has this bite left a cut or puncture wound that might require a physician's attention?

yes →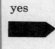

Consult **Cuts** (Problem 2) or **Puncture Wounds** (Problem 3).

no ↓

APPLY HOME TREATMENT

Consult **Tetanus Shots** (Problem 6).

5 Scrapes and Abrasions

Scrapes and abrasions are shallow. Several layers of the skin may be torn or even totally scraped off, but the wound does not go far beneath the skin. Abrasions are usually caused by falls onto the hands, elbows, or knees, but skateboard and bicycle riders can get abrasions on just about any part of the body. Since abrasions expose millions of nerve endings, all of which send pain impulses to the brain, they are usually much more painful than cuts.

Home Treatment

Remove all dirt and foreign matter. Washing the wound with soap and warm water is the most important step in treatment. Hydrogen peroxide (3%) may also be used to cleanse the wound. Most scrapes will "scab" rather quickly; this is nature's way of "dressing" the wound. The use of Mercurochrome, iodine, and other antiseptics does little good and is usually painful. The use of adhesive bandages may be necessary for a wound that continues to ooze blood, but it should be discontinued as soon as possible to allow exposure of the wound to the air and sun.

Loose skin flaps, if they are not dirty, may be left to help form a natural dressing. If the skin flap is dirty, cut it off carefully with nail scissors. (If it hurts, stop! You're cutting the wrong tissue.) Watch the wound for signs of infection—pus, a fever, or severe redness or swelling—but don't be worried by redness around the edges; this is an indication of normal healing. Infection will not be obvious in the first twenty-four hours; fever may indicate a serious infection.

Pain can be treated for the first few minutes with an ice pack in a plastic bag or towel applied over the wounds as needed. The worst pain subsides fairly quickly, and aspirin or acetaminophen can then be used if necessary.

See the doctor if signs of infection appear or if the scrape or abrasion is not healed within two weeks.

What to Expect at the Doctor's Office

The physician will make sure that the wound is free of dirt and foreign matter. Soap and water and hydrogen peroxide (3%) will often be used. Sometimes a local anesthetic is required to reduce the pain of the cleansing process. An antibacterial ointment such as Neosporin or Bacitracin is sometimes applied after cleansing the wound. Betadine is a painless iodine preparation that is also occasionally used. Tetanus shots are not required for simple scrapes, but if the patient is overdue, it is a good chance to get caught up.

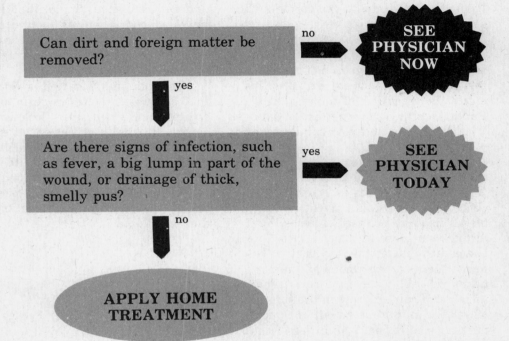

Can dirt and foreign matter be removed?

no → **SEE PHYSICIAN NOW**

yes ↓

Are there signs of infection, such as fever, a big lump in part of the wound, or drainage of thick, smelly pus?

yes → **SEE PHYSICIAN TODAY**

no ↓

APPLY HOME TREATMENT

6 Tetanus Shots

Patients often come to the doctor's office or emergency room simply to get a tetanus shot. Often the wound is minor and needs only some soap and water. If the shot is not needed, you don't need a doctor. The chart on the facing page illustrates the essentials of the current U.S. Public Health Service recommendations. It can save you and your family several visits to the doctor.

The question of whether or not a wound is "clean" and "minor" may be troublesome. Wounds caused by sharp, clean objects such as knives or razor blades have less chance of becoming infected than those in which dirt or foreign bodies have penetrated and lodged beneath the skin. Abrasions and minor burns will not result in tetanus. The tetanus germ cannot grow in the presence of air; the skin must be cut or punctured for the germ to reach an airless location.

If you have never received a basic series of three tetanus shots, you should see the doctor. Sometimes a different kind of tetanus shot is required if you have not been adequately immunized. This shot is called "tetanus immune globulin," and is used when immunization is not complete and there is a significant risk of tetanus. It is more expensive, more painful, and more likely to cause an allergic reaction than the tetanus booster. So keep a record of your family's immunizations in the back of this book and know the dates.

During the first tetanus shots (usually a series of three injections given in early childhood), immunity to tetanus develops over a three-week period. This immunity then slowly declines over many months. After each booster, immunity develops more rapidly and lasts longer. If you have had an initial series of five tetanus injections, immunity will usually last at least ten years after every booster injection. Nevertheless, if a wound has contaminated material beneath the skin and not exposed to the air, and if you have not had a tetanus shot within the past five years, a booster shot is advised to keep the level of immunity as high as possible.

Tetanus immunization is very important because the tetanus germ is quite common and the disease (lockjaw) is so severe. Be absolutely sure that each of your children has had the basic series of three injections and appropriate boosters. Since the immunity lasts so long, adults usually get away with a long period between boosters, but immunization of children should be "by the book."

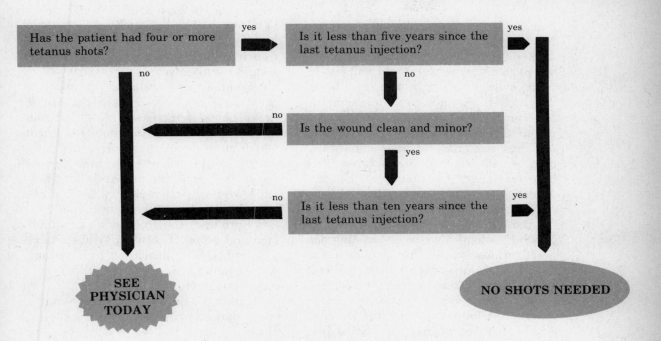

7 Is a Bone Broken?

Neither patient nor doctor can always tell by eye whether or not a bone is broken. We have found fractures when we were not expecting them and not found them when we were sure a bone was broken. So an X-ray is necessary any time that there is a reasonable suspicion of a fracture. The chart on the facing page is a guide to "reasonable suspicion." In the majority of fractures, the bone fragments are already aligned for good healing. Thus prompt manipulation of the fragments is not necessary. If the injured part is protected and resting, a delay of several days before casting does no harm. Remember that the cast does not have healing properties; it just keeps the fragments from getting joggled too much during the healing process. Possible fractures are discussed further in **Ankle Injuries** (Problem 8), **Knee Injuries** (Problem 9), and **Wrist, Elbow, and Shoulder Injuries** (Problem 10).

A fracture can injure nearby nerves and arteries. If the limb is cold, blue, or numb, see the doctor now! Fractures of the pelvis or thigh are particularly serious. Check out all injuries to these areas with the doctor. Fortunately, these fractures are relatively rare except when great force is involved, as in automobile accidents. In these situations the need for immediate help is obvious. For head injuries, see Problem 11.

Paleness, sweating, dizziness, and thirst can indicate shock, and immediate attention is needed.

A crooked limb is an obvious reason to check for fracture. A fracture is clearly indicated when the arm is bent halfway between the elbow and wrist or the leg is bent at midcalf. Pain that prevents use of the injured limb suggests the need for an X-ray. Soft-tissue injuries usually allow some use of the limb, although there are exceptions to this rule.

Although large bruises under the skin are usually caused by soft-tissue injuries alone, marked bruising in a limb that may have a fracture means that you should see the doctor.

Common sense tells us that when great force is involved the possibility of a broken bone is increased. The most common example is the automobile accident, which often gives us the unwanted opportunity to witness the results of great forces applied to the human body. The child who has fallen twenty feet out of a tree is much more likely to have a broken limb than the child who has stumbled and fallen. The severity of the accident is helpful information to have, but some bones break with very little provocation.

Children's bones are younger and hence more flexible and resilient than those of adults. Instead of outright breaks, young bones often bend or splinter like young tree limbs and hence are called "greenstick" fractures. Young bones are also still growing. The growth plates of all bones are at the ends. Consequently, an injury to a bone near the end must be treated more cautiously since growth plate damage may stop limb growth.

Home Treatment

Apply ice packs. The immediate application of cold will help to decrease swelling and inflammation. If a broken bone is suspected, the involved limb should be protected and rested for at least forty-eight hours. To rest a bone effectively, the joint above and below the bone should be immobilized. For example, if

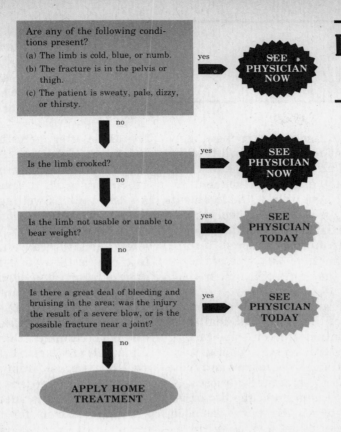

Are any of the following conditions present?
(a) The limb is cold, blue, or numb.
(b) The fracture is in the pelvis or thigh.
(c) The patient is sweaty, pale, dizzy, or thirsty.

yes → **SEE PHYSICIAN NOW**

no ↓

Is the limb crooked?

yes → **SEE PHYSICIAN NOW**

no ↓

Is the limb not usable or unable to bear weight?

yes → **SEE PHYSICIAN TODAY**

no ↓

Is there a great deal of bleeding and bruising in the area; was the injury the result of a severe blow, or is the possible fracture near a joint?

yes → **SEE PHYSICIAN TODAY**

no ↓

APPLY HOME TREATMENT

you suspect a fracture of the lower arm, the splint should prevent the wrist and elbow from moving. Magazines, cardboard, or rolled newspaper can be used. Do not wrap tightly or circulation will be cut off. During this time the limb should be cautiously tested to determine persistence of pain with movement and the return of function. A limb that cannot be used at all is more likely to be broken.

Any injury that is still painful after forty-eight hours should be examined by a physician. Minutes and hours are *not* crucial unless the limb is crooked or there is injury to arteries or nerves. A limb that is adequately protected and rested is likely to have a good outcome even if a fracture is present and casting or splinting is delayed. Aspirin or acetaminophen can be used for pain.

What to Expect at the Doctor's Office

Usually an X-ray will be required. In many offices and emergency rooms, a nurse or physician's assistant will order the X-ray before the patient is even seen by a physician. In other instances, the physician will examine the injury before ordering the X-ray. In a small number of cases, it is possible to be relatively sure that an X-ray is not needed from the history and physical examination. A crooked limb must be "set," which sometimes requires general anesthesia. Pinning the fragments together surgically so that they will heal well is required for certain fractures, such as those of the elbow.

8 Ankle Injuries

Ligaments are tissues that connect the bones of a joint to provide stability during the joint's action. When the ankle is twisted severely, either the ligament or the bone must give way. If the ligaments give way, they may be stretched (strained), partially torn (sprained), or completely torn (torn ligaments). If the ligaments do not give way, one of the bones around the ankle will break (fracture).

Strains, sprains, and even some minor fractures of the ankle will heal well with home treatment. Even some torn ligaments may do well without a great deal of medical care; operations to repair them are rare. For practical purposes, the immediate attention of the doctor is only necessary when the injury has been severe enough to cause obvious fracture to the bones around the ankle or to cause a completely torn ligament. This is indicated by a deformed joint with abnormal motion. Fractures are more likely in a fall from a considerable height, or in automobile or bicycle accidents. They are less likely to happen when the ankle is twisted while walking or running.

The typical ankle sprain swells either around the bony bump at the outside of the ankle or about two inches in front of and below it. The usual sprain does not need prolonged rest, casting, or X-rays. Except for obvious deformities of the ankle suggesting a severe fracture, home treatment should be started promptly. Detection of any damage to the ligaments is difficult immediately after the injury because of the amount of swelling that may be present. Since it is easier to do an adequate examination of the foot after the swelling has gone down, and since no damage is done by resting a mild fracture or torn ligament, there is no need to rush to the doctor.

Pain "tells" you what to do (or not do) with ankle injuries. If it hurts, don't do it. If pain prevents *any* standing on the ankle after more than twenty-four hours, see the doctor. If little progress is being made so that pain makes weight bearing difficult at seventy-two hours, see the doctor. Swelling is not a good guide as to what to do with an ankle injury. Sprains and torn ligaments usually swell quickly because there is bleeding into the tissue around the ankle. The skin will turn blue-black in the area as the blood is broken down by the body. The amount of swelling does not differentiate between sprains, tears, and fractures. The common chip fractures around the ankle are variable, and often the swelling is considerably less than with a sprain. Remember these basic facts: Home treatment is adequate for all ankle injuries except for some fractures and complete ligament tears. Even if a fracture is present, if the ankle is rested and protected, no harm will be done by waiting and watching it.

Home Treatment

RIP is your key word: rest, ice, and protection. Rest the ankle and keep it elevated. Apply ice in a towel to the injured area and leave it there for at least thirty minutes. If there is any evidence of swelling after the first thirty minutes, then ice should be applied for thirty minutes on and fifteen minutes off through the next few hours. If pain subsides completely in the elevated position, weight bearing may be attempted cautiously. If pain is present when bearing weight, weight bearing should be avoided for the first twenty-four hours. Heat may be applied, but only after twenty-four hours.

Is the ankle deformed or bending in an abnormal fashion?

yes 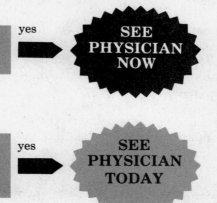 **SEE PHYSICIAN NOW**

no

Has pain prevented the ankle from bearing any weight for more than twenty-four hours?

yes **SEE PHYSICIAN TODAY**

no

Has pain made weight bearing difficult for more than seventy-two hours?

yes 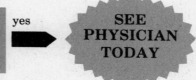 **SEE PHYSICIAN TODAY**

no

APPLY HOME TREATMENT

An elastic bandage can be used but will not prevent reinjury if full activity is resumed. Do not stretch the bandage so that it is very tight and interferes with blood circulation. Taping generally should not be attempted on children; if it is done incorrectly, it may cut off circulation to the foot. The ankle should feel relatively normal by about ten days. Be warned, however, that full healing will not take place for four to six weeks. If strenuous activity, such as organized athletics, is to be pursued during this time, the ankle should be taped by someone experienced in this technique.

What to Expect at the Doctor's Office

The doctor will examine the motions of the ankle to see if they are abnormal and may take an X-ray. If there is no fracture, it is likely that a continuation of home treatment will be recommended. Home treatment may also be recommended if a minor chip fracture is noted. For other fractures, a cast will be necessary or, rarely, an operation to put the bones back together. Depending on the nature of a ligament injury, an operation may be required to repair a completely torn ligament.

9 Knee Injuries

The ligaments of the knee may be stretched (strained), partially torn (sprained), or completely torn (torn ligament). Unlike the ankle, torn ligaments in the knee need to be repaired surgically as soon as possible after the injury occurs. If surgery is delayed, the operation is more difficult and less likely to be successful. For this reason, the approach to knee injuries is more cautious than for ankle injuries. If there is any possibility of a torn ligament, go to the doctor. Fractures in the area of the knee are less common than around the ankle and need to be cared for by a doctor.

Significant knee injuries usually occur during a sports activity, when the knee is more likely to experience twisting and side contact; these are responsible for most ligament injuries. (Deep knee bends stretch knee ligaments and may contribute to knee injuries; they should be practiced cautiously, if at all.) Serious knee injuries occur when the leg is planted on the ground and a blow is received to the knee from the side. If the foot cannot give way, the knee will. There is no way to totally avoid this possibility in athletics. The use of shorter spikes and cleats help, but elastic knee supports and wraps give virtually no protection.

When ligaments are completely torn, the lower leg can be wiggled from side to side when the leg is straight. Compare the injured knee to the opposite knee to get some idea of what amount of side-to-side motion is normal. Your examination will not be as skilled as that of the doctor, but if you think that the motion may be abnormally loose, see the doctor.

If the cartilage within the knee has been torn, the normal motion of the knee may be blocked, preventing it from being straightened. Although a torn cartilage does not need immediate surgery, it deserves prompt medical attention. The amount of pain and swelling does not indicate the severity of the injury. The ability to bear weight, to move the knee through the normal range of motion, and to keep the knee stable when wiggled is more important. Typically, strains and sprains hurt immediately and continue to hurt for hours and even days after the injury. Swelling tends to come on rather slowly over a period of hours, but may reach rather large proportions. When a ligament is completely torn, there is intense pain immediately, which subsides until the knee may hurt little or not at all for a while. Usually, there is significant bleeding into the tissues around the joint when a ligament is torn so that swelling tends to come on quickly and be impressive in its quantity. The best policy when there is a potential injury to the ligament is to avoid any major activity until it is clear that this is a minor strain or sprain. Home treatment is intended only for minor strains and sprains.

Home Treatment

RIP is again the key word—rest, ice, and protection. Rest the knee and elevate it. Apply an ice pack for at least thirty minutes to minimize swelling. If there is more than slight swelling or pain, despite the fact that the knee was immediately rested and ice was applied, see the doctor. If this is not the case, apply the ice treatment on the knee for thirty minutes and then off for fifteen minutes for the next several hours. Limited weight bearing may be attempted during this time with a close watch for increased swelling and pain. Heat may be applied

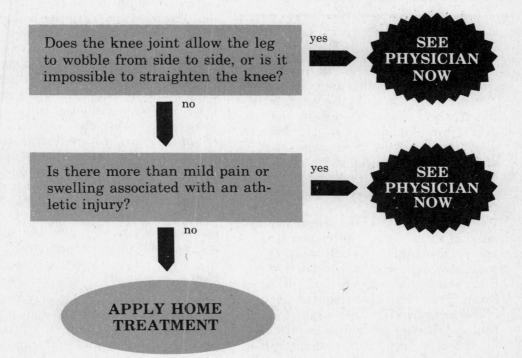

Does the knee joint allow the leg to wobble from side to side, or is it impossible to straighten the knee? **yes →** SEE PHYSICIAN NOW

no ↓

Is there more than mild pain or swelling associated with an athletic injury? **yes →** SEE PHYSICIAN NOW

no ↓

APPLY HOME TREATMENT

after twenty-four hours. By then, the knee should look and feel relatively normal, and after seventy-two hours this should clearly be the case. Remember, however, that a strain or sprain is not completely healed for four to six weeks and requires protection during this healing period. Elastic bandages will not give adequate support but will ease symptoms a bit and remind the patient to be careful with the knee.

What to Expect at the Doctor's Office

The knee will be examined for range of motion, and the lateral stability will be tested by stressing the knee from side to side. A massively swollen knee may have blood removed from the joint with a needle. Torn ligaments need surgical repair. X-rays may be taken but are not always helpful. For injuries that appear minor, home treatment will be advised. Pain medications are sometimes, but not often, required.

10 Wrist, Elbow, and Shoulder Injuries

The ligaments of these joints may be stretched (strained) or partially torn (sprained), but complete tears are rare. Fractures may occur at the wrist, are less frequent around the elbow, and are uncommon around the shoulder. Injuries to wrists and elbows occur most often during a fall, when the weight of the body is caught on the outstretched arm. Injuries to the shoulder usually result from direct blows.

The wrist is the most frequently injured of these joints. Strains and sprains are common, and the small bones in the wrist may be fractured. Fractures of these small bones may be difficult to see on an X-ray. The most frequent fracture of the wrist involves the ends of the long bones of the forearm and is easily recognized because it causes an unnatural bend near the wrist. Physicians refer to this as the "silver fork deformity."

"Tennis elbow" is the most frequent elbow injury; if you think this is the problem, consult **Tennis Elbow** (Problem 65). Other injuries are much less frequent and usually result from falls, automobile accidents, or contact sports. A common problem in children under five years of age is minor dislocations due to pulling on the arm (see Robert Pantell, James Fries, and Donald Vickery, *Taking Care of Your Child,* Reading, Mass.: Addison-Wesley Publishing Co., 1977).

The collarbone (clavicle) is a frequently fractured bone; fortunately, it has remarkable healing powers. An inability to raise the arm on the affected side is common; the shoulders may also appear uneven. Bandaging is the only treatment required.

The shoulder separation often seen in athletes is perhaps the most common injury of the shoulder. It is a stretching or tearing of the ligament that attaches the collarbone to one of the bones that forms the shoulder joint. It causes a slight deformity and extreme tenderness at the end of the collarbone. Sprains and strains of other ligaments occur but complete tearing is rare, as are fractures. Dislocations of the shoulder are rare outside of organized athletics but are best treated early when they do occur.

In summary, severe fractures and dislocations are best treated early. These usually cause deformity, severe pain, and limitation of movement. Other fractures will not be harmed if the injured limb is rested and protected. Complete tears of ligaments are rare; strains and sprains will heal with home treatment.

Home Treatment

RIP is the key word—rest, ice, and protection. Rest the arm and apply ice wrapped in a towel for at least thirty minutes. If the pain is gone and there is no swelling at the end of this time, the ice treatment may be discontinued. A sling for shoulder and elbow injuries and a partial splint for wrist injuries will give protection and rest to the injury while allowing the patient to move around. Continue ice treatment for thirty minutes on and fifteen minutes off through the first eight hours if swelling appears. Heat may be applied after twenty-four hours. The injured joint should be usable with little pain within twenty-four hours and should be almost normal by seventy-two hours. If not, see the doctor. Complete healing takes from four to six weeks and activities with a likelihood of reinjury should be avoided by the patient if possible during this time.

Wrist, Elbow, and Shoulder Injuries

10

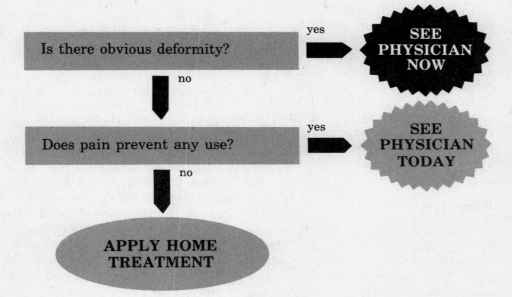

Is there obvious deformity? — yes → **SEE PHYSICIAN NOW**

no ↓

Does pain prevent any use? — yes → **SEE PHYSICIAN TODAY**

no ↓

APPLY HOME TREATMENT

What to Expect at the Doctor's Office

An examination and sometimes X-rays will be performed. A broken bone may require a cast. A sling may be devised. Pain medication is sometimes given, but aspirin or acetaminophen are about as good and are less hazardous. Certain fractures, especially those around the elbow, may require surgery.

11 Head Injuries

Head injuries are potentially serious but few ever lead to problems. The major concern in a head injury in which the skull is not clearly and obviously damaged is the occurrence of bleeding inside the skull. The accumulation of blood inside the skull will eventually put pressure on the brain and cause damage. Fortunately the valuable contents of the skull are carefully cushioned. Careful observation is the most valuable tool for diagnosing serious head injury. This can be done as well at home as at the hospital; there is some risk either way, so it is your choice.

Home Treatment

Ice applied to a bruised area may minimize swelling, but "goose eggs" often develop anyway. The size of the bump does not indicate the severity of the injury.

The initial observation period is crucial. Bleeding inside the head may be rapid within the first twenty-four hours and may continue for as long as seventy-two hours or more. Some bleeding may occur very slowly; this is called a *subdural hematoma* and may produce chronic headache, persistent vomiting, or personality changes months after the injury.

Check the patient every two hours during the first twenty-four-hour period, every four hours during the second period, and every eight hours during the third. Look for the following:

Alertness: Increasing lethargy, unresponsiveness, and *abnormally* deep sleep can precede coma. The seriously affected patient *cannot* be easily roused.

Unequal pupil size: This *can* be caused by increased internal pressure. About 25 percent of the population have pupils that are unequal all the time—this is normal for them. If pupils become unequal *after* the injury, this is a serious sign.

Severe vomiting: Forceful vomiting may occur, and the vomit may be ejected several feet. If significant, repeated vomiting occurs, see the physician.

A typical minor head injury generally occurs when a child falls off a table or tree and bangs his or her head. A bump immediately begins to develop. The child remains conscious, although initially stunned. For a few minutes the child is unconsolable and may vomit once or twice during the first couple of hours. Some sleepiness due to the excitement may be noted; the child may nap but is easily aroused. Neither pupil is enlarged and the vomiting ceases shortly. Within eight hours, the child is back to normal except for the tender and often prominent "goose egg."

In a more severe head injury, symptoms usually take longer to develop. Two or more of the danger signs often are present at the same time. The patient remains lethargic and is not easily aroused. A pupil may enlarge. Vomiting is usually violent, repeated, and progressively worse.

A critical sign of a serious complication will not be present one minute and gone the next. But, if you have any doubt, call your physician.

Since most accidents occur in the evening hours, patients will generally be asleep several hours after most accidents; you can look in on them periodically to check their pulse, pupils, and arousability if you are concerned. With minor head bumps, nighttime checking is usually not necessary.

What to Expect at the Doctor's Office

The diagnosis of bleeding within the skull cannot be made with great accuracy. Skull X-rays are seldom helpful except in detecting whether a fragment of

120

Have any of the following occurred?

(a) Unconsciousness

(b) Patient cannot remember injury

(c) Seizure

yes →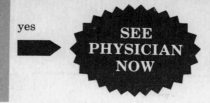
SEE PHYSICIAN NOW

no

Are any of the following present?

(a) Visual problems

(b) Bleeding from eyes, ears, or mouth

(c) Black eyes or blackness behind ears

(d) Change in behavior (sleep, irritability, lethargy)

(e) Fluid draining from nose

(f) Persistent vomiting

(g) Irregular breathing or heart rate

yes →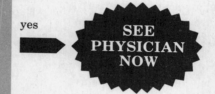
SEE PHYSICIAN NOW

no

Is there a cut?   yes → See **Cuts** (Problem 2).

no

APPLY HOME TREATMENT

bone from the skull has been pushed into the brain, but this situation is rare. With severe injuries, neck X-rays may occasionally be required. The physician will ask for a complete description of the accident, assess the patient's general appearance, and take repeated blood pressures and pulse rates. In addition, the head, eyes, ears, nose, throat, neck, and nervous system will be examined. The physician will also check for other possible sites of injury such as the chest, abdomen, and arms and legs. When internal bleeding is likely but not certain, the patient may be hospitalized for observation. During this observation period, the pulse, pupils, and blood pressure will be checked periodically. In short, the doctor will observe and wait, much as would be done at home. Use of medications, which may obscure the situation, will be avoided.

121

12 Burns

How bad is a burn? Burns are classified as first, second, or third degree, according to the depth of the burn. **First-degree burns** are superficial and cause the skin to turn red. A sunburn is usually a first-degree burn. **Second-degree burns** are deeper and result in splitting of the skin layers or blistering. Scalding with hot water or a very severe sunburn with blisters are common instances of second-degree burns. **Third-degree burns** destroy all layers of the skin and extend into the deeper tissues. They are *painless* because nerve endings have been destroyed. Charring of the burned tissue is usually present.

First-degree burns may cause a lot of pain but are not a major medical problem. Even when they are extensive, they seldom result in lasting problems and seldom need a doctor's attention.

Second-degree burns are also painful and if extensive, may cause significant fluid loss. Scarring, however, is usually minimal, and infection usually is not a problem. Second-degree burns can be treated at home if they are not extensive. Any second-degree burn that involves an area larger than the patient's hand should be seen by a doctor. In addition, a second-degree burn that involves the face or hands should be seen by a physician; these might result in cosmetic problems or loss of function.

Third-degree burns result in scarring and present frequent problems with infection and fluid loss. The more extensive the burn, the more difficult these problems. All third-degree burns should be seen by a physician because they may lead to scarring and infection and skin grafts are often needed.

Home Treatment

Apply cold water or ice immediately. This reduces the amount of skin damage caused by the burn and also eases pain. The cold should be applied for at least five minutes and continued until pain is relieved or for one hour, whichever comes first. Be careful not to apply cold so long that the burned area turns numb, since frostbite can occur! Reapply treatment if pain returns. Aspirin or acetaminophen may be used to reduce pain. Blisters should not be broken. If they burst by themselves, as they often do, the overlying skin should be allowed to remain as a wet dressing. The use of local anesthetic creams or sprays is not recommended, since they may slow healing. Also, some patients develop an irritation or allergy to these drugs. Any burn that continues to be painful for more than forty-eight hours should be seen by a physician.

Do not use butter, cream, or ointments (such as Vaseline). They may slow healing and increase the possibility of infection. Antibiotic creams (such as Neosporin, Bacitracin) probably neither help nor hurt minor burns but are expensive.

What to Expect at the Doctor's Office

The physician will establish the extent and degree of the burn and will determine the need for antibiotics, hospitalization, and skin grafting. An antibacterial ointment and dressing will often be recommended; it must be frequently changed while checking the burn for infection. Extensive burns may require hospitalization, and third-degree burns may eventually require skin grafts.

Is this a second-degree burn that is

(a) extensive, or

(b) on the face or hands?

Or is it a third-degree burn?

yes →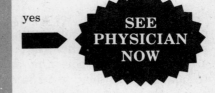

SEE PHYSICIAN NOW

no ↓

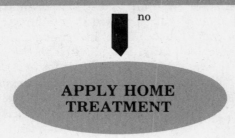

APPLY HOME TREATMENT

13 Infected Wounds and Blood Poisoning

"Blood poisoning" is not a current medical term. There is a folk saying that red streaks running up the arm or leg from a wound are blood poisoning and that the patient will die when the streaks reach the heart. In fact, such streaks are only an inflammation of the lymph channels carrying away the debris from the wound. They will stop when they reach local lymph nodes in the armpit or groin and do not, by themselves, indicate blood poisoning. Check by phone with the doctor if you are unsure.

Blood poisoning, to a physician, means bacterial infection in the bloodstream and is termed *septicemia*. Fever is a better indication of this rare occurrence. A local wound should only give a very minor temperature elevation unless infected. If there is a fever, see the doctor.

An infected wound usually festers beneath the surface of the skin, resulting in pain and swelling. Bacterial infection requires at least a day, and usually two or three days, to develop. Therefore, a late increase in pain or swelling is a legitimate cause for concern. If the festering wound bursts open, pus will drain out. This is good, and the wound will usually heal well. Still, this demonstrates that an infection was present, and the doctor should evaluate the situation unless it is clearly minor.

An explanation of normal wound healing will be helpful. First, the body pours out serum into a wound area. Serum is yellowish and clear, and later turns into a scab. *Serum is frequently mistaken for pus, which is thick, cheesy, smelly, and never seen in the first day or so.* Second, inflammation around a wound is normal. In order to heal an area, the body must remove the debris and bring in new materials. Thus, the edges of a wound will be pink or red, and the wound area may be warm. Third, the lymphatic system is actively involved in debris clearance, and pain along lymph channels or in the lymph nodes can occur without infection.

Home Treatment

Keep a wound clean. Leave it open to the air unless it is unsightly or in a location where it gets dirty easily; if so, bandage it, but change the bandage daily. Soak and clean the wound gently with warm water for short periods, three or four times daily, to remove debris and keep the scab soft. Children like to pick at scabs and often fall on a scab. In these instances, a bandage is useful. The simplest wound of the face requires three to five days for healing. The healing period for the chest and arms is five to nine days, for the legs it is seven to twelve days. Larger wounds, or those that have gaped open and must heal across a space, require correspondingly longer periods to heal. Children heal more rapidly than adults. If a wound fails to heal within the expected time, call the doctor.

What to Expect at the Doctor's Office

An examination of the wound and regional lymph nodes will be done, and the patient's temperature will be taken. Sometimes cultures of the blood or the wound are performed, and antibiotics may be prescribed. If there is a suspicion of bacterial infection, cultures may be taken before the antibiotics are given. If a wound is festering, it may be drained either with a needle or a scalpel. This procedure is not very painful and actually relieves discomfort. For severe wound infections, hospitalization may be needed.

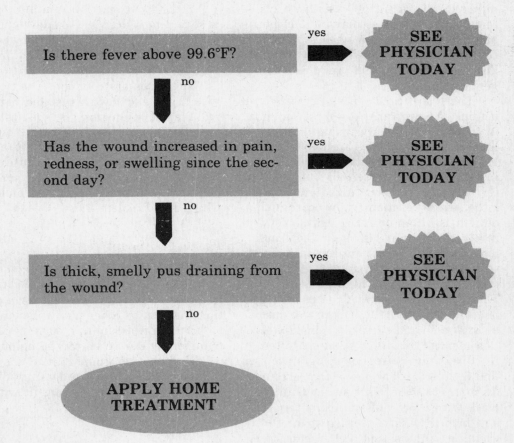

Is there fever above 99.6°F?

yes → **SEE PHYSICIAN TODAY**

no

Has the wound increased in pain, redness, or swelling since the second day?

yes → **SEE PHYSICIAN TODAY**

no

Is thick, smelly pus draining from the wound?

yes → **SEE PHYSICIAN TODAY**

no

APPLY HOME TREATMENT

14 Insect Bites or Stings

Most insect bites are trivial, but some insect bites or stings may cause reactions either locally or in the basic body systems. *Local reactions* may be uncomfortable but do not pose a serious hazard. In contrast, *systemic reactions* may occasionally be serious and may require emergency treatment.

There are three types of systemic reactions. All are rare. The most common is an asthma attack, causing difficulty in breathing and perhaps audible wheezing. Hives or extensive skin rashes following insect bites are less serious but indicate that a reaction has occurred and that a more severe reaction might occur if the patient is bitten or stung again. Very rarely, fainting or loss of consciousness may occur. If the patient has lost consciousness, you must assume that the collapse is due to an allergic reaction. This is an emergency. If the patient has had any of these reactions in the past, he or she should be taken immediately to a medical facility if stung or bitten.

Bites from poisonous spiders are rare. The female black widow spider accounts for many of them. This spider is glossy black with a body of approximately one-half inch in diameter, a leg span of about two inches, and a characteristic red hourglass mark on the abdomen. The black widow spider is found in woodpiles, sheds, basements, or outdoor privies. The bite is often painless, and the first sign may be cramping abdominal pain. The abdomen becomes hard and boardlike as the waves of pain become severe. Breathing is difficult and accompanied by grunting. There may be nausea, vomiting, headaches, sweating, twitching,

shaking, and tingling sensations of the hand. The bite itself may not be prominent and may be overshadowed by the systemic reaction. Brown recluse spiders, which are slightly smaller than black widows and have a white "violin" pattern on their backs, cause painful bites and serious local reaction but are not as dangerous as black widows.

If the local reaction to a bite or sting is severe or a deep sore is developing, a physician should be consulted by telephone. Children frequently have more severe local reactions than adults.

Tick bites are common. The tick lives in tall grass or low shrubs and hops on and off passing mammals, such as deer or dogs. In some localities, ticks may carry Rocky Mountain spotted fever, but most tick bites are not complicated by subsequent illness. Ticks will commonly be found in the scalp. Consult **Ticks and Chiggers** (Problem 49).

Home Treatment

Apply something cold promptly, such as ice or cold packs. Delay in application of cold results in a more severe local reaction. Aspirin or other pain relievers may be used. Antihistamines, such as Chlortrimeton or Benadryl, can be helpful in relieving the itch somewhat. If the reaction is severe, or if pain does not diminish in forty-eight hours, consult with the physician by telephone.

What to Expect at the Doctor's Office

The physician will inquire what sort of insect or spider has inflicted the wound and will search for signs of systemic reaction. If a systemic reaction is present, adrenalin by injection is usually necessary. Rarely, measures to support breathing or blood pressure will be needed; these measures require the facilities of an emergency room or hospital.

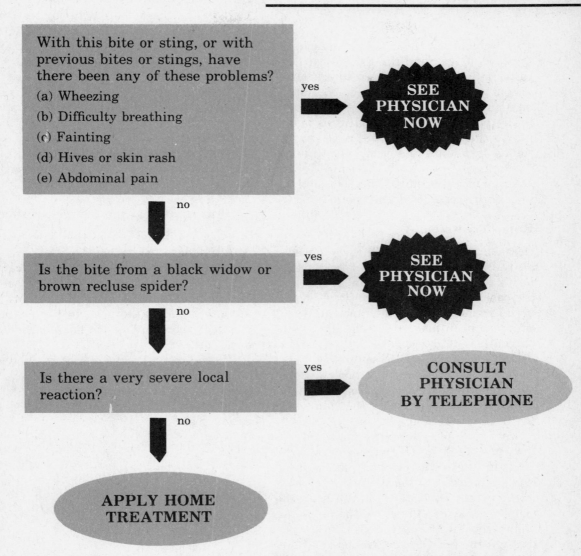

With this bite or sting, or with previous bites or stings, have there been any of these problems?
(a) Wheezing
(b) Difficulty breathing
(c) Fainting
(d) Hives or skin rash
(e) Abdominal pain

yes → **SEE PHYSICIAN NOW**

no

Is the bite from a black widow or brown recluse spider?

yes → **SEE PHYSICIAN NOW**

no

Is there a very severe local reaction?

yes → **CONSULT PHYSICIAN BY TELEPHONE**

no

APPLY HOME TREATMENT

If the problem is a local reaction, the physician will examine the wound for signs of death of tissue or infection. Occasionally, surgical drainage of the wound will be needed. In other cases, pain relievers or antihistamines may make the patient more comfortable.

Adrenalin injections are occasionally used for very severe local reactions.

If a systemic reaction has occurred, desensitization shots may be initiated. In addition, emergency kits can be purchased to help the person with a serious allergy.

127

15 Fishhooks

The problem with fishhooks is, of course, the barb. If you and the patient can keep calm, you can remove the fishhook, unless it is in the eye. (No attempt should be made to remove hooks that have actually penetrated the eyeball; this is a job for the doctor.) You will need the patient's confidence and cooperation in order to avoid a visit to the doctor. The advantage of the doctor's office is the availability of a local anesthetic.

Home Treatment

Occasionally the hook will have moved all the way around so that it lies just beneath the surface of the skin. If this is the case, often the best technique is simply to push the hook on through the skin, cut it off just behind the barb with wirecutters, and remove it by pulling it back through the way it entered.

On other occasions, the hook will be embedded only slightly and can be removed by simply grasping the shank of the hook (pliers help), pushing slightly forward and away from the barb, and then pulling it out. If the barb is not near the surface or you don't have pliers or wirecutters, use the method illustrated on the opposite page; the hook is usually removed quickly and almost painlessly. First, a loop of fish line is put through the bend of the fishhook so that, at the appropriate time, a quick jerk can be applied and the hook can be pulled out directly in line with the shaft of the hook. (a) Holding onto the shaft, push the hook slightly in and away from the barb so as to disengage the barb. (b and c) Holding this pressure constant to keep the barb disengaged, give a quick jerk on the fish line and the hook will pop out. If you are successful, be sure that the patient's tetanus shots are up to date (see **Tetanus Shots**, Problem 6). Treat the wound as in the home treatment section for **Puncture Wounds** (Problem 3). If you are not successful, push the hook all the way through and out so that the barb can be cut off with wirecutters as described above. However, this may be a bit more painful; the average child may not be able to tolerate it. If all else fails, a visit to the doctor should solve the problem. A pair of electrician's pliers with a wire-cutting blade should be part of your fishing equipment.

What to Expect at the Doctor's Office

The doctor will use one of the three methods above to remove the hook. If necessary, the area around the hook can be infiltrated with a local anesthetic before the hook is removed. Often the injection of a local anesthetic is more painful than just removing the hook without the anesthetic.

If the hook is in the eye, it is likely that the help of an ophthalmologist (eye specialist) will be needed, and it may be necessary to remove the hook in the operating room.

Is the hook in the eye? — yes → SEE PHYSICIAN NOW

no ↓

APPLY HOME TREATMENT

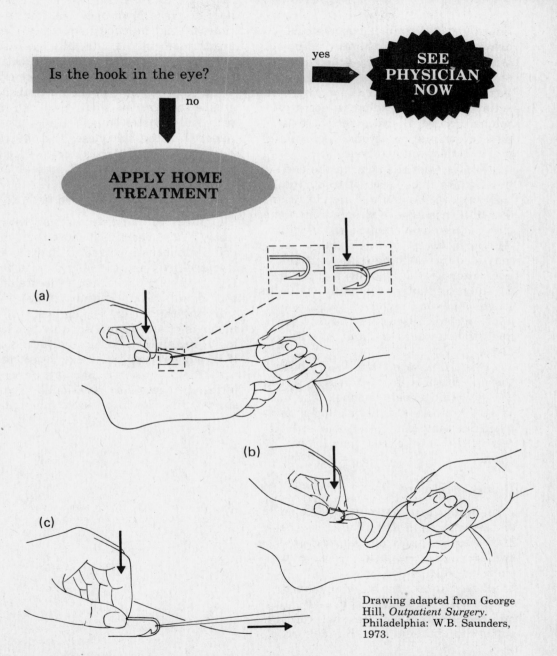

(a)

(b)

(c)

Drawing adapted from George Hill, *Outpatient Surgery*. Philadelphia: W.B. Saunders, 1973.

129

16 Smashed Fingers

Smashing fingers in car doors or desk drawers, or with hammers or baseballs, is all too common. If the injury involves only the end segment of the finger (the terminal phalanx) and does not involve a significant cut, the help of a doctor is seldom needed. Blood under the fingernail (subungual hematoma) is a painful problem that you can treat.

Fractures of the bone in the end segment of the finger are not treated unless they involve the joint. Many physicians feel that it is unwise to splint the finger even if there is a fracture of the joint. Although the splint will decrease pain, it may also increase the stiffness of the joint after healing. However, if the fracture is not splinted, the pain may persist longer and you may end up with a stiff joint anyway. Discuss the advantages and disadvantages of splinting with your doctor.

Fingernails are often dislocated in these injuries. It is not necessary to have the entire fingernail removed. The nail that is detached should be clipped off to avoid catching it on other objects. Nail regrowth will take from four to six weeks.

Home Treatment

If the injury does not involve other parts of the finger, and if the finger can be moved easily, apply an ice pack for swelling and use aspirin or acetaminophen for pain.

Pain caused by a large amount of blood under the fingernail can often be relieved simply. Bend open an ordinary paper clip and hold it with a pair of pliers. Heat one end with a candle flame, steadying the hand holding the pliers with the opposite hand. When the tip is quite hot, touch it to the nail and it will melt its way through the fingernail, leaving a clean, small hole. There is no need to press down hard. Take your time, lifting the paper clip to see if you are through the nail; usually the blood will spurt a little when you are through. Reheat the paper clip if necessary. The blood trapped beneath the nail can now escape through the small hole, and the pain will be relieved as the pressure is released. If the hole closes and the blood reaccumulates, the procedure can be repeated using the same hole once again.

What to Expect at the Doctor's Office

The finger will be examined; an X-ray is likely if it appears that more than the end segment is involved. If there is a fracture involving the last joint on the finger, you should expect a discussion of the advantages and disadvantages of splinting the finger. The splinting of one finger is often accomplished by bandaging it together with the adjacent finger. If the finger is splinted, exercise it periodically to preserve mobility. Severe injuries of fingers may occasionally require surgery in order to preserve function.

Is the injury limited to the end section of the finger?

yes → **SEE PHYSICIAN TODAY**

no ↓

Is the end of the finger deformed?

yes → **SEE PHYSICIAN TODAY**

no ↓

APPLY HOME TREATMENT

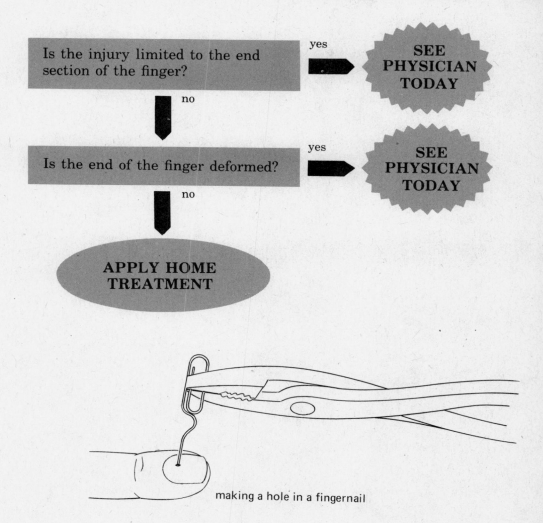

making a hole in a fingernail

E Fever

17 Fever

Many people, including physicians, speak of fever and illness as if they were one and the same. Surprisingly, an elevated temperature is not necessarily a sign of illness. Normal body temperature varies from individual to individual. If we measured the body temperatures of a large number of healthy people while they were resting, we would find a difference of 1.5°F between the lowest and highest temperatures. We are all individuals, and there is nothing absolute about a 98.6°F (37°C) temperature.

Normal body temperature varies greatly during the day. Temperature is generally lowest in the morning upon awakening. Food, excess clothing, excitement, and anxiety can all elevate body temperature. Vigorous exercise can raise body temperature to as much as 103°F. Severe exercise, without water or salt, can result in a condition known as heat stroke, with temperatures about 106°F. Other mechanisms also influence body temperature. Hormones, for example, account for a monthly variation of body temperature in ovulating women. The normal temperature is 1° to 1.5°F higher in the second half of the menstrual cycle. In general, children have higher body temperatures than adults and seem to have greater daily variation because of their greater amounts of excitement and activity.

Having said all this, we know you would like a rule to follow. If the temperature is 99° to 100°F, start thinking about the possibility of fever; if it is 100°F or above, it's a fever.

The most common causes for persistent fevers are viral and bacterial infections, such as colds, sore throats, earaches, diarrhea, urinary infections, roseola, chickenpox, mumps, measles, and occasionally pneumonia, appendicitis, and meningitis.

A viral infection can result in a normal temperature or a temperature of 105°F. The height of the temperature is *not* a reliable indicator of the seriousness of the underlying infection.

Taking A Temperature

Both Fahrenheit and centigrade thermometers are acceptable. Rectal temperatures are usually more accurate and are about 0.5°F higher than oral temperatures. Oral temperature can be affected by hot or cold foods, routine breathing, and smoking. Generally, oral thermometers can be recognized by the longer bulb at the business end of the thermometer. The longer length of the bulb provides a greater surface area and a faster, more accurate reading. Rectal thermometers have a shorter, rounder bulb to facilitate entry into the rectum.

Rectal thermometers can be used to take oral temperatures but require a longer period in the mouth to achieve the same degree of accuracy as the oral thermometer. While oral thermometers can be used to take rectal temperatures, we do not recommend their use in children, because their shape is not ideal for younger children.

Rectal thermometers are best for young children. Lubricants can make insertion of rectal thermometers easier. Place the child on his or her stomach and hold one hand on the buttocks to prevent movement. Insert the thermometer only an inch or so inside the rectum. On a rectal thermometer the mercury will rise within seconds because the rectum closely contacts the thermometer. Remove the thermometer when the mercury is no longer rising after a minute or two.

We are frequently asked what temperature should be considered dangerous, or at what temperature a child should be brought to the doctor if no other symptoms are present. Consult a doctor for the following:

- Fever in a child less than four months old.
- Fever associated with a severe stiff neck.
- Fever of more than 105°F if the home treatment measures described below fail to reduce the temperature at least partly. This is not because this temperature signifies a serious underlying condition, but because a temperature that is higher than 105°F may be potentially damaging if it persists. Any temperature of 106°F should be promptly evaluated by a physician.
- Fever persisting for more than five days.
- If there are other symptoms with a fever, consult the appropriate section of this book.

Febrile Seizures (Fever Fits)

The danger of an extremely high temperature is the possibility that the fever will cause a seizure (convulsion). All of us are capable of "seizing" if our body temperatures become too high. Febrile seizures are relatively common in normal, healthy children; about 3 to 5 percent will experience a febrile seizure. However, although common, they must be treated with respect.

Febrile seizures occur most often in children between the ages of six months and four years. Illnesses that cause rapid elevations to high temperatures, such as roseola, have been frequently associated with febrile seizure. Rarely, a seizure is the first sign of a serious underlying problem such as meningitis.

The brain, which is normally transmitting electrical impulses at a fairly regular rhythm, begins misfiring during a seizure because of overheating and causes involuntary muscular responses, termed a seizure, convulsion, fit, or "falling out spell." The first sign may be a stiffening of the entire body. Children may have rhythmic beating of a single hand or foot, or any combination of the hands and feet. The eyes may roll back and the head may jerk. Urine and feces may pass involuntarily.

Most seizures last only from one to five minutes. There is very little evidence that such a short seizure is of any long-term consequence. On the other hand, prolonged seizures of more than 30 minutes are often a sign of a more serious underlying problem. Less than half of all children who have a short febrile seizure will ever experience a second, and less than half who experience a second will ever have a third.

Although a "seizing" child is a terrifying sight to a parent, the dangers to the child during a seizure are small. The following commonsense rules should be followed during a seizure.

- Protect your child's head from hitting anything hard. Place the child on a bed.
- Considerable damage can be done by forcing objects into the child's mouth to prevent biting of the tongue. Surprisingly, cut tongues are uncommon and they heal quickly.
- Make sure the child's breathing passage is open. Forcing a stick in your child's mouth does not ensure an open airway. In order to facilitate breathing, (1) clear the nose and mouth of vomitus or other material, and (2) pull the head backward slightly to "hyperextend" the neck. Artificial respiration is almost never necessary. These techniques are best

135

learned in demonstrations. In a true emergency, hyperextend the neck and breathe ten times each minute through the child's nose while keeping the mouth covered (or through the child's mouth while keeping the nose pinched with your finger). Only blow air in; the child will blow the air out naturally.

• Begin fever reduction (discussed below) and seek medical attention immediately. Fortunately, once the seizure has stopped the child is usually temporarily resistant to a second seizure. However, since there are exceptions to this rule, medical attention is critical.

After the seizure has subsided, the child may be very groggy and have no recollection of what has occurred. Others may show signs of extreme weakness and even paralysis of an arm or leg. This paralysis is almost always temporary but must be carefully evaluated.

A good physician will do a careful study to determine the cause of a febrile seizure. For the first febrile seizure, this will usually include a spinal tap (lumbar puncture) and fluid analysis to make certain that the seizure was not caused by meningitis. Following the termination of the fever, the physician will stress the importance of fever control for the next few days and will often place the child on anticonvulsant medications.

The Meaning of a Chill

A chill is another symptom of a fever. The feeling of being hot or cold is maintained by a complex system of nerve receptors in our skin and in a part of our brain known as the hypothalamus. This system is sensitive to the difference between the body temperature and the temperature outside. Cold can be sensed in two different ways, either by lowering the environmental temperature or by raising the body temperature. The body responds in a similar manner to a fever as it would if the outside temperature dropped. All of the normal systems that increase heat production, such as shivering, become active.

Because eating is a means of increasing heat production, hunger may be experienced. The body tries to conserve heat by causing constriction of the blood vessels near the skin. Children will sometimes curl up in a ball to conserve heat. Goose bumps are intended to raise the hairs on our body to form a layer of insulation. Don't bundle up the patient in blankets if he or she shivers or becomes chilled; this will only cause the fever to go higher. Use home treatment as described below.

Home Treatment

There are two ways to reduce a fever: sponging and medication.

Sponging. Evaporation has a cooling effect on the skin and hence on the body temperature. Evaporation can be enhanced by sponging the skin with water. Although alcohol evaporates more rapidly, it is somewhat uncomfortable and the vapors can be dangerous. Generally, sponging with tepid water (water that is comfortable to the touch) will be sufficient. Heat is also lost by conduction when a patient is sponged or sitting in a tub. Conduction is the process in which heat is lost to a cooler environment (the bathwater or air) from the warmer environment of the body. A comfortable tub of water (70°F) is sufficiently lower than the body temperature to encourage conduction. Although cold water will work somewhat faster, the discomfort makes this less desirable. A child will tolerate cold bathing and sponging for a much shorter period.

Medication. Medication should not be given by mouth to a seizing or unconscious child. A child who has just had a seizure can be given an aspirin suppository. Most aspirin suppositories come in 5-grain sizes, and approximately 1¼ to 1½ grains per year of age can be given—somewhat higher than the recommended dose for oral aspirin. To give the proper dose, the suppository can be cut lengthwise using a warm knife.

Temperature can be controlled in the conscious, alert patient with either aspirin or acetaminophen (Tylenol, Tempra, Liquiprin, Valadol, Datril, Tenlap, and so on). Remember that fever is the body's way of naturally responding to a variety of conditions, including infection. A fever may signify the response of a body's immune system to an infection and thus be the visible manifestation of a beneficial effect. Nonetheless, fevers are uncomfortable. Controlling a fever that is sufficiently high to interfere with eating, drinking, sleeping, or other important activities will make the patient feel better. In short, if the patient is suffering from the fever, treat it. If the fever is mild and the patient shows no effects, it may be unnecessary to treat.

Aspirin is universally familiar, effective, and reliable. It does *not* come in a liquid preparation. A few individuals are allergic to aspirin and may experience severe skin rashes or gastrointestinal bleeding. All people will suffer if they take too much aspirin. Early signs of excess aspirin include rapid breathing and ringing in the ears. All aspirin kept at home should be in child-proof bottles. Since there really are no totally child-proof bottles, aspirin should be kept out of the child's reach. An excessive dose of aspirin can be fatal and has in fact been responsible for more childhood deaths than any other medication.

"Baby aspirin" contains 1¼ grains (75 mg) per tablet. Children can take approximately 1 grain (60 mg) per year of age, up to ten years, and 10 grains every four to six hours after age ten. By the time a child is five, an adult aspirin or four baby aspirin (5 grains) can be given. Toxic effects will begin to develop at less than twice the recommended dosage so you must handle this medication with respect.

In adults, the standard dose for pain relief is two tablets taken every three to four hours as required. The maximum effect occurs in about two hours. Each standard tablet is five grains (300 mg or 0.3 g). If you use a nonstandard concoction, you will have to do the arithmetic to calculate equivalent doses. The terms "extra-strength," "arthritis pain formula," and the like indicate a greater amount of aspirin per tablet. This is medically trivial. You can take more tablets of the cheaper aspirin and still save money. When you read that a product "contains more of the ingredient that doctors recommend most," you may be sure that the product contains a little bit more aspirin per tablet; perhaps 325 to 350 mg instead of 300.

Acetaminophen unfortunately carries the nickname of "liquid aspirin," but it is a completely different medication. The advantage of acetaminophen is that it can be given in either liquid or tablet form. Acetaminophen is as effective as aspirin in fever reduction. It is not as effective as aspirin for other purposes, such as reducing inflammation, and hence is not recommended for conditions like arthritis. Fewer people are allergic to acetaminophen, and it does not cause as many gastrointestinal disturbances. However, if the patient has never had nausea, abdominal pain, or other gastrointestinal problems with aspirin, this is probably not an important consideration. Although acetaminophen carries the reputation of being safer than aspirin, overdoses can be fatal. There are no

137

"safe" drugs. Acetaminophen causes liver damage at high doses and consequently can cause death.

Acetaminophen is available in drops, suspension, tablets, or capsules. The concentration of the drops is much higher than the suspension and therefore must be administered cautiously. An unsuspecting person used to a different preparation of acetaminophen can create a problem by using the wrong dosage on your child. The recommended dosage is 60 mg per year of age every four to six hours, the same as aspirin. Again this means that the adult dose of two tablets or capsules every four hours can be taken at age ten. Again, "extra strength" just means more drug per tablet or capsule.

Since aspirin and acetaminophen are different medications that exert their effects in slightly different manners, they can be used together when one is not effective in maintaining proper tempera-, ture control. The dosages are the same but the aspirin and acetaminophen are given together every six hours or staggered so that one or the other is given every three hours.

Feed a Cold, Starve a Fever?

This folk remedy probably originated from individuals who were observant enough to notice the relationship between food and temperature elevation. However, there are many reasons why patients should eat during a fever. The increased heat increases caloric requirements since calories are being consumed rapidly at the higher body temperature. More important, there is an increased demand for fluid. Liquids should never be withheld from a feverish patient. If a patient will not eat because of the discomfort caused by fever, it is still essential to encourage that he or she drink fluids.

What to Expect at the Doctor's Office

Treatment depends on how long you have had a fever and how sick you appear. To determine whether an infection is present, the doctor will examine the skin, eyes, ears, nose, throat, neck, chest, and belly. If no other symptoms are present and the exam does not reveal an infection, watchful waiting may be advised. If the fever has been prolonged or the patient appears ill, tests of the blood and urine may be done. A chest X-ray or spinal tap may be needed. Specific infections will be treated appropriately; fever will be treated as discussed in "Home Treatment."

Is this a temperature of 101°F or more in a child less than three months of age?)

yes → **SEE PHYSICIAN NOW**

no ↓

Is there stiffness of the neck, confusion, marked irritability, lethargy? Has there been a seizure or is breathing rapid?

yes → **SEE PHYSICIAN NOW**

no ↓

In a child between three months and one year of age, has fever lasted more than twenty-four hours?

yes → **CALL PHYSICIAN TODAY**

no ↓

Has fever shown no improvement in seventy-two hours or has it lasted more than five days?

yes → **SEE PHYSICIAN TODAY**

no ↓

Is there sore throat, ear pain, cough, abdominal pains, skin rash, diarrhea, urinary frequency, or other symptoms?

yes → See discussions of these problems.

no ↓

APPLY HOME TREATMENT

F The Ears, Nose, and Throat

Is It A Virus, Bacteria, Or An Allergy?

The following sections discuss upper respiratory problems, including colds and "flu," sore throats, ear pain or stuffiness, runny nose, cough, hoarseness, swollen glands, nosebleeds. A central question is important to each of these complaints: Is it caused by a virus, bacteria, or an allergic reaction? In general, the doctor has more effective treatment than is available at home only for bacterial infection. Remember that viral infections and allergies do *not* improve with treatment by penicillin or other antibiotics. To demand a "penicillin shot" for a cold or allergy is to ask for a drug reaction, risk a more serious "super-infection," and to waste time and money. Among common problems well treated at home are:

- The common cold—often termed "viral URI (Upper Respiratory Infection)" by doctors.
- The flu, when uncomplicated.
- Hay fever.
- Mononucleosis—infectious mononucleosis or "mono."

Medical treatment *is* commonly required for:

- Strep throat.
- Ear infection.

How can you tell these conditions apart? Table 1 and the charts for the following problems will usually suffice. Here are some brief descriptions:

Viral syndromes—Viruses usually involve several portions of the body and cause many different symptoms. Three basic patterns (or syndromes) are common in viral illnesses; however, overlap between these three syndromes is not unusual. Your illness may sometimes have features of each.

Viral URI—This is the "common cold." It includes some combination of the following: sore throat, runny nose, stuffy or congested ears, hoarseness, swollen glands, and fever. One symptom usually precedes the others, and another symptom (usually hoarseness or cough) may remain after the others have disappeared.

The flu—Fever may be quite high. Headache can be excruciating, muscle aches and pain (especially in the lower back and eye muscles) are equally troublesome.

Viral gastroenteritis—This is the "stomach flu" with nausea, vomiting, diarrhea, and crampy abdominal pain. It may be incapacitating and can mimic a variety of other more serious conditions including appendicitis.

Hay fever—The seasonal runny nose and itchy eyes are well known. Patients usually diagnose this condition accurately themselves. As with viruses, this disorder is treated simply to relieve symptoms; given enough time the condition runs its course without doing any permanent harm. Allergies tend to recur whenever the pollen or other allergic substance is encountered.

Strep throat—Bacterial infections tend to localize at a single point. Involvement of the respiratory tract by strep is usually limited to the throat. However, symptoms outside the respiratory tract can occur, most commonly fever and swollen lymph glands (from draining the infected material) in the neck. The rash of scarlet fever sometimes may help to distinguish a streptococcal (strep) from a viral infection. In children, abdominal pain may be associated with a strep throat. This disorder must be diagnosed and treated, since serious heart and kid-

TABLE 1

Is It a Virus, Bacteria, or an Allergy?		**Virus**	**Bacteria**	**Allergy**
	Runny nose?	Often	Rare	Often
	Aching muscles?	Usual	Rare	No
	Headache?	Often	Rare	No
	Dizzy?	Often	Rare	Rare
	Fever?	Often	Often	No
	Cough?	Often	Sometimes	Rare
	Dry cough?	Often	Rare	Sometimes
	Raising sputum?	Rare	Often	Rare
	Hoarseness?	Often	Rare	Sometimes
	Recurs at a particular season?	No	No	Often
	Only a single complaint (sore throat, earache, sinus pain, or cough)?	Unusual	Usual	Unusual
	Do antibiotics help?	No	Yes	No
	Can the doctor help?	Seldom	Yes	Sometimes

Remember, viral infections and allergies *do not* improve with treatment by penicillin or other antibiotics.

ney complications can follow if adequate antibiotic therapy is not given.

Other conditions—Factors other than diseases may cause or contribute to upper respiratory symptoms. Smoking accounts for a large number of coughs and sore throats. Pollution (smog) can produce the same problems. Tumor and other frightening conditions account for only a very small number. Complaints lasting beyond two weeks without one of the common diseases as the obvious cause are not alarming but should be investigated on a routine basis by the doctor.

18 Colds and Flu

Most doctors believe that colds and the flu account for more unnecessary visits than any other group of problems. Since these are viral illnesses, they cannot be cured by antibiotics or any other drugs. However, there are nonprescription drugs—aspirin, decongestants, antihistamines—that may help to relieve symptoms while these problems cure themselves.

There seem to be three main reasons why these unnecessary visits are made. First, some patients are not sure that their illness is a cold or the flu, although this seems to be a relatively small part of the problem. Most patients state clearly that they know they have a cold or the flu. Second, many come seeking a cure. There are still large numbers of people who believe that penicillin or other antibiotics are necessary to recover from these problems. Finally, there are many patients who feel so sick that they feel that the doctor *must* be able to do something. Faced with this expectation, doctors sometimes try too hard to satisfy the patient. A physician may even give an antibiotic if it is requested, or fail to fully inform the patient as to the limitations of the drugs prescribed. This is understandable; who wants to tell a sick patient that they have wasted their time and money by coming to the doctor?

Of course colds and flu do lead to necessary visits as well. These visits from the complications of colds and the flu, primarily bacterial ear infections and bacterial pneumonia. In very young children, viral infections of the lung may lead to complications. The questions in the chart will help you look for the complications of colds and the flu.

Home Treatment

"Take two aspirin and call me in the morning." This familiar phrase does *not* indicate neglect or lack of sympathy for your problem. Aspirin is the best available medicine for the fever and muscular aches of the common cold. For adults, two five-grain aspirin tablets every four hours is standard treatment. The fever, aches, and prostration are most pronounced in the afternoon and evening: take the aspirin regularly over this period. If you have trouble tolerating aspirin, use acetaminophen in the same dose. If you want to spend money, buy a patent cold formula, but remember that the important ingredient that "doctors recommend most" is aspirin; check labels for equivalent dosage.

"Drink a lot of liquid." This is insurance. The body requires more fluid when you have a fever. Be sure you get enough. Fluids help to keep the mucus more liquid, and help prevent complications such as bronchitis and ear infection. A vaporizer (particularly in the winter if you have forced-air heat) will help liquefy secretions.

"Rest." How you feel is an indication of your need to rest. If you don't have fever and feel like being up and about, go ahead. It won't prolong your illness, and your friends and family were exposed during the incubation period, before you had symptoms.

A word about chicken soup: dizziness when standing up is common with colds and is helped by drinking salty liquids; bouillon and chicken soup are excellent.

For relief of particular symptoms, see the appropriate section of this book: **Runny Nose** (Problem 23), **Ear Pain and Stuffiness** (Problem 20), **Sore Throat** (Problem 19), **Cough** (Problem 24), **Nausea and Vomiting** (Problem 82), **Diarrhea** (Problem 83), and so on.

If symptoms persist beyond two weeks, call the doctor.

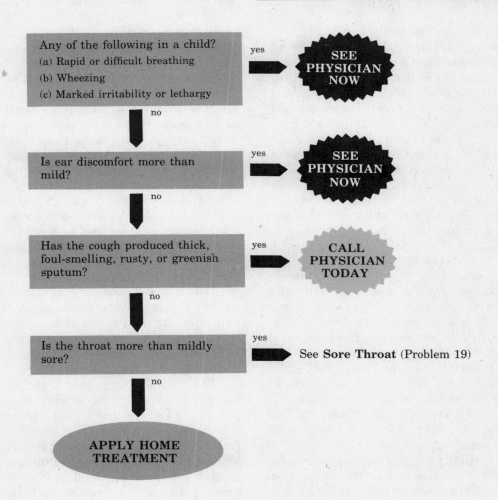

Any of the following in a child?
(a) Rapid or difficult breathing
(b) Wheezing
(c) Marked irritability or lethargy

yes → **SEE PHYSICIAN NOW**

no ↓

Is ear discomfort more than mild?

yes → **SEE PHYSICIAN NOW**

no ↓

Has the cough produced thick, foul-smelling, rusty, or greenish sputum?

yes → **CALL PHYSICIAN TODAY**

no ↓

Is the throat more than mildly sore?

yes → See **Sore Throat** (Problem 19)

no ↓

APPLY HOME TREATMENT

What to Expect at the Doctor's Office

The ears, nose, throat, and chest will be examined routinely, and the abdomen may be examined. If a bacterial pneumonia is suspected, a chest X-ray may be done, but studies have indicated that X-rays are rarely of help. If a bacterial infection is present as a complication, antibiotics will be prescribed.

If the cold or flu is uncomplicated, the physician should explain this and prescribe home treatment. The unnecessary use of antibiotics invites unnecessary complications, such as reaction to the antibiotics and "super infections" by bacteria that are resistant to antibiotics.

145

19 Sore Throat

Sore throats can be caused by either viruses or bacteria. Often, especially in the winter, breathing through the mouth can cause drying and irritation of the throat. This type of irritation always subsides quickly after the throat becomes moist again.

Viral sore throats, like other viral infections, cannot be treated successfully with antibiotics; they must run their course. Cold liquids for pain, and aspirin or acetaminophen for pain and fever are often helpful. Older children and adolescents frequently develop a viral sore throat known as infectious mononucleosis or "mono." Despite the formidable sounding name of this illness, complications seldom occur. The "mono" sore throat is often more severe and is often prolonged beyond a week, and the patient may feel particularly weak. The spleen, one of the internal organs in the abdomen may enlarge during mononucleosis; resting will be important. A viral sore throat that does not resolve within a week might be caused by the virus responsible for mononucleosis. Again, there is no antibiotic cure for mononucleosis.

Virtually all sore throats caused by bacteria are due to the streptococcal bacteria. These sore throats are commonly referred to as "strep throat." A strep throat should be treated with an antibiotic because of two types of complications. First, an abscess may form in the throat. This is an extremely rare complication but should be suspected if there is extreme difficulty in swallowing, difficulty opening the mouth, or excessive drooling in a child. The second and most significant complications occur from one to four weeks after the pain in the throat has disappeared. One of these complications, called acute glomerulonephritis, causes an inflammation of the kidney. It is not certain that antibiotics will prevent this complication, but they may prevent the strep from spreading to other family members or friends. Of greatest concern is the complication of rheumatic fever which is much less common today than in the past but is still a significant problem in some parts of the country. Rheumatic fever is a complicated disease that causes painful swollen joints, unusual skin rashes, and results in heart damage in half of its victims. Rheumatic fever can be prevented by antibiotic treatment of a strep throat.

Strep throat is much less frequent in adults than in children, and rheumatic fever is very rare in adults. Strep throat is unlikely if the sore throat is a minor part of a typical cold (runny nose, stuffy ears, cough, and so on).

If you or someone in your family has had rheumatic fever or acute glomerulonephritis, preventive use of antibiotics ("prophylaxis") as prescribed by the physician should be followed instead of the instructions given here.

The choice of when to use antibiotics for sore throats is controversial. Many physicians believe that throat cultures are the best way to determine the need for antibiotics; this is a reasonable approach, especially if throat cultures are available without a full office visit. More recently, physicians have begun to rely on studies that indicate that many patients do not need a culture, either because the risk of rheumatic fever is almost nil, or because this risk is high enough to justify the use of antibiotics without waiting two days for the culture results. The decision chart uses this last approach (the symptoms that lead to "Call physician today" are those that make antibiotic use likely).

146

We feel strongly that throat cultures should be available without a full office visit. We are especially impressed with home throat-culture programs which demonstrate that you, the public, can perform this test with somewhat greater yield than the physician's office staff. If your physician believes that every sore throat should be cultured, express your belief that cultures should be easily available and inexpensive.

Frequent and recurrent sore throats are common, especially in children between the ages of five and ten. There is no evidence that removing the tonsils decreases this frequency. Tonsillectomy is an operation that is very seldom indicated.

Home Treatment

Cold liquids, aspirin, and acetaminophen are effective for the pain and fever. Home remedies that may help include saltwater gargles and honey or lemon in tea. Time is the most important healer for pain; a vaporizer makes the waiting more comfortable for some.

What to Expect at the Doctor's Office

A throat culture usually will be taken. Many physicians will delay treating a sore throat until the culture results are known; delaying treatment by one or two days does not seem to increase the risk of developing rheumatic fever. Further, antibiotic treatment has been shown to be effective in reducing only the complications and not the discomfort of a sore throat. Since the majority of sore throats are due to viruses, treating all sore throats with antibiotics would needlessly expose patients to the risks of allergic reactions from the drugs. Physicians often will begin treatment with antibiotics immediately if there is a family history of rheumatic fever, or if the patient has scarlet fever (the rash described in the decision chart), or if rheumatic fever

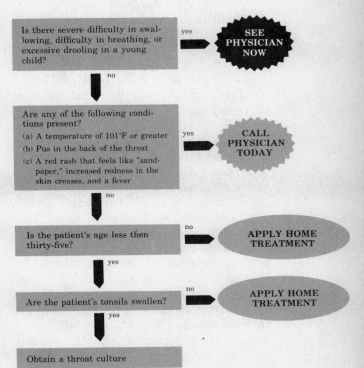

Is there severe difficulty in swallowing, difficulty in breathing, or excessive drooling in a young child? — yes → **SEE PHYSICIAN NOW**

no ↓

Are any of the following conditions present?
(a) A temperature of 101°F or greater
(b) Pus in the back of the throat
(c) A red rash that feels like "sandpaper," increased redness in the skin creases, and a fever
— yes → **CALL PHYSICIAN TODAY**

no ↓

Is the patient's age less then thirty-five? — no → **APPLY HOME TREATMENT**

yes ↓

Are the patient's tonsils swollen? — no → **APPLY HOME TREATMENT**

yes ↓

Obtain a throat culture

is commonly occurring in the community at the time. If one child has a strep throat, the chances are very good that other family members will also have a strep throat, and it is common for physicians to take cultures from brothers and sisters.

147

20 Ear Pain and Stuffiness

Ear pain is caused by a buildup of fluid and pressure in the middle ear (the portion of the ear behind the eardrum). Under normal circumstances, the middle ear is drained by a short narrow tube (the eustachian tube) into the nasal passages. Often during a cold or allergy, the eustachian tube will become swollen shut; this occurs most easily in small children in whom the tube is smaller. When the tube closes, the normal flow of fluid from the middle ear is prevented and the fluid begins to accumulate; this causes stuffiness and decreased hearing.

The stagnant fluid provides a good place for the start of a bacterial infection. A bacterial infection usually results in pain and fever, often in one ear only.

The symptoms of an ear infection in children may include fever, ear pain, fussiness, increased crying, irritability, or pulling at the ears. Since infants cannot tell you that their ears hurt, increased irritability or ear pulling should make a parent suspicious of ear infection.

Ear pain and ear stuffiness can also result from high altitudes, as when descending in an airplane. Here again, the mechanism for the stuffiness or pain is obstruction of the eustachian tube. Swallowing will frequently relieve this pressure. Closing the mouth and holding the nose closed while pretending to blow one's nose is another method of opening the eustachian tube.

Parents are often concerned about hearing impairment after ear infections. While most children will have a temporary and minor hearing loss during and immediately following an ear infection, there is seldom any permanent hearing loss with adequate medical management.

Home Treatment

Moisture and humidity are important in keeping the mucus thin. Use a vaporizer if you have one. Curious maneuvers (such as hopping up and down in a steamy shower while shaking the head and swallowing) are sometimes dramatically successful in clearing out mucus.

Aspirin or acetaminophen (Tylenol) will provide partial pain relief. Antihistamines, decongestants, and nose drops are used to decrease the amount of nasal secretion and shrink the mucus membranes in order to open the eustachian tube. Fluid in the ear will often respond to home treatment alone. See Chapter 9, "The Home Pharmacy," for information on these drugs.

If symptoms continue beyond two weeks, see the doctor.

What to Expect at the Doctor's Office

An examination of the ear, nose, and throat as well as the bony portion of the skull behind the ears, known as the mastoid, will be performed. Pain, tenderness, or redness of the mastoid signifies a serious infection.

Therapy will generally consist of an antibiotic as well as an attempt to open the eustachian tube by medication. Nose drops, decongestants, and antihistamines can be used for this purpose. Antibiotic therapy generally will be prescribed for at least a week, while other treatments will usually be given for a shorter period. Be sure to give all of the antibiotic prescribed, and on schedule.

Occasionally fluid in the middle ear will persist for a long period without infection. In this case, there may be a slight decrease in hearing. This condition, known as *serous otitis media,* is

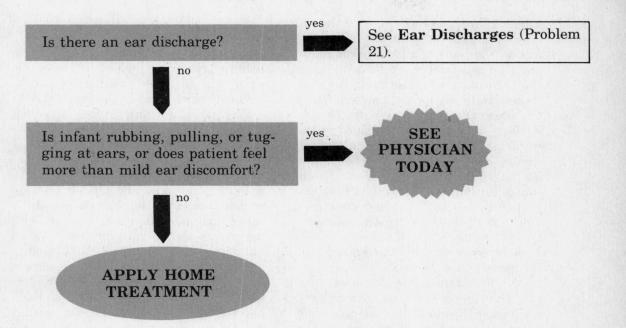

Is there an ear discharge?

yes → See **Ear Discharges** (Problem 21).

no

Is infant rubbing, pulling, or tugging at ears, or does patient feel more than mild ear discomfort?

yes → SEE PHYSICIAN TODAY

no

APPLY HOME TREATMENT

usually treated by attempting to open the eustachian tube and allow drainage; it is not treated with antibiotics. If this condition persists the physician may resort to placement of ear tubes in order to reestablish proper functioning of the middle ear. Placing ear tubes sounds frightening, but this is actually a simple and very effective procedure.

21 Ear Discharges

Ear discharges are usually just wax but may be caused by minor irritation or infection. Ear wax is almost never a problem unless attempts are made to "clean" the ear canals. Ear wax functions as a protective lining for the ear canal. Taking warm showers or washing the external ears with washcloths dipped in warm water usually provides enough vapor to prevent the buildup of wax that is thick and caked. Children often like to push things in their ear canal, and they may pack the wax tightly enough to prevent vibration of the eardrum and hence interfere with hearing. Adults armed with a cotton swab on a stick often accomplish the same awkward result.

In the summertime, ear discharges are commonly caused by "swimmer's ear," an irritation of the ear canal and not a problem of the middle ear or eardrum. Children will often complain that their ears are itchy. In addition, tugging on the ear will often cause pain; this can be a helpful clue to an inflammation of the outer ear and canal, such as swimmer's ear. The urge to scratch inside the ear is very tempting but must be resisted. We especially caution against the use of hairpins or other such instruments to accomplish the scratching, since injury to the eardrum can result.

In a young child or in an older child who has been complaining of ear pain, relief of pain accompanied by a white or yellow discharge may be the sign of a ruptured eardrum. Sometimes the parents will find that there is dry crusted material on the child's pillow; here again, a ruptured eardrum should be suspected. The child should be taken to a physician for antibiotic therapy. Do not be unduly alarmed; the ruptured eardrum is actually the first stage of a natural healing process which the antibiotics will help. Children have remarkable healing powers and most eardrums will heal completely within a matter of weeks.

Home Treatment

Packed-down ear wax can be removed by using warm water flushed in gently with a syringe, available at drugstores. A water jet that is set *at the very lowest setting* can also be useful, but it can be frightening to young children and is dangerous at higher settings. We do not advise that parents attempt to remove impacted ear wax unless they are dealing with an older child and can see the impacted, blackened ear wax. Wax softeners such as ordinary olive oil or Cerumenex are useful; however, all of the commercial products can be irritating if not used properly. Cerumenex, for example, must be flushed out of the ear within thirty minutes. Washing should never be attempted if there is a possibility of a ruptured eardrum.

Although swimmer's ear (or other causes of similar "otitis externa") is often caused by a bacterial infection, the infection is very shallow and does not often require antibiotic treatment. The infection can be effectively treated by placing a cotton wick soaked in Burrow's solution in the ear canal overnight, followed by a brief irrigation with 3% hydrogen peroxide followed by warm water. Success has also been reported with Merthiolate mixed with mineral oil (enough to make it pink), followed by the hydrogen peroxide and warm water rinse. For particularly severe or itching cases or persistence beyond five days, a doctor's visit is advisable.

What to Expect at the Doctor's Office

A thorough examination of the ear will be performed. In severe cases a culture

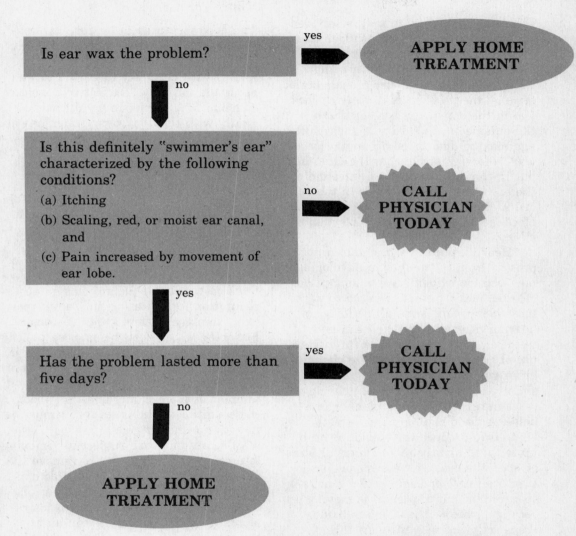

Is ear wax the problem? — yes → **APPLY HOME TREATMENT**

no ↓

Is this definitely "swimmer's ear" characterized by the following conditions?
(a) Itching
(b) Scaling, red, or moist ear canal, and
(c) Pain increased by movement of ear lobe.

— no → **CALL PHYSICIAN TODAY**

yes ↓

Has the problem lasted more than five days? — yes → **CALL PHYSICIAN TODAY**

no ↓

APPLY HOME TREATMENT

for bacteria may be taken. Corticosteroid and antibiotic preparations which are placed in the ear canal may be prescribed, or one of the regimens described above under "Home Treatment" may be advised. Oral antibiotics will usually be given if a perforated eardrum is causing the discharge.

22 Hearing Loss

Problems with hearing may be divided into two broad categories: sudden and slow. When a child of age five or older complains of a difficulty in hearing which has developed over a short period of time, the problem is usually a blockage in the ear of one type or another. On the outside of the eardrum, such blockage may be due to the accumulation of wax, a foreign object that the child has put in the ear canal, or an infection of the ear canal. On the inside of the eardrum, fluid may accumulate and cause blockage because of an ear infection or allergy.

Hearing problems in children may be present from birth, slow in developing, or may become evident over a long period of time. Many parents become concerned that their infant or small child is not hearing normally. Hearing can now be tested in a child of any age through the use of computers that analyze changes in brain waves in response to sounds. More simply, a child with normal hearing will react in a characteristic manner to a noise. A hand clap, horn, or whistle may be used to produce the sound. From birth up to three months, an infant will blink or open the eyes, move arms or legs, turn the head, or begin sucking in response to sound. If a child is moving or vocalizing before the sound is made, these activities may stop. At three months, children begin to attempt to find a sound by moving the head and looking for it. The ability to find the sound no matter where it is (below, behind, or above the child) may not be fully developed until the age of two.

Normal speech development relies upon hearing. A child whose speech is developing slowly or not at all may, in fact, have difficulty in hearing. Children who babble continually beyond a year without forming words should also be suspected of hearing difficulties.

Home Treatment

The need for an accurate ear examination usually necessitates a trip to the doctor. However, a problem that is known with certainty to be due to wax accumulation may be effectively treated at home. The ear is simply flushed gently with tepid or warm water to wash out the wax. Ear syringes or other devices for squirting water into the ear canal are available in drugstores. A water jet set at the *very lowest setting* can be used with considerable success, but we do not recommend the use of it for young children because of the frightening noise. Wax softeners, such as Cerumenex, may be needed when the wax is hard and impacted; follow the instructions on the label. (Debrox has gained a reputation for irritating ear canals, perhaps unjustly.) A few words of warning: First, the water must be as close to body temperature as possible; the use of cold water may result in dizziness and vomiting. Second, washing should never be attempted if there is any question about the condition of the eardrum; it must be intact and undamaged.

Be cautious with respect to removing foreign bodies. Do not try to remove the object unless it is easily accessible and removing it clearly poses no threat of damage to ear structures. Sharp instruments should never be used in an attempt to remove foreign bodies. Many times, efforts to remove an object push it further into the ear or damage the eardrum.

What to Expect at the Doctor's Office

A thorough examination of both ears often reveals the cause of the hearing

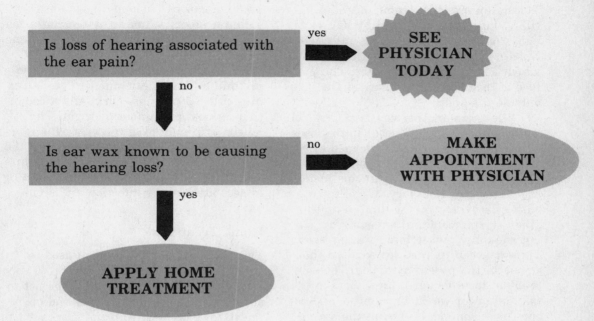

Is loss of hearing associated with the ear pain?

yes → SEE PHYSICIAN TODAY

no

Is ear wax known to be causing the hearing loss?

no → MAKE APPOINTMENT WITH PHYSICIAN

yes

APPLY HOME TREATMENT

loss. If it does not, the physician may recommend audiometry (an electronic hearing test) or other tests. Some decrease in hearing is normal after the age of twenty. If this becomes a problem in later life, it is time to visit the physician. Hearing can often be improved by a variety of methods.

23 Runny Nose

The hallmark of the common cold is the runny nose. It is intended by nature to help the body fight the virus infection. Nasal secretions contain antibodies, which act against the viruses. The profuse outpouring of fluid carries the virus outside the body.

Allergy is another common cause of runny noses. People whose runny noses are due to an allergy are deemed to have *allergic rhinitis,* better known as hay fever. The nasal secretions in this instance are often clear and very thin. People with allergic rhinitis will often have other symptoms simultaneously, including sneezing, and itching, watery eyes. They will rub their noses so often that a crease in the nose may appear. This problem lasts longer than a viral infection, often for weeks or months, and occurs most commonly during the spring and fall when pollen particles or other allergens are in the air. A great many other substances may aggravate allergic rhinitis, including house dusts, molds, and animal danders.

Once in a great while a head injury causes the fluid around the brain to leak down into the nose. This results in a clear, watery discharge, often one-sided and requires a doctor's attention.

Bacterial infections may cause a foul-smelling discharge which is often rusty or green in color. Antibiotics may help in this case.

The runny nose may also be due to a small object that a young child has pushed into the nose. Usually, but not always, this will produce a discharge from only one nostril. Often the discharge will be foul smelling and yellow or green.

Another common cause of runny noses as well as stuffy noses is prolonged use of nose drops. This problem of excess medication is known as *rhinitis medicamentosum.* Nose drops containing substances like ephedrine should never be used for longer than three days. This problem can be avoided by switching to saline nose drops (made by placing a teaspoon of salt in a pint of water) over the next few days.

Complications from the runny nose are due to the excess mucus. The mucus may cause a postnasal drip and a cough that is most prominent at night. The mucus drip may plug the eustachian tube between the nasal passages and the ear, resulting in ear infection and pain. It may plug the sinus passages, resulting in secondary sinus infection and sinus pain.

Home Treatment

Two major types of drugs are used to control a runny nose. Decongestants such as pseudoephedrine and ephedrine act to shrink the mucus membranes and open the nasal passages. Antihistamines act to block allergic reactions and decrease the amount of secretion. Decongestants make some children overly active. Antihistamines may cause drowsiness as well as interfere with sleep. Because of the complications of the medications, runny noses should be treated only when they are severely impairing comfort. Using a facial tissue is often the best approach—it has no side effects, costs less, and helps get the virus outside the body!

If you choose to treat a runny nose with medication, nose drops are suitable. Saline nose drops are fine for young infants. Older children and adults may use drops containing decongestants. See Chapter 9, "The Home Pharmacy," for information on decongestants, antihistamines, and nose drops.

Complications such as ear and sinus infection may be prevented by ensuring

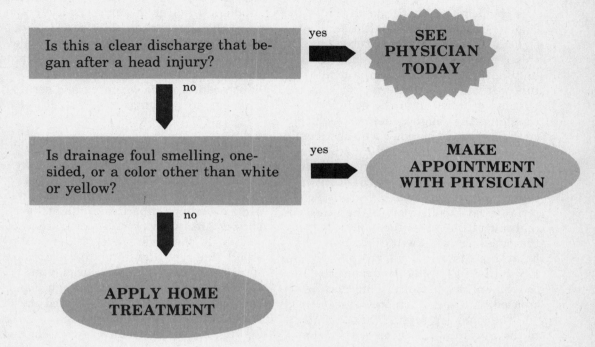

Is this a clear discharge that began after a head injury?

yes → **SEE PHYSICIAN TODAY**

no ↓

Is drainage foul smelling, one-sided, or a color other than white or yellow?

yes → **MAKE APPOINTMENT WITH PHYSICIAN**

no ↓

APPLY HOME TREATMENT

that the mucus is thin rather than thick and sticky. This helps to prevent plugging of the nasal passages. Increasing the humidity in the air with a vaporizer or humidifier helps to liquefy the mucus. Heated air inside a house is often very dry; cooler air contains more moisture and is preferable. Drinking a large amount of liquid will also help liquefy the secretions.

If symptoms persist beyond three weeks, your physician should be contacted.

What to Expect at the Doctor's Office

The doctor will thoroughly examine the ears, nose, and throat and will check for tenderness over the sinuses. Often, a swab of the nasal secretions will be taken and examined under a microscope. The presence of certain types of cells, known as eosinophils, will indicate the presence of hay fever (allergic rhinitis). If allergic rhinitis is found, antihistamines may be prescribed and an avoidance program of dust, mold, dander, and pollen will be explained, similar to that described in Section G (Allergies).

24 Cough

The cough reflex is one of the body's best "defense mechanisms." Irritation or obstruction in the breathing tubes triggers this reflex, and the violent rush of air helps clear material from the breathing tubes. If abnormal material, such as pus, is being expelled from the body by coughing, the cough is desirable. Such a cough is termed "productive" and should usually not be suppressed by drugs.

Often, a minor irritation or a healing area in a breathing tube will start the cough reflex even though there is no material to be expelled, other than the normal mucus. At other times, mucus from the nasal passages will drain into breathing tubes at night (postnasal drip) and initiate the cough reflex. Such coughs are not beneficial and may be decreased with cough suppressants.

The smoker's cough bears testimony to the continual irritation of the breathing tubes. The smoke also poisons the cells that line these tubes so that mucus cannot be expelled normally. Smoker's cough is a sign of the deadly diseases yet to come.

Next to smoking, viral infections are the most common causes of coughs. These coughs usually bring up only yellow or white mucus. In contrast, coughs producing mucus that is rusty or green and looks like it contains pus are most likely to be caused by a bacterial infection. Bacterial infections require the doctor's help and antibiotics.

The term "pneumonia" is most often used to mean a bacterial infection of the lung but can be used for viral infection and other problems as well. In fact, a "chest cold" is a viral pneumonia and the terms "double pneumonia" and "walking pneumonia" usually indicate a viral pneumonia. So don't panic when you hear "pneumonia"—it is not a very precise term.

In very young infants, coughing is unusual and may indicate a serious lung problem. In older infants, who are prone to swallowing foreign objects, an object may become lodged in the windpipe and cause coughing. Young children also tend to inhale bits of peanut and popcorn, which can produce coughing and serious problems in the lung.

Home Treatment

The mucus in the breathing tubes may be made thinner and less sticky by several means. Increased humidity in the air will help; a vaporizer and a steamy shower are two ways to increase the humidity. In the severe "croup" cough of small children, high humidity is absolutely essential. Drinking large quantities of fluids is helpful for cough, particularly if a fever has dehydrated the body. Glycerol guaiacolate (Robitussin or 2G) is available without prescription and may help to liquefy the secretions. The liberal use of such common home substances as pepper and garlic also liquefies the secretions and may help relieve the cough.

Decongestants and/or antihistamines may help if a postnasal drip is causing the cough. Otherwise, avoid drugs that contain antihistamines because they tend to dry the secretions and make them thicker.

Various over-the-counter cough preparations will give relief from a bothersome cough. Dry, tickling coughs are often relieved by cough lozenges or sucking on hard candy. Dextromethorphan (Romilar, St. Joseph's Cough Syrup, etc.) is an effective cough suppressant, available without prescription. Adults may re-

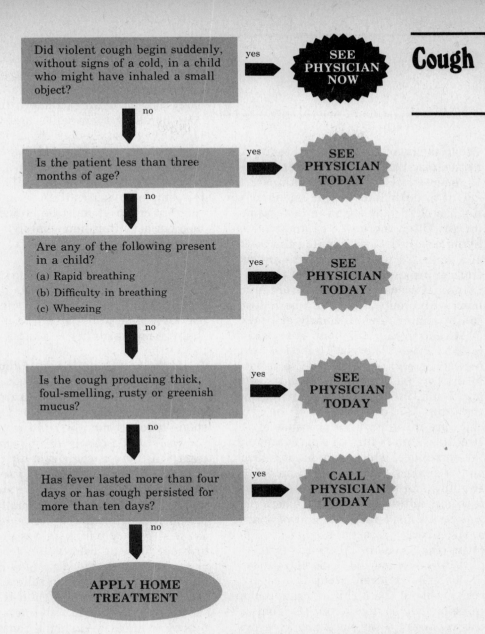

Did violent cough begin suddenly, without signs of a cold, in a child who might have inhaled a small object? — yes → **SEE PHYSICIAN NOW**

no ↓

Is the patient less than three months of age? — yes → **SEE PHYSICIAN TODAY**

no ↓

Are any of the following present in a child?
(a) Rapid breathing
(b) Difficulty in breathing
(c) Wheezing
— yes → **SEE PHYSICIAN TODAY**

no ↓

Is the cough producing thick, foul-smelling, rusty or greenish mucus? — yes → **SEE PHYSICIAN TODAY**

no ↓

Has fever lasted more than four days or has cough persisted for more than ten days? — yes → **CALL PHYSICIAN TODAY**

no ↓

APPLY HOME TREATMENT

quire up to twice the dosage recommended in the package instructions. Do not exceed this amount; neither dextromethorphan nor codeine will completely eliminate most coughs at any dosage, and side effects of drowsiness or constipation can occur.

See Chapter 9, The Home Pharmacy, for more information.

What to Expect at the Doctor's Office

The doctor will examine the ears, nose, throat, and chest; a chest X-ray may be taken in some instances. Do not expect antibiotics to be prescribed for a routine viral or allergic cough; they do not help.

25 Croup

Croup is one of the most frightening illnesses that parents will ever encounter. It generally occurs in children under the age of three or four. In the middle of the night a child may sit up in bed gasping for air. Often there will be an accompanying cough that sounds like the barking of a seal. The child's symptoms are so frightening that panic is often the response. However, the most severe problems with croup usually can be relieved safely, simply, and efficiently at home.

Croup is caused by one of several different viruses. The viral infection causes a swelling and outpouring of secretions in the larynx (voice box), trachea (windpipe), and the larger airways going to the lungs. The air passages of the young child are made narrower because of the swelling. This is further aggravated by the secretions, which may become dried out and caked. This combination of swelling and thickened, dried secretions makes it difficult to breathe. There may also be a considerable amount of spasm of the airway passages, further complicating the problem. Treatment is designed to dissolve the dried secretions.

In some children, croup is a recurring problem; these children may have three or four bouts of croup. Seldom does this represent a serious underlying problem, but a physician's advice should be sought. Croup will be outgrown as the airway passages grow larger; it is unusual after the age of seven.

Occasionally, a more serious obstruction caused by a bacterial infection and known as epiglottitis can be confused with croup. Epiglottitis is more common in children over the age of three, but there is considerable overlap in the ages of children affected by these two conditions. Children with epiglottitis often have more serious difficulty in breathing. They may have an extremely difficult time handling their saliva and will drool. Often they assume a characteristic position with their head tilted forward and their jaw pointed out and will gasp for air. Epiglottitis will not be relieved by the simple measures that bring prompt relief of croup. It must be brought to medical attention immediately.

Home Treatment

Mist is the backbone of therapy for croup and can be supplied efficiently by a cold steam vaporizer. Cold steam vaporizers are preferable to hot steam ones because there is no possibility of scalding from hot water.

If the breathing is very difficult, you can obtain faster results by taking the child to the bathroom and turning on the hot shower to make thick clouds of steam. (Do not put the child in the hot shower!) Steam can be created more efficiently if there is some cold air in the room. Remember that steam rises, so the child will not benefit from the steam by sitting on the floor. Relief usually occurs promptly and should be noticeable within the first twenty minutes. It is important to keep the child calm and not become alarmed; holding the child may comfort him or her and may help relieve some of the airway spasm. If the child is not showing significant improvement within twenty minutes, you should contact your physician or the local emergency room immediately. They will want to see the child and will make arrangements in advance while you are in transit. Unfortunately, few emergency rooms can provide steam as easily as the home shower.

If improvement is significant but the problem persists for more than an hour, call the doctor.

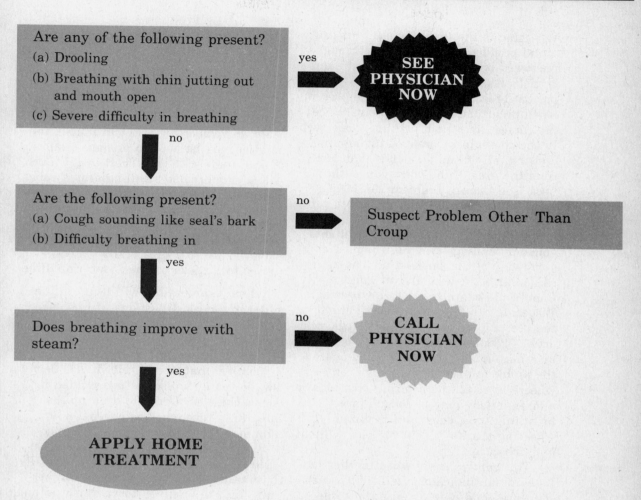

Are any of the following present?
(a) Drooling
(b) Breathing with chin jutting out and mouth open
(c) Severe difficulty in breathing

yes → **SEE PHYSICIAN NOW**

no

Are the following present?
(a) Cough sounding like seal's bark
(b) Difficulty breathing in

no → Suspect Problem Other Than Croup

yes

Does breathing improve with steam?

no → **CALL PHYSICIAN NOW**

yes

APPLY HOME TREATMENT

What to Expect at the Doctor's Office

If the physician feels confident that this is croup, further use of mist will be tried. In difficult cases, X-rays of the neck are a reliable way of differentiating croup from epiglottitis. A swollen epiglottis often can be seen in the back of the throat, but this examination has its risks and should not be tried at home. If epi-glottitis is diagnosed, the child will be admitted to the hospital; an airway will be placed in the child's trachea to enable the child to breathe, and intravenous antibiotics directed at curing the bacterial infection will be started. In the case of croup, the trip to the doctor often cures the problem that was resistant to steam at home; keep the car windows open a bit and let the cool night air in.

26 Wheezing

Wheezing is the high-pitched whistling sound produced by air flowing through narrowed breathing tubes (bronchi and bronchioles). It is most obvious when the patient breathes out but may be present when breathing both in and out. Wheezing comes from the breathing tubes deep in the chest, in contrast to the croupy, crowing, or whooping sounds that come from the area of the voice box in the neck (see **Croup**, Problem 25). Most often, a narrowing of the breathing tubes is due to a viral infection or to an allergic reaction as in asthma. In infants younger than age two, bronchiolitis or narrowing of the smallest air passages can occur because of a viral infection. Pneumonia can also produce wheezing. Wheezing can follow an insect sting or the use of a medicine; these allergic reactions require that the patient be seen by a doctor. Any medication can cause the problem; some individuals even wheeze after taking aspirin. Occasionally a foreign body may be lodged in a breathing tube, causing a localized wheezing that is difficult to hear without a stethoscope.

The importance of wheezing lies in its being an indicator of difficult breathing. In a child with a respiratory infection, wheezing may occur before shortness of breath is marked. Therefore, when wheezing appears in the presence of a fever, early consultation with a physician is advisable, even though the illness seldom turns out to be serious.

Treatment of wheezing is symptomatic; there are no drugs that cure viral illnesses or asthma. Home treatment is an important part of this approach. However, the physician's help is needed so that drugs that widen the breathing passages can be used. Intravenous fluids may be required on some occasions.

Home Treatment

Hydration by drinking fluids is very important. It is best to drink water, but fruit juices or soft drinks may be used if this will increase the amount taken. The use of a vaporizer, preferably one that produces a cold mist, may sometimes help. If a vaporizer is not available, the shower may be used to produce a mist. Unfortunately, it is difficult to get much vapor down to the small breathing tubes. These measures will be part of the therapy that the doctor recommends and may be begun immediately, even though a visit to the doctor will be necessary.

What to Expect at the Doctor's Office

Physical examination will focus on the chest and neck. Questions will be asked not only about the current illness but also about a past history of allergies either in the patient or the family. The possibility that a foreign body has been swallowed may also be investigated in small children. Drugs to open up the breathing tube, such as adrenalin or aminophylline, may be given by injection, by mouth, or by rectal suppository. (See **Asthma**, pp. 177–179.) Occasionally hospitalization will be necessary to permit fluids to be given through a vein and for effective humidification of the air to be achieved. Most important, the patient can be closely watched; the hospital is used as a precautionary measure to prevent the condition from getting worse before it gets better.

Is this a recurrent problem due to asthma?

no → **SEE PHYSICIAN TODAY**

yes ↓

APPLY TREATMENT RECOMMENDED BY PHYSICIAN

27 Hoarseness

Hoarseness is usually caused by a problem in the vocal cords. In infants under three months of age, this can be due to a serious problem such as a birth defect or thyroid disorder. In young children, hoarseness is more often due to prolonged or excessive crying, which puts a strain on the vocal cords.

In older children, viral infections are the most common cause of hoarseness. If the hoarseness is accompanied by difficulty in breathing or a cough that sounds like a barking seal, the hoarseness is considered a symptom of croup (see Problem 25). Croup is characteristic in children under the age of four, while the symptom of hoarseness by itself is more common in older children.

If hoarseness is accompanied by difficulty in breathing or swallowing, drooling, gasping for air, or breathing with the mouth wide open and the chin jutting forward, a physician must be seen immediately—this is a medical emergency. This problem is known as *epiglottitis* and is a bacterial infection that affects the entrance to the airway.

In adults, a virus is most often responsible for the development of hoarseness or laryngitis without any other symptoms. As with any symptom of an upper respiratory tract infection, hoarseness may linger after other symptoms disappear. When hoarseness is mild, the most common cause is cigarette smoke. If persistent hoarseness is *not* associated with either a viral infection or with smoking, it should be investigated by a physician. The length of the wait is controversial; we suggest one month. If you are a smoker, stop smoking and wait one month. Persistent hoarseness has many causes; the most common are cysts or polyps on the vocal chords. Cancer is also a cause but is relatively rare.

Home Treatment

Hoarseness, unassociated with other symptoms, is very resistant to medical therapy. Nature must heal the inflamed area. Humidifying the air with a vaporizer or taking in fluids can offer some relief. However, healing may not occur for several days. Resting the vocal cords is sensible; crying or shouting makes the situation worse. For the treatment of hoarseness associated with coughs, see **Cough** (Problem 24).

What to Expect at the Doctor's Office

If a child has severe difficulty in breathing, the first priority is to ensure that the air passage is adequate. This may require the placement of a breathing tube, performed in the emergency room, hospital, or physician's office. If X-rays of the neck are taken, a physician should accompany the child at all times.

In uncomplicated hoarseness that has persisted for a long period of time, a physician will look at the vocal cords with the aid of a small mirror. Occasionally more extensive physical examination and blood tests will be performed.

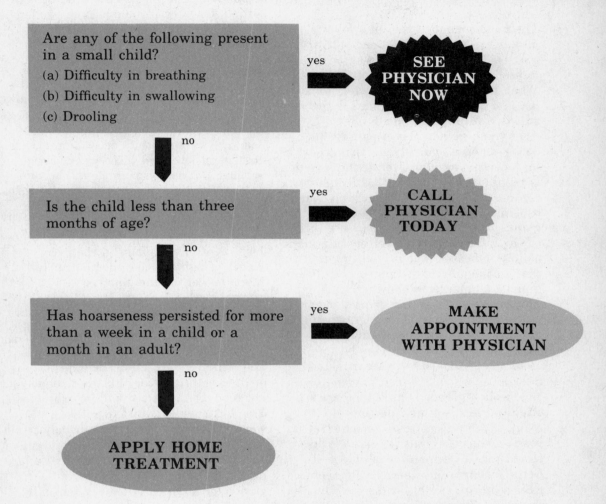

Are any of the following present in a small child?
(a) Difficulty in breathing
(b) Difficulty in swallowing
(c) Drooling

yes → **SEE PHYSICIAN NOW**

no

Is the child less than three months of age?

yes → **CALL PHYSICIAN TODAY**

no

Has hoarseness persisted for more than a week in a child or a month in an adult?

yes → **MAKE APPOINTMENT WITH PHYSICIAN**

no

APPLY HOME TREATMENT

28 Swollen Glands

The most common types of swollen glands are lymph glands and salivary glands. The biggest salivary glands are located below and in front of the ears. When they swell, the characteristic swollen jaw appearance of mumps is the result (see **Mumps**, Problem 53).

Lymph glands play a part in the body's defense against infection. They may become swollen even if the infection is trivial or not apparent, although you can usually identify the infection that is causing the swelling. Swollen neck glands frequently accompany sore throats or ear infections. The swelling of a gland simply indicates that it is taking part in the fight against infection. Glands in the groin are enlarged when there is infection in the feet, legs, or genital region; these glands are often swollen when no obvious infection can be found. Sometimes the basic problem may be so minor as to be overlooked (as with athlete's foot).

Swollen glands behind the ears are often the result of an infection in the scalp. If there is no scalp infection, it is possible that the patient currently has or recently had German measles (see **Rubella**, Problem 56). Infectious mononucleosis (mono) can also cause swelling of the glands behind the ears.

If a swollen gland is red and tender, there may be a bacterial infection within the gland itself that requires antibiotic treatment. Swollen glands otherwise require no treatment, since they are merely fighting infections elsewhere. If there is an accompanying sore throat or earache, these should be treated as described in Problems 19 and 20, respectively. However, the swollen glands are usually the result of multiple viral infections that require no treatment. If you have noticed one or several glands progressively enlarging over a period of three weeks, a physician should be consulted. On very rare occasions, swollen glands can signal serious underlying problems.

Home Treatment

Merely observe the glands over several weeks to see if they are continuing to enlarge or if other glands become swollen. The vast majority of swollen glands that persist beyond three weeks are not serious, but a physician should be consulted if the glands show no tendency to become smaller. Soreness in the glands will usually disappear in a couple of days; the pain results from the rapid enlargement of the gland in the early stages of fighting the infection. It takes much longer for the gland to return to normal size.

What to Expect at the Doctor's Office

The physician will examine the glands and search for infections or other causes of the swelling. Other glands that may not have been noticed will be examined. The doctor will inquire about fever, weight loss, or other symptoms associated with the swelling of the glands. The physician may decide that blood tests are indicated or will simply observe the glands for a period of time. Eventually, it might be necessary to remove (biopsy) the gland for examination under the microscope, but this is very seldom required.

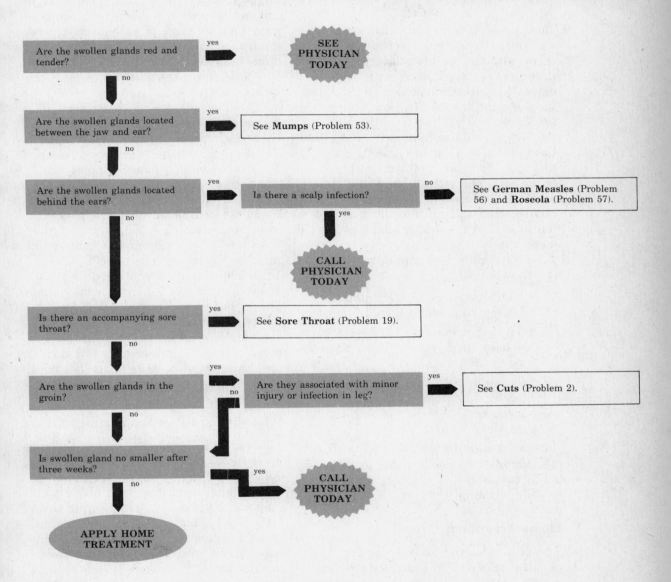

Are the swollen glands red and tender?

yes → **SEE PHYSICIAN TODAY**

no ↓

Are the swollen glands located between the jaw and ear?

yes → See **Mumps** (Problem 53).

no ↓

Are the swollen glands located behind the ears?

yes → Is there a scalp infection?

no → See **German Measles** (Problem 56) and **Roseola** (Problem 57).

yes → **CALL PHYSICIAN TODAY**

no ↓

Is there an accompanying sore throat?

yes → See **Sore Throat** (Problem 19).

no ↓

Are the swollen glands in the groin?

yes → Are they associated with minor injury or infection in leg?

yes → See **Cuts** (Problem 2).

no →

no ↓

Is swollen gland no smaller after three weeks?

yes → **CALL PHYSICIAN TODAY**

no ↓

APPLY HOME TREATMENT

29 Nosebleeds

The blood vessels within the nose lie very near the surface, and bleeding may occur with the slightest injury. In children, picking the nose is a common cause. Keeping their fingernails cut and discouraging the habit is good preventive medicine.

Nosebleeds are frequently due to irritation by a virus or to vigorous nose blowing. The main problem in this case is the cold, and treatment of cold symptoms will reduce the probability of the nosebleed. If the mucous membrane of the nose is dry, cracking and bleeding is more likely.

These key points should be remembered:

- You can almost always stop the bleeding yourself.
- The great majority of nosebleeds are associated with colds or minor injury to the nose.
- Treatment such as packing the nose with gauze has significant drawbacks and should be avoided if possible.
- Investigation into the cause of recurrent nosebleeds is not urgent and is best accomplished when the nose is *not* bleeding.

Home Treatment

The nose consists of a bony part and a cartilaginous part: a "hard" portion and a "soft" portion. The area of the nose that usually bleeds lies within the "soft" portion, and compression will control the nosebleed. Simply squeeze the nose between thumb and forefinger just below the hard portion of the nose. Pressure should be applied for at least five minutes. The patient should be seated. Holding the head back is not necessary. It merely directs the blood flow backward rather than forward. Cold compresses or ice applied across the bridge of the nose may help. Almost all nosebleeds can be controlled in this manner if *sufficient time* is allowed for the bleeding to stop.

Nosebleeds are more common in the winter when viruses and dry, heated air indoors are common. A cooler house and a vaporizer to return humidity to the air help many people.

If nosebleeds are a recurrent problem, are becoming more frequent, and are not associated with a cold or other minor irritation, a physician should be consulted, without urgency. A physician need not be seen immediately after the nosebleed since examination at that time may simply restart the nosebleed.

Medical opinion is divided as to whether high blood pressure causes nosebleeds, but most physicians believe that the two conditions are seldom related. As a precaution, an individual with high blood pressure who experiences a nosebleed may want to have his or her blood pressure taken within a few days.

What to Expect at the Doctor's Office

The doctor will seat the patient and compress his or her nostrils. This will be done even if the patient has been doing this at home, and it will usually work. Packing the nose or attempting to cauterize a bleeding point is less desirable. If the nosebleed cannot be stopped, the nose will be examined to see if a bleeding point can be identified. If a bleeding point is seen, coagulation by either electrical or chemical cauterization may be attempted. If this is not successful, packing of the nose may be unavoidable. Such packing is uncomfortable and may

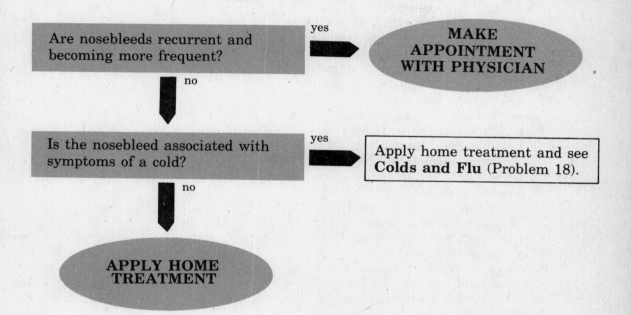

Are nosebleeds recurrent and becoming more frequent? — yes → **MAKE APPOINTMENT WITH PHYSICIAN**

no ↓

Is the nosebleed associated with symptoms of a cold? — yes → Apply home treatment and see **Colds and Flu** (Problem 18).

no ↓

APPLY HOME TREATMENT

lead to infection; thus the patient must be carefully observed.

If a physician is seen because of recurrent nosebleeds, questions about events preceding the nosebleeds and a careful examination of the nose itself should be expected. Depending on the history and the physical examination, blood-clotting tests may be ordered on rare occasions.

30 Bad Breath

Poor dental hygiene and smoking cause most cases of bad breath in adults. Infections of the mouth, including sore throats, may also be a cause of bad breath. Recently it has been suggested that bad breath is occasionally due to gases absorbed from the intestine and released through the lungs. Unfortunately, even if this is correct, it is not clear what can be done about it.

Children seldom have the problem with bad breath in the morning that is so common with adults; regular tooth brushing should eliminate this problem.

A rare cause of prolonged bad breath in a child is a foreign body in the nose. This is especially common in toddlers, who have inserted some small object which remains unnoticed. Often, but not always, there is a white, yellowish, or bloody discharge from one nostril.

Finally, unusual problems such as abscesses of the lung or heavy worm infestations have been reported to cause bad breath, although we have not seen these in our practices.

Home Treatment

Proper dental hygiene and not smoking will prevent most cases of bad breath. If this does not eliminate the odor, a visit to the doctor or dentist may be helpful.

Do not use mouthwash to perfume the breath; these cover up but do not treat the underlying problem.

What to Expect at the Doctor's Office

The doctor will thoroughly examine the mouth and the nose. A culture may be taken if the patient has a sore throat or mouth sores; antibiotics may be prescribed. If there is an object in the nose, the physician will use a special instrument to remove it.

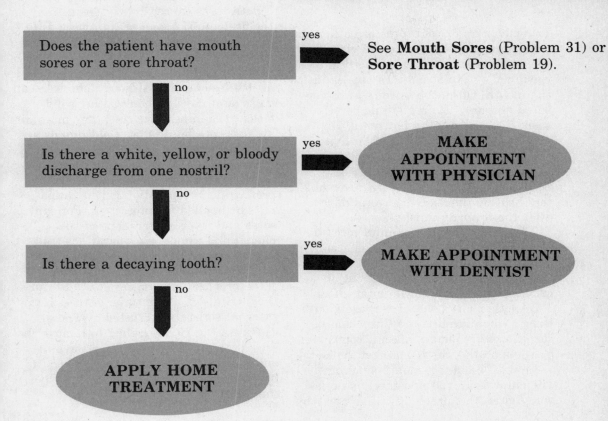

Does the patient have mouth sores or a sore throat? — **yes** → See **Mouth Sores** (Problem 31) or **Sore Throat** (Problem 19).

no ↓

Is there a white, yellow, or bloody discharge from one nostril? — **yes** → **MAKE APPOINTMENT WITH PHYSICIAN**

no ↓

Is there a decaying tooth? — **yes** → **MAKE APPOINTMENT WITH DENTIST**

no ↓

APPLY HOME TREATMENT

31 Mouth Sores

Fever blisters or cold sores are a familiar problem caused by the herpes virus. They are usually found on the lips, although they can sometimes appear inside the mouth. Often the blisters have ruptured and only the remaining sore is seen. Fever is usually but not always present. The herpes virus often lives in the body for years, causing trouble only when another illness causes a rise in body temperature. Generally, fever blisters heal by themselves several days after the fever diminishes.

A canker sore is a painful ulcer that often follows an injury, such as accidently biting the inside of the lip or the tongue, or it may appear without obvious cause. Eventually it heals by itself.

Another virus that can cause mouth lesions in children is the Coxsackie virus. These lesions are often accompanied by spots on the hands and feet; hence the name "hand-foot-mouth syndrome." The child feels well and there is no fever. Again, this problem will go away by itself.

Allergic reactions to drugs may cause mouth ulcers. In such cases a skin rash may be present on other parts of the body as well, and a physician must be contacted.

A cancer of the lip or gum is rare; it does not need to be treated in the first few days. Syphilis transmitted by oral sexual contact may produce a mouth sore. Both of these problems are usually painless. There are other conditions that may also cause mouth ulcers, but they also cause problems with eyes, joints, or other organs. Rarely, allergic reactions to drugs may cause mouth ulcers. In such cases a skin rash usually will be present on other parts of the body as well; a physician must be seen.

Home Treatment

Mouth sores caused by viruses heal by themselves. The goal of treatment is to reduce fever, relieve pain, and maintain adequate fluid intake. Children will seldom want to eat when they have painful mouth lesions, and although children can go several days without taking solid foods, it is imperative that they maintain an adequate liquid diet. Cold liquids are the most soothing and Popsicles® or iced frozen juices often are helpful. For sores inside the lip and on the gums, a non-prescription preparation called Orabase may be applied for protection. For canker sores and fever blisters, one of the phenol and camphor preparations (Blistex, Campho-Phenique) may provide relief, especially if applied early. If one of these preparations appears to cause further irritation, discontinue its use. If the external sores have crusted over, cool compresses may be applied to remove the crusts. Mouth sores usually resolve in one to two weeks; any sore that persists beyond three weeks should be seen by the physician.

What to Expect at the Doctor's Office

A thorough examination of the mouth will be done. A drug called Nystatin will usually be prescribed for thrush, a yeast infection. For viral infections, physicians have no more to offer than home remedies. We caution against the use of oral anesthetics, such as viscous Xylocaine in children. This anesthetic can interfere with proper swallowing and can lead to inhalation of food into the lungs.

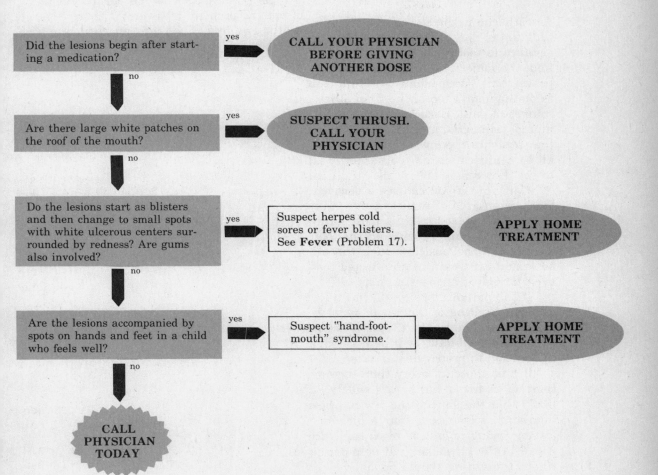

Did the lesions begin after starting a medication? — **yes** → CALL YOUR PHYSICIAN BEFORE GIVING ANOTHER DOSE

no

Are there large white patches on the roof of the mouth? — **yes** → SUSPECT THRUSH. CALL YOUR PHYSICIAN

no

Do the lesions start as blisters and then change to small spots with white ulcerous centers surrounded by redness? Are gums also involved? — **yes** → Suspect herpes cold sores or fever blisters. See **Fever** (Problem 17). → APPLY HOME TREATMENT

no

Are the lesions accompanied by spots on hands and feet in a child who feels well? — **yes** → Suspect "hand-foot-mouth" syndrome. → APPLY HOME TREATMENT

no

CALL PHYSICIAN TODAY

32 Toothaches

A toothache is the sad result of a poor program of dental hygiene. Although resistance to tooth decay is partly inherited, the majority of dental problems are preventable. Occasionally, it is difficult to distinguish a toothache from other sources of pain. Earaches, sore throats, mumps, sinusitis, and injury to the joint that attaches the jaw to the skull may all be confused with a toothache. A call to the doctor may clarify the situation.

Certainly if you can see a decayed tooth or an area of redness surrounding a tooth, a diseased tooth is most likely the cause of pain. Tapping on the teeth with a wooden Popsicle® stick will often accentuate the pain in an affected tooth, even though it appears normal.

If the patient appears ill, has a fever, and has swelling of the jaw or redness surrounding the tooth, a tooth abscess is likely and antibiotics will be necessary in addition to proper dental care.

If a pain occurs every time the patient opens his or her mouth widely, it is likely that the joint of the jaw has been injured; this can occur from a blow or just by trying to eat too big a sandwich. A call to the physician will help decide what, if anything should be done.

Home Treatment

Aspirin or acetaminophen may be used for pain when a toothache is suspected and while a dental appointment is being arranged. Aspirin is also helpful for problems in the joint of the jaw.

What to Expect at the Dentist's Office

At the dentist's office, fillings or extractions will be performed. Often in baby teeth, an extraction will be most likely. Root canals as opposed to extraction are generally performed on permanent teeth if the problem is severe. If there is fever or swelling of the jaw, an antibiotic will usually be prescribed.

Are any of the following present?

(a) Fever

(b) Earache

(c) Pain upon opening the mouth widely

yes →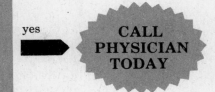

CALL PHYSICIAN TODAY

no

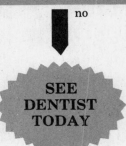

SEE DENTIST TODAY

G Allergies

Allergy was first described at the turn of the century by a pediatrician named Clemens von Pirquet. The term *allergy* meant "changed activity" and described changes that occurred after contacting a foreign substance. Two types of change were noticed, one of which was beneficial. The benefit occurred from the development of protection against a foreign substance after having been once exposed to it. This response prevents us from developing many infectious diseases for a second time and provides the scientific basis for most immunizations. The other type of response generally not beneficial, was known as a hypersensitivity response, and it is the response for which the term *allergy* is generally used.

Allergy is now known to be possible even without previous exposure to the substance. All persons are capable of allergic responses; for example, anyone given a transfusion with the wrong type of blood will have an allergic reaction.

However, the term *allergy* is overused. When your eyes smart in Los Angeles, they are not allergic to the air but are experiencing a direct chemical irritation from the pollutants. Similarly, skin coming in contact with some plants or chemicals experiences direct damage and not an allergic response. Physicians often blame milk or food allergy for vomiting, diarrhea, colic, crying, irritability, fretfulness, or sneezing in infants. While allergy can cause these symptoms, countless other things can also.

Over the next few pages we will discuss common allergies (such as those to food, insects, drugs, pets, pollen, and dust), the common allergic problems (such as asthma, hay fever, hives, and other skin problems), and the medical treatments available.

FOOD ALLERGY

Food allergy occurs at all ages, but is of most concern in children. Almost any food can produce an allergic response; only breast milk appears to be incapable of causing an allergy. Even in this case, a 1928 report incriminates beans in a mother's diet, detected in the breast milk, as a cause of allergy in an infant. Food allergy is not the only cause of digestive upsets

175

but is blamed for much that it does not cause. For example, some children are born without an important digestive enzyme, known as lactase, which is necessary to digest the sugars present in milk. Other children lose the ability to make lactase after the age of three or four. Many adults have a relative deficiency of lactase. The absence of lactase can produce diarrhea, abdominal pain, and vomiting after the drinking of milk. This is only one example of a digestive problem that can be confused with food allergy; there are many others.

Symptoms of Food Allergy

Food allergy may produce swelling of the mouth and lips, hives, skin rashes, vomiting, diarrhea, asthma, runny nose, and other problems. Of course, many other allergens besides food can cause these problems, making it difficult to prove that a particular food is the culprit. The best approach for detecting food allergy is to think like Sherlock Holmes. If the lips swell only after eating strawberries, you have your suspect!

Foods Responsible for Allergy

Cow's milk is frequently blamed for food allergy in small children. Since almost any symptom can be blamed on allergy, and since infants consume so much cow's milk, it is easy to see why milk is so quickly blamed. Infant intestines are capable of absorbing proteins that older children's digestive tracts would not absorb. These proteins may set up altered reactions or allergies.

Controversy exists over the relationship of early exposure to cow's milk and the later development of asthma. Some physicians have maintained that avoidance of cow's milk will delay or eliminate the development of asthma. Others have found the opposite. The only agreement is that the children most likely to develop allergies, including asthma, come from families that have other allergic members. Cow's milk may have some effects on children who are likely to develop allergies but probably should not be of particular concern in children with no family history of allergy.

Cow's milk can cause allergic responses in infants, with diarrhea and even blood loss through the intestines, but very rarely. This situation is a clear indication for removal of cow's milk, if the severe diarrhea is documented by a physician. The necessary tests are simple and require analysis of the stools (feces). Stool analysis should be repeated after the child has been taken off cow's milk.

Other foods that have been associated with allergic reactions in children include wheat, eggs, citrus fruits, beef and veal, fish, and nuts. Severe reactions are very rare in children; parents need not be anxious about giving their children new foods. Families with a strong history of allergy can introduce one new food to an infant every few days so that if an allergy develops, the cause is obvious.

Soybean Substitutes for Milk

The amount of soybean formula produced in this country exceeds the amount necessary to provide for children with cow's milk allergy. Milk allergy consists of an altered response to the cow's milk protein, producing vomiting and/or diarrhea, and is extremely rare. Intolerance to cow's milk because of lack of the enzyme lactase to digest the sugar lactose will produce bloating, abdominal pain, vomiting, and/or diarrhea. This intolerance is also rare.

There are two possible explanations for the purchase of soybean preparations. First, parents may buy them because they like them. They are nutritious and children tolerate them well. However, they tend to be more expensive than cow's milk. The other reason for the high consumption of soybean formula is that parents have been instructed to substitute for cow's milk at the slightest suspicion of an allergy. Every childhood symptom known has been attributed to cow's milk allergy—but the condition is rare.

Before you spend money on a soybean formula, make sure that your physician has determined that the child really needs it. Many stories of children getting better on a soybean preparation result from the child spontaneously recovering from whatever was formerly producing the troublesome symptom.

ASTHMA

Asthma is a severe allergic disorder which is most common in children and adolescents. It is discussed further in the description of its most prominent symptom—wheezing (see Problem 26). The wheezing in asthma is caused by spasm of the muscles in the walls of the smaller air passages in the lungs. An excess amount of mucus production further narrows the air passages and can aggravate the difficulty in getting the air out. Infections and foreign bodies in the air passages can mimic asthma. All wheezing in children is potentially serious and should be evaluated by a medical professional, at least for the first few occurrences. Asthma tends to occur in families where other members have either asthma, hay fever, or eczema.

An attack can be triggered by an infection, by an emotionally upsetting event, or by exposure to an *allergen*. Common allergens include house dust, pollen, mold, food, and shed animal materials or "animal danders." It is sometimes easy to identify airborne allergens to which a person is susceptible. Some people will wheeze only around cats, others only during a particular pollen season. (Pollens most often cause seasonal hay fever, or allergic rhinitis, rather than asthma.) Most often, there is no clear reason for a particular asthmatic attack. If asthma is severe, it is desirable to identify the offending allergens if possible.

177

Treatment of Asthma

The treatment of asthma varies according to the severity of the problem. Some people have only one or two episodes of asthma and are never troubled again. We wonder if these episodes should even be called asthma attacks. Other people will have daily attacks, which severely compromise their ability to function normally.

While some doctors maintain that children never truly outgrow asthma, the evidence is otherwise. More than half of the children diagnosed as having asthma will never have an asthmatic attack as an adult. Another 10 percent will have only occasional attacks during adult life.

Therapy provides relief of symptoms, often dramatically so, but must also work to remove the cause, whether it is allergic, infectious, or emotional. Symptomatic relief of asthma is provided through a variety of prescription medications, including epinephrine, isoproterenol, ephedrine, aminophylline, prednisone, and others.

Several different prescription drugs are often combined, but we see no reason to begin treatment with such combination drugs. Many of these compounds have phenobarbital added to counteract some of the stimulating effects of the other medicines included; new medications to counteract the side effects of the previous medication could be added continually. All of these drugs are powerful, and all cause side effects. Minimal side effects may be acceptable to relieve major symptoms. If side effects are intolerable, a new treatment plan can be made. Try to avoid combination drugs.

Corticosteroid drugs (steroids, prednisone) are effective in severe asthmatic patients. They block the smooth muscle contractions that narrow the airway passages. They have many side effects, including growth retardation, and should be used only after full discussion with your physician.

Antihistamines are not useful in the treatment of asthma. In fact, the drying of secretions by antihistamines may actually cause airway plugging.

Nebulizers (spray medicines) can be potentially abused and can even have fatal reactions. They should be used sparingly in children, and only in those not responding to medication by mouth. Freon-containing nebulizers should not be used.

Cromolyn is a relatively new drug that is taken by inhalation. Unlike other inhaled drugs, it is not useful during an attack but can prevent future attacks. Cromolyn should be used only in patients with severe asthma who are requiring high dosages of oral medications. Many patients on corticosteroid drugs have been able to reduce steroid dosage by using Cromolyn. Cromolyn seems to work particularly well in patients sensitive to inhaled allergens and in patients who develop asthma after exercise.

Asthma is a complicated subject. If you or a family member is asthmatic, your physician will need to thoroughly discuss management of the illness with you. You cannot manage this problem entirely by yourself.

Allergen Avoidance

A relatively clean and dust-free house is healthy for all people but essential for the allergic. Rugs, furniture, drapes, bedspreads, and other items that are particular dust-catchers should be vacuumed regularly. An asthmatic's room should be particularly allergen-free, since sleeping requires that eight to ten hours be spent in the room. Except in very severe cases we do not recommend changing the entire household furnishings to reduce potential allergen exposure. Even then, removal of items should progress on a rational basis after suspected allergens have been identified. Patients and pets may do fine together, although it is best not to allow pets to sleep in an allergic patient's room. Toy animals should be kept clean; washable ones are the best. Avoid products that may be stuffed with animal hair. Finally, don't forget to change heating filters and air-conditioner filters regularly.

Infection Control

Since infections can trigger asthma, a physical examination is important during any first or frequently recurring attacks. Antibiotics should be not be given unless a definite infection is present.

Hydration Therapy

Water and other fluids taken by mouth are very important. Water can help loosen the mucus in the lungs and make breathing easier. Mist is not too helpful during asthmatic attacks because the affected airway passages are beyond the reach of the mist. Vaporizers are most useful for problems of the upper air passages of ears, nose, sinuses, mouth, and throat.

Supportive Therapy

Severe asthma is strenuous for the asthmatic and his or her family. Assistance is often required to manage the emotional consequences of asthma for the whole family. Do not hesitate to seek this assistance; social workers and other counselors can be invaluable.

Exercise and Asthma

Asthmatics can participate in athletics; five athletes with asthma recently have won gold medals in Olympic swimming. Swimming appears to be far and away the best exercise and best sport for the asthmatic. Exercise programs with long and steady energy requirements seem to work the best, and swimmers have the advantage of an environment that has very high humidity.

ALLERGIC RHINITIS (HAY FEVER)

Allergic rhinitis is the most common allergic problem. A stuffy, runny nose, watering itchy eyes, headache, and sneezing are all common. The cause in infants is often dust or food, and in adults, it is dust or pollens. Most individuals are troubled only in pollen season; ragweed is particularly troublesome. The problem seems to run in families.

Treatment is directed toward both symptomatic relief and avoidance of the offending allergen. The use of tissues or handkerchiefs for symptomatic relief is often not enough. Drugs that will reduce symptoms may be prescribed or purchased over the counter, but all have some side effects.

Antihistamines block the action of histamine, a substance released during allergic reactions. They also have a drying effect and improve nasal stuffiness. They also may be useful in reducing itching, helping motion sickness, or decreasing vomiting. The antihistamines used most often in allergic rhinitis are diphenhydramine (Benadryl), chlorpheniramine maleate (Chlor-Trimeton), tripelennamine (Pyribenzamine), and brompheniramine (Dimetane). These four drugs are from three different classes of antihistamine compounds. Individuals respond differently to different drugs and a trial of the different types of antihistamines may be necessary to determine the most effective type.

The most common side effect of antihistamines is drowsiness, and this may interfere with work or school. Antihistamines should not be used as sleeping pills because the drowsiness they produce *decreases* the amount of deep sleep, which is necessary for normal rest.

ATOPIC DERMATITIS (ECZEMA)

Atopic dermatitis, known commonly as eczema, is an allergic skin condition characterized by dry, itching skin. This itching often leads to scratching. The scratching then produces weeping, infected skin. Dried weepings lead to crusting. Sufficient scratching will produce a thickened, rough skin, which is characteristic of long-standing atopic dermatitis.

Atopic dermatitis runs in families with asthma and allergic rhinitis. Like asthma, a variety of conditions can aggravate it. These conditions include infection, emotional stress, food allergy, and sweating.

Infants seldom exhibit any signs of this problem at birth. The first signs may be red, chapped cheeks. Often infants can rub these itchy areas and cause secondary infections.

As the child grows older, the atopic dermatitis can spread. It may be found on the back of the legs and front of the arms. Adults often have problems with their hands; this is especially true of people whose hands are in frequent contact with water. Water tends to have a drying effect on the skin and tends to aggravate the dry skin-itch-scratch-weep-crust cycle.

Therapy is based upon avoidance of allergens and maintenance of good skin care.

• Avoid wool, which tends to aggravate itching.

• Avoid excessively warm clothing, which will cause sweat retention and aggravate itching.

• Keep a child's fingernails clipped short.

• Avoid bathing with soap and water, since these tend to dry the skin. Instead use non-lipid containing cleansers. Some cleansers with cetyl alcohol aid in preventing drying of the skin (Cetaphil lotion).

• Avoid all oil or grease preparations. They occlude the skin and increase sweat retention and itching.

• Avoiding cow's milk is often suggested particularly for children; make sure this really works for your child before permanently changing to more expensive feedings. When trying your child on any milk avoidance diet, make *no* other changes in food or other care for a full two weeks unless absolutely necessary.

• Itching is often worse at bedtime. Aspirin is an effective and inexpensive medication for reducing itching. Antihistamines also reduce itching but should be used only if necessary.

• Steroid creams are useful in severe cases. When possible, steroids should be used only for a short period of time. Prolonged use of steroids on the skin can produce numerous side effects.

• Antibiotics are sometimes necessary to clear up badly infected skin.

• Emotional factors may need attention; they may be the key to successful therapy.

• There has been no benefit demonstrated from either skin testing or hyposensitization.

ALLERGY TESTING AND HYPOSENSITIZATION

The purpose of allergy testing is to help decide what is causing the allergy; it is not a treatment, and as a test it is not always accurate. Once an allergy test is positive, there are two treatment approaches: avoidance and hyposensitization (desensitization).

Avoidance is sometimes, though not usually, possible. Seldom is a person allergic to cats and nothing else, and usually such an isolated allergy is noted by an alert patient or family. Avoiding dusts, pollens, trees, and flowers is next to impossible, so hyposensitization is sometimes reasonable if the problem is severe. Hyposensitization involves injecting a tiny amount of the offending allergen. Gradually larger and larger amounts are injected until the patient is able to tolerate exposure to the allergen with only mild symptoms.

Hyposensitization works in many cases, but there are many problems. Local reactions at the site of the injection are common but can be minimized by injecting through a different needle from the one used to withdraw the material from the bottle. Hyposensitization requires weekly injections for months or years. It may be considered for patients with moderate or severe asthma or severe hay fever but appears unwarranted, as does the preliminary skin testing, for patients with mild asthma or mild allergic rhinitis.

181

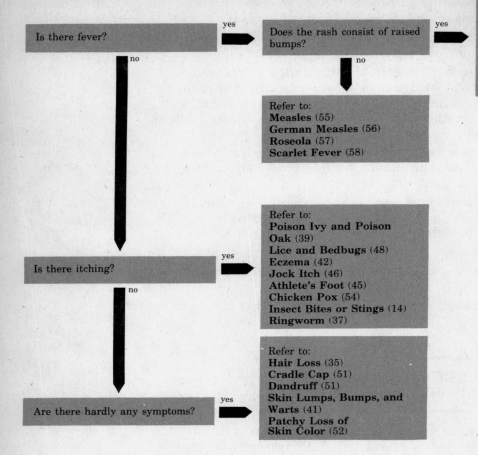

Is there fever? — yes → Does the rash consist of raised bumps? — yes → Refer to:
Chicken Pox (54)
Mouth Sores (31)
Impetigo (36)
Boils (43)
Insect Bites or Stings (14)
Hives (38)
If none of these,
suspect drug reaction.

Does the rash consist of raised bumps? — no → Refer to:
Measles (55)
German Measles (56)
Roseola (57)
Scarlet Fever (58)

Is there fever? — no

Is there itching? — yes → Refer to:
Poison Ivy and Poison Oak (39)
Lice and Bedbugs (48)
Eczema (42)
Jock Itch (46)
Athlete's Foot (45)
Chicken Pox (54)
Insect Bites or Stings (14)
Ringworm (37)

Is there itching? — no

Are there hardly any symptoms? — yes → Refer to:
Hair Loss (35)
Cradle Cap (51)
Dandruff (51)
Skin Lumps, Bumps, and Warts (41)
Patchy Loss of Skin Color (52)

H Common Skin Problems

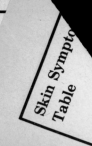

	Fever	Itching	Elevation
Baby rashes (33)	No	Sometimes	Slightly raised dots
Diaper rash (34)	No	No	Only if infected
Impetigo (36)	Sometimes	Occasionally	Crusts on sores
Ringworm (37)	No	Occasionally	Slightly raised rings
Hives (38)	No	Intense	Raised with flat tops
Poison ivy (39)	No	Intense	Blisters are elevated
Rashes caused by chemicals (40)	No	Moderate to intense	Sometimes blisters
Eczema (42)	No	Moderate to intense	Occasional blisters when infected
Acne (44)	No	No	Pimples, cysts
Athlete's foot (45)	No	Mild to intense	No
Dandruff and Cradle Cap (51)	No	Occasionally	Some crusting
Chicken pox (54)	Yes	Intense during pustular stage	Flat, then raised, then blisters, then crusts
Measles (55)	Yes	None to mild	Flat
German Measles (Rubella) (56)	Yes	No	Flat or slightly raised
Roseola (57)	Yes	No	Flat, occasionally with a few bumps

Color	Location	Duration of Problem	Other Symptoms
White or red dots; surrounding skin may be red	Trunk, neck, skin folds on arms and legs	Until controlled	
Red	Under diaper	Until controlled	
"Golden crusts on red sores"	Arms, legs, face first; then most of body	Until controlled	
Red	Anywhere, including scalp and nails	Until controlled	Flaking or scaling
Pale raised lesions surrounded by red	Anywhere	Minutes to days	
Red	Exposed areas	7 to 14 days	Oozing; some swelling
Red	Areas exposed to chemicals	Until exposure to chemical stopped	Some oozing and/or swelling
Red	Elbows, wrists, knees, cheeks	Until controlled	Moist; oozing
Red	Face, back, chest	Until controlled	Blackheads
Colorless to red	Between toes	Until controlled	Cracks; scaling; oozing blisters
White to yellow to red	Scalp, eyebrows, behind ears, groin	Until controlled	Fine, oily scales
Red	May start anywhere; most prominent on trunk and face	4 to 10 days	Lesions progress from flat to tiny blisters, then become crusted.
Pink; then red	First face; then chest and abdomen; then arms and legs	4 to 7 days	Preceded by fever, cough, red eyes.
Red	First face; then trunk; then extremities	2 to 4 days	Swollen glands behind ears. Occasional joint pains in older children and adults
Pink	First trunk; then arms and neck; very little on face and legs	1 to 2 days	High fever for three days which disappears with rash

Skin Symptom Table Cont.

	Fever	Itching	Elevation
Scarlet fever (58)	Yes	No	Flat; feels like sandpaper
Fifth disease (59)	No	No	Flat; lacy appearance

Skin problems must be approached somewhat differently from other medical problems. Decision charts that proceed from complaints such as "red bumps" can be developed, but the charts are complicated and somewhat unsatisfactory. This is because most people, including doctors, identify skin diseases by recognizing a particular pattern. This pattern is composed of not only what the skin problem looks like at a particular time but also how it began, where it spread, and whether it is associated with other symptoms such as itching or fever. Also important are elements of the medical history that may suggest an illness to which the patient has been exposed. Fortunately, many times you already have a good idea of the problem, and it is possible to proceed immediately with the question of whether this is poison ivy, ringworm, or something else.

If you are confused about what skin problem is present, we have provided two tables that will help you find a place to start. Each decision chart in this section begins with the question of whether the problem is compatible with the pattern for that skin disease. (Note that a more com-

Color	Location	Duration of Problem	Other Symptoms
Red	First face; then elbows; spreads rapidly to entire body in twenty-four hours.	5 to 7 days	Sore throat. Skin peeling afterwards, especially palms
Red	First face; then arms and legs; then rest of body	3 to 7 days	"Slapped-cheek" appearance. Rash comes and goes.

plete description of the pattern is given on the left-hand page.) If it is not, you are directed to reconsider the problem and consult the tables.

Most cases of a particular skin disease do not look exactly as a textbook says they should, so we have not provided you with pictures. We have tried to allow for a reasonable amount of variation in the descriptions, and often you will have to exercise your common sense. Don't be afraid to ask for other opinions; grandparents or others have seen a lot of skin problems over the years and know what the problems look like. We have listed some of the more common problems, but by no means all. If your problem doesn't seem to fit any of the descriptions use common sense as to whether the problem is serious, and call the doctor if it is.

Finally, because every case is at least a little bit different, even the best doctors will not be able to immediately identify all skin problems. Simple office laboratory methods can help sort out the possibilities. Fortunately, the vast majority of skin problems are minor, self-limited, and pose no major threat to health. Usually it is reasonable for you to wait quite some time to see if the problem goes away by itself.

33 Baby Rashes

The skin of the newborn child may exhibit a wide variety of bumps and blotches. Fortunately, almost all of these are harmless and clear up by themselves. The most common of these conditions are addressed in this section and only one, heat rash, requires any treatment. If the baby was delivered in a hospital, many of these conditions may occur before discharge so that advice will be readily available from nurses or physicians.

Heat rash is caused by blockage of the pores that lead to the sweat glands. It actually can occur at any age but is most common in the very young child in which the sweat glands are still developing. When heat and humidity rise, these glands attempt to provide sweat as they would normally, but because of the blockage, this sweat is held within the skin and forms little red bumps. It is also knowns as "prickly heat" or "miliaria."

On the other hand, the "little white bumps of milia" are composed of normal skin cells that have overaccumulated in some spots. As many as 40 percent of children have these bumps at birth. Eventually the bumps break open, the trapped material escapes, and the bumps disappear without requiring any treatment.

Erythema toxicum is an unnecessarily long and frightening term for the flat red splotches that appear in up to 50 percent of all babies. These seldom appear after five days of age and have usually disappeared by seven days. The children involved are perfectly normal, and whether or not any real toxin is involved is not clear.

Because the baby is exposed to the mother's adult hormones, a mild case of acne may develop, which may also occur when a child begins to produce adult hormones during adolescence. (The little white dots often seen on a newborn's nose represent an excess amount of normal skin oil, *sebaceous gland hyperplasia*, that has been produced by the hormones.) Acne usually becomes evident at between two and four weeks of age and clears up spontaneously within six months to a year. It virtually never requires treatment.

Home Treatment

Heat rash is effectively treated simply by providing a cooler and less humid environment. Powders carefully applied do no harm, but are unlikely to help. Ointments and creams should be avoided since they tend to keep the skin warmer and block the pores.

Acne should *not* be treated with the medicines used by adolescents and adults. Normal washing usually is all that is required.

None of these problems should be associated with fever and, with the exception of minor discomfort in heat rash, should be painless. If any question should arise about these conditions, a telephone call to the physician's office often will answer your questions.

What to Expect at the Doctor's Office

Discussion of these problems can usually wait until the regular scheduled well-baby visit. The physician can confirm your diagnosis at that time.

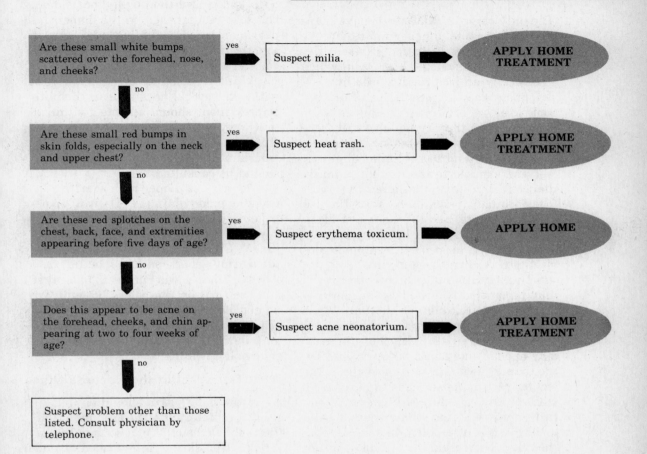

Are these small white bumps scattered over the forehead, nose, and cheeks? — **yes** → Suspect milia. → **APPLY HOME TREATMENT**

no ↓

Are these small red bumps in skin folds, especially on the neck and upper chest? — **yes** → Suspect heat rash. → **APPLY HOME TREATMENT**

no ↓

Are these red splotches on the chest, back, face, and extremities appearing before five days of age? — **yes** → Suspect erythema toxicum. → **APPLY HOME**

no ↓

Does this appear to be acne on the forehead, cheeks, and chin appearing at two to four weeks of age? — **yes** → Suspect acne neonatorium. → **APPLY HOME TREATMENT**

no ↓

Suspect problem other than those listed. Consult physician by telephone.

34 Diaper Rash

The only children who never have diaper rash are those who never wear diapers. An infant's skin is particularly sensitive and likely to develop diaper rash, which is basically an irritation caused by dampness and the interaction of urine and skin. An additional irritant is thought to be the ammonia in urine and often its odor is unmistakably present. Factors that tend to keep the baby's skin wet and exposed to the irritant promote diaper rash; commonly there are three: (1) continuously wet diapers, (2) the use of plastic pants, and (3) the use of disposable diapers, which have a plastic cover. For the most part, treatment consists of reversing these factors.

The irritation of simple diaper rash may become complicated by an infection due to yeast (candida) or bacteria. When yeast is the culprit, small red spots may be seen. Also, small patches of the rash may appear outside the area covered by the diaper, as far away as the chest. Infection with bacteria leads to development of large fluid-filled blisters. If the rash is worse in the skin creases, a mild underlying skin problem known as seborrhea may be present. This skin condition is also responsible for cradle cap and dandruff.

Occasionally parents will notice blood or what appear to be blood spots when boys have diaper rash. This is due to a similar rash at the urinary opening at the end of the penis. This problem will clear up as the diaper rash clears up.

Home Treatment

Treatment of diaper rash is aimed at keeping the skin dry and exposed to air. As implied above, the first things to do are to change the diapers frequently and to discontinue the use of plastic pants or disposable diapers with a heavy plastic coating. Leaving the diapers off altogether for as long as possible will also help. Diapers should be washed in a mild soap and rinsed thoroughly; occasionally the soap residues left in the diapers will act as an irritant. Adding a half cup of vinegar to the last rinse cycle may help counter the irritating ammonia.

While complete clearing of the rash will take several days at least, definite improvement should be noted within the first forty-eight to seventy-two hours. If this is not the case or if the rash is extraordinarily severe, the physician should be consulted.

To prevent diaper rash some parents use zinc oxide ointment (Desitin) or petroleum jelly (Vaseline). Others use baby powders (**caution**: talc dust can injure lungs). Caldesene powder is helpful in preventing seborrhea and monilial rashes. Always place powder in your hand first and then pat on the baby's bottom. We do not feel that all babies need the use of powders and creams. If a rash has begun, ointments should *not* be used, since they delay healing.

What to Expect at the Doctor's Office

All of the baby's skin should be inspected to determine the true extent of the rash. Occasionally, a scraping from the involved skin will be looked at under the microscope. If a yeast (monilial) infection has complicated the simple diaper rash, the doctor will prescribe home treatment plus the use of a medication to kill the yeast (Nystatin cream and occasionally oral Nystatin). If a bacterial infection has occurred, then an antibiotic to be taken by mouth will be recommended. If the rash is very severe or seborrhea is suspected, then a steroid cream (usually stronger than 0.5% hydrocortisone) may be advised. In any case, home therapy may be begun safely before seeing the doctor.

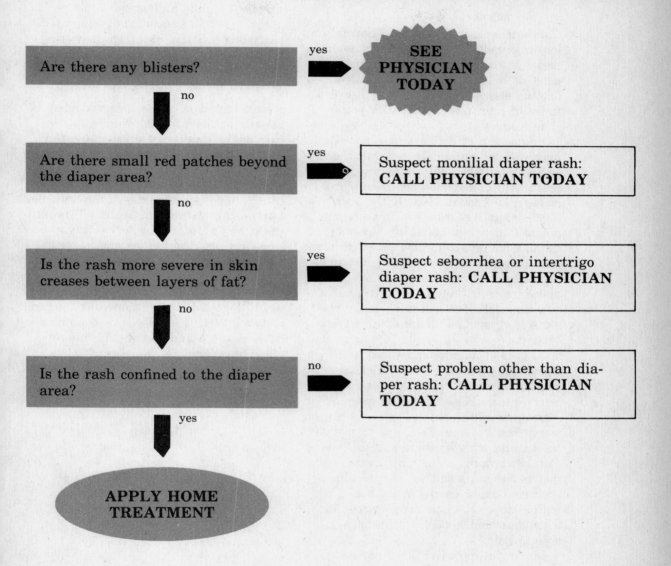

Are there any blisters? — yes → **SEE PHYSICIAN TODAY**

no ↓

Are there small red patches beyond the diaper area? — yes → Suspect monilial diaper rash: **CALL PHYSICIAN TODAY**

no ↓

Is the rash more severe in skin creases between layers of fat? — yes → Suspect seborrhea or intertrigo diaper rash: **CALL PHYSICIAN TODAY**

no ↓

Is the rash confined to the diaper area? — no → Suspect problem other than diaper rash: **CALL PHYSICIAN TODAY**

yes ↓

APPLY HOME TREATMENT

35 Hair Loss

This section is not about the normal hair loss that most men and many women experience as they get older. We have no cure for baldness, and we don't think anyone else does. But there are several kinds of hair loss about which you should know.

Sometimes all the hair in one small area will be completely lost, but the scalp underneath will be normal. This problem is called *alopecia areata*, and its cause is unknown. Usually the hair will be completely regrown within twelve months, although about 40 percent of patients will have a similar loss within the next four to five years. This problem resolves by itself. Cortisone creams will make the hair grow back faster, but the new hair falls out again when the treatment is stopped, so these creams are of little use.

Types of hair loss that may need treatment by a physician are characterized by abnormalities in the scalp skin or the hairs themselves. The most frequent problem in this category is ringworm (see Problem 37). Ringworm may be red and scaly or there may be pustules with oozing. The ringworm fungus infects the hairs so they become thickened and break easily. Whenever the scalp skin or the hairs themselves appear abnormal, the physician may be able to help.

Hair pulling by children, or occasionally a friend, often is responsible for hair loss. Tight braids or ponytails may also cause some hair loss. If a child constantly pulls out his or her hair, you should consider this unusual behavior and discuss it with a physician.

Home Treatment

In this instance, home treatment is reserved for presumed alopecia areata and consists of watchful waiting. The skin in the involved area must be completely normal to make a diagnosis of alopecia areata. If the appearance of scalp or hairs becomes abnormal, the physician should be consulted.

What to Expect at the Doctor's Office

An examination of the hair and scalp is usually sufficient to determine the nature of the problem. Occasionally, the hairs themselves may be examined under the microscope. Certain types of ringworm of the scalp can be identified because they fluoresce under an ultraviolet lamp. Ringworm of the scalp will require the use of an oral drug, griseofulvin, because creams and lotions applied to the affected area will not penetrate into the hair follicles to kill the fungus. We hope that no physician would recommend the use of X-rays today as some did a decade or two ago. If it is offered, it should be flatly rejected and you should find another physician.

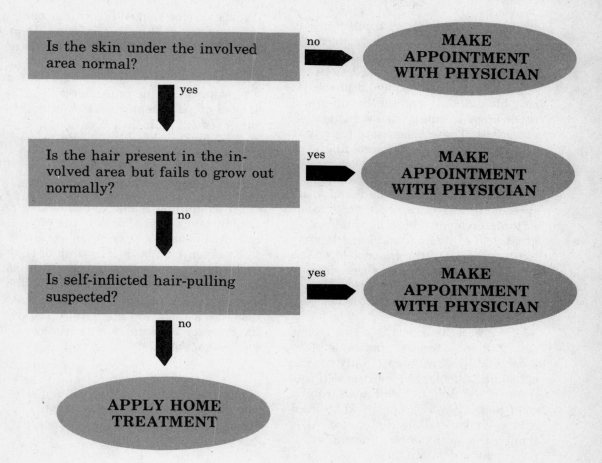

Is the skin under the involved area normal?

no → MAKE APPOINTMENT WITH PHYSICIAN

yes ↓

Is the hair present in the involved area but fails to grow out normally?

yes → MAKE APPOINTMENT WITH PHYSICIAN

no ↓

Is self-inflicted hair-pulling suspected?

yes → MAKE APPOINTMENT WITH PHYSICIAN

no ↓

APPLY HOME TREATMENT

36 Impetigo

Impetigo is particularly troublesome in the summer, especially in warm, moist climates. It can be recognized by the characteristic appearance of lesions that begin as small red spots and progress to tiny blisters that eventually rupture, producing an oozing, sticky, honey-colored crust. These lesions are usually spread very quickly by scratching.

Impetigo is a skin infection caused by streptococcal bacteria; occasionally other bacteria may also be found. If it spreads, impetigo, can be a very uncomfortable problem. There is usually a great deal of itching, and scratching hastens spreading of the lesions. After the sores heal, there may be slight decrease in skin color at the site. Skin color usually returns to normal, so this need not concern you.

Of greatest concern is a rare, complicating, kidney problem known as *glomerulonephritis*, which occasionally occurs in epidemics. Glomerulonephritis will cause the urine to turn a dark brown (cola) color and is often accompanied by headache and elevated blood pressure. Although this problem has a formidible name, the kidney problem is short-lived and heals completely in most people.

Unfortunately, antibiotics will not prevent glomerulonephritis but may help prevent the impetigo from spreading to other people, thus protecting them from both impetigo and glomerulonephritis. They are effective in healing the impetigo.

Although there is some debate on this matter, many physicians believe that if only one or two lesions are present and the lesions are not progressing, home treatment may be used for impetigo. The exception to this rule is if an epidemic of glomerulonephritis is occurring within your community.

Home Treatment

Crusts may be soaked off with either warm water or Burrow's Solution (Domeboro, Bluboro). Antibiotic ointments are no more effective than soap and water. The lesions should be scrubbed with soap and water after the crusts have been soaked off. If lesions do not show prompt improvement or if they seem to be spreading, the physician should be seen without delay.

What to Expect at the Doctor's Office

After examining the sores and taking an appropriate medical history, the physician will usually prescribe an antibiotic to be taken by mouth. The drug of choice is penicillin unless there is penicillin allergy, in which case erythromycin will usually be prescribed. Some physicians may check the blood pressure or the urine in order to examine for early signs of glomerulonephritis.

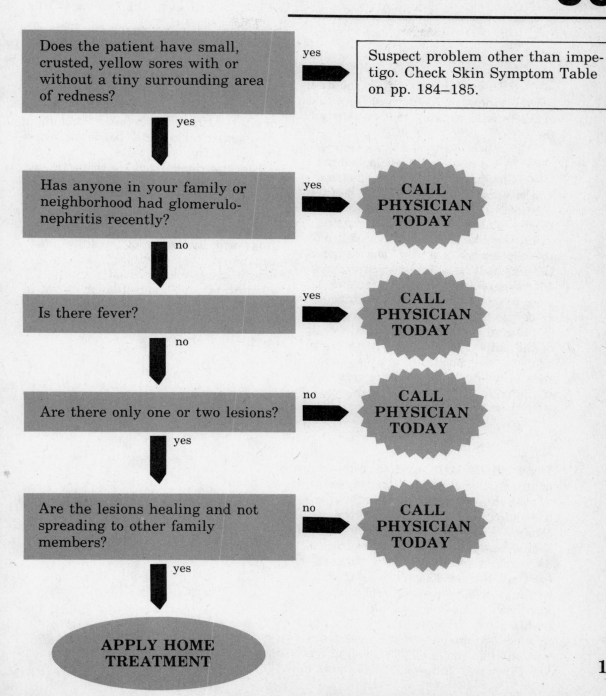

Does the patient have small, crusted, yellow sores with or without a tiny surrounding area of redness? — yes → Suspect problem other than impetigo. Check Skin Symptom Table on pp. 184–185.

yes ↓

Has anyone in your family or neighborhood had glomerulonephritis recently? — yes → **CALL PHYSICIAN TODAY**

no ↓

Is there fever? — yes → **CALL PHYSICIAN TODAY**

no ↓

Are there only one or two lesions? — no → **CALL PHYSICIAN TODAY**

yes ↓

Are the lesions healing and not spreading to other family members? — no → **CALL PHYSICIAN TODAY**

yes ↓

APPLY HOME TREATMENT

195

37 Ringworm

Ringworm is a shallow fungus infection of the skin. Worms have nothing whatsoever to do with this condition; the designation "ringworm" is derived from the characteristic red ring that appears on the skin.

Ringworm can generally be recognized by its pattern of development. The lesions begin as small, round, red spots and get progressively larger. When they are about the size of a pea, the center begins to clear. When the lesions are about the size of a dime, they will have the appearance of a ring. The border of the ring will be red, elevated, and scaly. Often there are groups of infections so close to one another that it is difficult to recognize them as individual rings.

Ringworm may also affect the scalp or the nails. The infections are more difficult to treat but fortunately are not seen very often. Epidemics of ringworm of the scalp were common many years ago.

Home Treatment

Tolnaftate (tinactin) applied to the skin is an effective treatment for ringworm. It is available in cream, solution, and powder and can be purchased over the counter. Either the cream or the solution should be applied two or three times a day. Only a small amount is required for each application. Resolution of the problem may require several weeks of therapy, but improvement should be noted within a week. Selsun Blue® shampoo, applied as a cream several times a day, will often do the job just as well and is less expensive. Ringworm that shows no improvement after a week of therapy or that continues to spread should be checked by a physician.

What to Expect at the Doctor's Office

The diagnosis of ringworm can be confirmed by scraping the scales, soaking them in a potassium hydroxide solution, and viewing them under the microscope. Some physicians may culture the scrapings. One of three agents usually will be present if tinactin has failed: haloprogin (Halotex), clotrimazole (Lotrimin), or miconazole (MicaTin).

In infections involving the scalp, an ultraviolet light (called a Wood's lamp) will cause affected hairs to become fluorescent. The Wood's lamp is used to make the diagnosis; it does not treat the ringworm. Ringworm of the scalp must be treated by griseofulvin, taken by mouth, usually for at least a month; this medication is also effective for fungal infections of the nails. Ringworm of the scalp should never be treated with X-rays.

Are all of the following conditions present?

(a) Rash begins as a small red, color-less, or depigmented circle that becomes progressively larger.

(b) The circular border is elevated and perhaps scaly.

(c) The center of the circle begins healing as the circle becomes larger.

no → Suspect problem other than ring-worm. Check Skin Symptom Table on pp. 184–185.

yes

Is the scalp infected?

yes → **MAKE APPOINTMENT WITH PHYSICIAN**

no

APPLY HOME TREATMENT

38 Hives

Hives are an allergic reaction. Unfortunately, the reaction can be to almost anything, including cold, heat, and even emotional tension. Unless you already have a good idea what is causing the hives or if a new drug has just been taken, the physician is unlikely to be able to determine the cause; most often, a search for a cause is fruitless. Here is a list of some of the things that are frequently mentioned as causes: drugs, eggs, milk, wheat, chocolate, pork, shellfish, freshwater fish, berries, cheese, nuts, pollens, and insect bites. The only sure way to know whether or not one of these is the culprit is to voluntarily expose the patient to it. The problem with this approach is that if an allergy does exist, the allergic reaction may include not only hives but a systemic reaction causing difficulty with breathing or circulation. As indicated by the decision chart, a systemic reaction is a potentially dangerous situation and the physician should be consulted immediately. Avoid exposure to a suspected cause to see if the attacks will cease. Such "tests" are difficult to interpret, since attacks of hives are often separated by long periods of time. Actually, most people have only one attack, lasting from a period of minutes to weeks.

You may want to read about allergies in Section G.

Home Treatment

Determine whether there has been any pattern to the appearance of the hives. Do they appear after meals? After exposure to the cold? During a particular season of the year? If there seem to be likely possibilities, eliminate these and see what happens. If the reactions seem to be related to foods, an alternative is available. Lamb and rice virtually never cause allergic reactions. The patient may be placed on a diet consisting only of lamb and rice until completely free of hives. Foods are then added back to the diet one at a time and the patient is observed for a development of hives.

Itching may be relieved by the application of cold compresses, the use of aspirin, or the use of antihistamines such as diphenhydramine (Benadryl) or chlorpheniramine (Chlortrimeton) (see Chapter 9, "The Home Pharmacy").

What to Expect at the Doctor's Office

If the patient is suffering a systemic reaction with difficulty breathing or dizziness, injections of adrenalin and other drugs may be given. In the more usual case of hives alone, the physician may do two things. First, the doctor can prescribe an antihistamine or use adrenalin injections to relieve swelling and itching. Second, the doctor can review the history of the reaction to try to find an offending agent and advise you as above. Remember that most often the cause of hives goes undetected, and usually they stop occurring after a while.

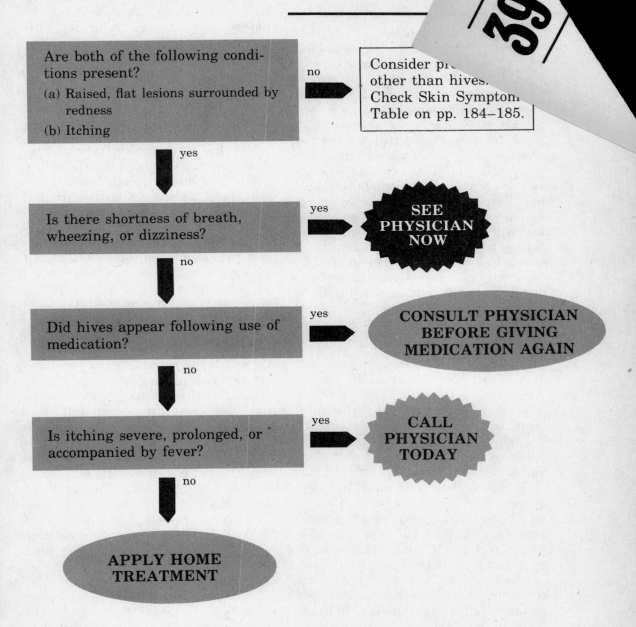

Are both of the following conditions present?

(a) Raised, flat lesions surrounded by redness

(b) Itching

no → Consider pr[...] other than hives[...] Check Skin Sympton[...] Table on pp. 184–185.

yes ↓

Is there shortness of breath, wheezing, or dizziness?

yes → **SEE PHYSICIAN NOW**

no ↓

Did hives appear following use of medication?

yes → **CONSULT PHYSICIAN BEFORE GIVING MEDICATION AGAIN**

no ↓

Is itching severe, prolonged, or accompanied by fever?

yes → **CALL PHYSICIAN TODAY**

no ↓

APPLY HOME TREATMENT

199

Poison Ivy and Poison Oak

Poison ivy and poison oak need little introduction. The itching skin lesions that follow contact with these and other plants of the *Rhus* plant family are the most common example of a larger category of skin problems known as *contact dermatitis*. Contact dermatitis simply means that something that has been applied to the skin has caused the skin to react to it. An initial exposure is necessary to "sensitize" the patient; a subsequent exposure will result in an allergic reaction if the plant oil remains in contact with skin for several hours. The resulting rash begins after a delay of twelve to forty-eight hours and persists for about two weeks. Contact may be indirect, from pets, contaminated clothing, or the smoke from burning *Rhus* plants. It can occur during any season.

Home Treatment

The best approach is to teach your children to recognize and avoid the plants, which are hazardous even in the winter when they have dropped their leaves. Next best is to remove the plant oil from the skin as soon as possible. If the oil has been on the skin for less than six hours, thorough cleansing with ordinary soap, repeated three times, will often prevent reaction. Alcohol-base cleansing tissues, available much more in prepackaged form (such as Alco-wipe) are effective in removing the oil. Rubbing alcohol on a washcloth is even better.

To relieve itching, many physicians recommend cool compresses of Burrow's solution (Domeboro, BurVeen, Bluboro) or baths with Aveeno or oatmeal (one cup to a tub full of water). Aspirin is also effective in reducing itching. The old standby, calamine lotion, is sometimes of help in early lesions but may spread the plant oil. (**Caution**: *Do not use Caladryl or Zyradryl. They cause allergic reactions in some people. Use only calamine lotion.*) Be sure to cleanse the skin, as above, even if you are too late to prevent the rash entirely. Another useful method of obtaining symptomatic relief is the use of a hot bath or hot shower. Heat releases histamine, the substance in the cells of the skin that causes the intense itching. Therefore, a hot shower or bath will cause intense itching as the histamine is released. The heat should be gradually increased to the maximum tolerable and continued until the itching has subsided. This process will deplete the cells of histamine and the patient will obtain up to eight hours of relief from the itching. This method has the advantage of not requiring frequent applications of ointments to the lesions and is a good way to get some sleep at night. Poison ivy and poison oak will persist for the same length of time despite any medication. If secondary bacterial infection occurs, healing will be delayed; hence scratching is not helpful. Cut the nails to avoid damage to the skin through scratching.

One-half percent hydrocortisone creams (Cortaid, Lanacort, etc.) are available without prescription. It will decrease inflammation and itching, but relief is not immediate and the cream must be applied often (four to six times a day). Do not use this cream for prolonged periods (see Chapter 9, "The Home Pharmacy").

Recently there has been enthusiasm (even among some doctors) for rubbing crushed plantain leaves on poison ivy rash. Quick relief of itching is reported; however, we know of no scientific studies of this treatment. Like so many home remedies, it seems to be low cost and to have few bad effects, but whether it really helps is unknown.

Poison ivy is not contagious; it cannot be spread once the oil has been absorbed by the skin or removed.

Are all of the following conditions present?

a) Itching
b) Redness, minor swelling, blisters, or oozing
c) Probably exposure to poison ivy, poison oak, or poison sumac

→ Suspect problem other than poison ivy or poison oak. Check the skin symptom table on pp. 184-185.

APPLY HOME TREATMENT

If the lesions are too extensive to be easily treated, if home treatment is ineffective, or if the itching is too severe that it can't be tolerated, a call to the physician may be necessary.

What to Expect at the Doctor's Office

After a history and physical examination, the physician may prescribe a steroid cream stronger than 0.5% hydrocortisone to be applied four to six times a day to the lesions. This is often of only moderate help. Another alternative is to give a steroid (such as prednisone) by mouth for short periods of time. A rather large dose is given the first day and the dose is then gradually reduced. We do not recommend oral steroids except when there have been previous severe reactions to poison ivy or poison oak, or extensive exposure. The itching may be treated symptomatically with either an antihistamine (Benadryl, Vistaril, etc.) or aspirin. The antihistamines may cause drowziness and interfere with sleep.

201

40 Rashes Caused by Chemicals — Contact Dermatitis

Chemicals may cause a rash (contact dermatitis) in two ways. The chemical may have a direct caustic effect that irritates the skin—a minor "chemical burn." More often the rash is due to an allergic reaction of the skin to the chemical. The most common allergic dermatitis is poison ivy; it is caused by an allergic reaction to chemicals in the leaves and stems of plants belonging to the Rhus family. If you see a rash that looks like poison ivy (Problem 39), but contact with poison ivy or poison oak seems impossible, consider other chemicals that can cause an allergic contact dermatitis and produce an identical rash.

The chemicals most frequently found to be causes of contact dermatitis are dyes and other chemicals found in clothing, chemicals used in elastic and rubber products, cosmetics, and deodorants including "feminine" deodorants.

Usually the tipoff to the cause of the rash is its location and shape. Sometimes this is very striking as the rash leaves a perfect outline of a bra or the elastic bands of underwear or some other article of clothing. More often the rash is not so distinct, but its location suggests the possible cause. The table on the opposite page suggests the possible source of offending chemicals according to the location of the rash on the body.

Home Treatment

If you have had difficulty with particular types of clothing, cosmetics, deodorants, etc., then avoiding contact is the best way to avoid a problem, of course.

Changing brands may also help. For example, some cosmetics are manufactured so as to have less chance of causing an allergic reaction ("hypoallergenic"). Rashes caused by deodorants are often of the direct caustic type so that using a milder preparation less often may solve the problem.

Once the rash has occurred, eliminating contact with the chemical is essential. Washing thoroughly with soap and water may remove chemicals on the skin and is especially important with materials such as cement dust. Oily substances may best be removed with rubbing alcohol, or by paint thinner quickly followed by soap and water to prevent contact dermatitis from the cleaner itself.

The remainder of home treatment is identical to that of poison ivy (see Problem 39) and consists of the use of Burrow's solution, hot water and hydrocortisone cream to achieve relief from itching. If the lesions are too extensive to be easily treated, if home treatment is ineffective, or if the itching is so severe that it can't be tolerated, a call to the physician may be necessary.

What to Expect at the Doctor's Office

The physician will examine the rash; the history will focus on possible exposure to substances such as those listed in the table. A steroid cream stronger than 0.5% hydrocortisone may be prescribed. Another alternative is to give a steroid (such as prednisone) for a short period of time; a rather large dose is given the first day and the dose is then gradually reduced. Itching may be treated symptomatically with either an antihistamine (Benadryl, Vistaryl) or aspirin. Antihistamines may cause drowsiness or interfere with sleep. Prevention is better.

202

Is this a red rash (sometimes with bumps or blisters and usually itchy or burning) that by its shape and location suggests contact with articles of clothing, cosmetics, deodorant or other chemicals?

no

Suspect problem other than contact dermatitis. Check Skin Symptom Table on pp. 184–185.

yes

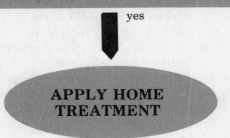

APPLY HOME TREATMENT

41 Skin Lumps, Bumps, and Warts

Lumps and bumps on the skin cause a great deal of unnecessary concern. Usually the worry is cancer. Only rarely is the problem serious, and treatment is seldom required. The lump may be above the skin, as in the case of warts and moles, within the skin as with boils and certain kinds of moles, or under the skin as in the case of small collections of fat called lipomas. If there is only one lump, and it is hot, red, swollen, and tender (inflamed), it should be considered a boil until proven otherwise (see **Boils**, Problem 43). A dark mole that appears to be enlarging or changing color might be melanoma, a kind of skin cancer. However, few skin lesions that appear to be enlarging and changing color are cancer. All moles must start small and grow larger, and the removal of all moles is impossible as well as undesirable. Unfortunately, there is no easy solution to this dilemma because there is no certain way for a patient to identify a melanoma without the aid of a physician.

The more common skin cancers are found in people of middle and older ages in sun-exposed areas of the skin. Usually skin cancer is not serious, but it may occasionally spread to other parts of the body. These cancers appear as nonhealing sores and should be shown to a physician. A more common recurrent problem in the same location and in the same age range is *actinic keratosis*, which is an irregular, brownish, raised, scaly lesion. Actinic keratosis is not cancerous, but on occasion, it will become malignant. Thus some physicians advocate observing these lesions for change or bleeding, while others recommend removal.

The most commonly found lumps in children are swollen lymph glands. These are discussed in more detail in (**Swollen Glands,** Problem 28).

Warts are caused by viral infections and often spontaneously resolve by themselves. However, warts can occasionally be troublesome, especially if they are on the fingers where they may interfere with writing, or on the face where they are cosmetically disturbing.

Home Treatment

Treatment of many lumps and bumps is discussed under **Insect Bites or Stings** (Problem 14). **Boils** (Problem 43), and **Swollen Glands** (Problem 28). Warts can be removed with over-the-counter medicines when used consistently and carefully. Available preparations include salicylic acid plasters, Compound W, and Vergo. On your next visit to the doctor you can ask about any skin lumps or warts that are of concern to you; these are seldom worth a special trip. However, if the problem has persisted for more than a month and you are not sure what it is, a visit may be helpful.

What to Expect at the Doctor's Office

The physician may be able to make the diagnosis simply by inspecting the wart or lump and obtaining a history. If a major question of diagnosis remains, a "punch" biopsy may be taken. This type of biopsy removes a portion of the bump for examination under the microscope. Alternatively, the entire lump may be removed. This approach may be desirable for cosmetic reasons or because of a potentially serious skin problem.

In treating warts, a prescription liquid such as Duo-Film, consisting of lactic and salicylic acid, may be tried. A wart

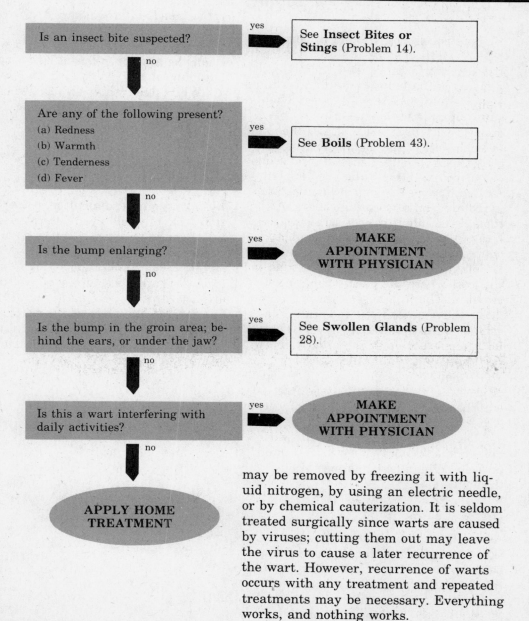

Is an insect bite suspected? — yes → See **Insect Bites or Stings** (Problem 14).

no ↓

Are any of the following present?
(a) Redness
(b) Warmth
(c) Tenderness
(d) Fever

— yes → See **Boils** (Problem 43).

no ↓

Is the bump enlarging? — yes → MAKE APPOINTMENT WITH PHYSICIAN

no ↓

Is the bump in the groin area; behind the ears, or under the jaw? — yes → See **Swollen Glands** (Problem 28).

no ↓

Is this a wart interfering with daily activities? — yes → MAKE APPOINTMENT WITH PHYSICIAN

no ↓

APPLY HOME TREATMENT

may be removed by freezing it with liquid nitrogen, by using an electric needle, or by chemical cauterization. It is seldom treated surgically since warts are caused by viruses; cutting them out may leave the virus to cause a later recurrence of the wart. However, recurrence of warts occurs with any treatment and repeated treatments may be necessary. Everything works, and nothing works.

42 Eczema (Atopic Dermatitis)

Eczema is commonly found in people with a family history of either eczema, hay fever, or asthma. The underlying problem is the inability of the skin to retain adequate amounts of water. The skin of people with eczema is consequently very dry, which causes the skin to itch. Most of the manifestations of eczema are a consequence of scratching.

In young infants who are unable to scratch, the most common manifestation is red, dry, mildly scaling cheeks. Although the infant cannot scratch his or her cheeks, the cheeks can be rubbed against the sheets and thus become red. In infants, eczema may also be found in the area where the plastic pants meet the skin. The tightness of the elastic produces the characteristic red scaling lesion. In older children, it is very common for eczema to involve the area behind the knees and behind the elbows.

If there is a large amount of weeping or crusting, the eczema may be infected with bacteria, and a call to the physician will most likely be required.

The course of eczema is quite variable. Some will only have a brief, mild problem; others have manifestations throughout life.

Home Treatment

Attempts must be made to prevent the skin from becoming too dry, and frequent bathings make the skin even dryer. Although the person will feel comfortable in the bath, itching will become more intense after the bath because of the drying effect.

Sweating aggravates eczema. Avoid overdressing. Light night clothing is important. Contact with wool and silk seems to aggravate eczema and should be avoided.

Nails should be kept trimmed short to minimize the effects of scratching. Rubber gloves can help prevent dryness of the hands after washing dishes or the car.

Washing is best accomplished with a cleansing and moisturizing agent such as Cetaphil lotion.

While fresh water or pool swimming can aggravate eczema by causing loss of skin moisture, ocean swimming does not do so and can be freely undertaken. (Also see Section G, Allergies.)

What to Expect at the Doctor's Office

By history and examination of the lesions, the physician can determine whether the problem is eczema. If home treatment has not improved the problem, steroid creams and lotions may be prescribed. While these are effective, they are not curative; eczema is characterized by repeated occurrences. If crusted or weeping lesions are present, bacterial infection is likely and an oral antibiotic will be prescribed.

Are the following conditions present (at least two of three)?

(a) Itching

(b) Flat red areas on cheeks, behind ears, on wrists, behind knees, or in front of elbows

(c) Family history of allergy

no → Suspect problem other than eczema. Check Skin Symptom Table on pp. 184–185.

yes ↓

Is there any crusting of lesions?

yes → **CALL PHYSICIAN TODAY**

no ↓

APPLY HOME TREATMENT

43 Boils

"Painful as a boil" is a familiar term and emphasizes the severe discomfort that can arise from this common skin problem. A boil is a localized infection usually due to the staphylococcus bacteria; often a particularly savage strain of the bacteria is responsible. When this particular germ inhabits the skin, recurrent problems with boils may persist for months or years. Often several family members will be affected at about the same time. Boils may be single or multiple, and they may occur anywhere on the body. They range from the size of a pea to the size of a walnut or larger. The surrounding red, thickened, and tender tissue increases the problem even further. The infection begins in the tissues beneath the skin and develops into an abscess pocket filled with pus. Eventually, the pus pocket "points" toward the skin surface and finally ruptures and drains. Then it heals. Boils often begin as infections around hair follicles, hence the term *folliculitis* for minor infections. Areas under pressure (such as the buttocks) are often likely spots for boils to begin. A boil that extends into the deeper layers of the skin is called a carbuncle.

Special consideration should be given to boils on the face, since they are more likely to lead to serious complicating infections.

Home Treatment

Boils are handled gently, because rough treatment can force the infection deeper inside the body. Warm, moist soaks are applied gently several times each day to speed the development of the pocket of pus and to soften the skin for the eventual rupture and drainage. Once drainage begins, the soaks will help keep the opening in the skin clear. The more drainage, the better. Frequent thorough soaping of the entire skin helps prevent reinfection. Ignore all temptation to squeeze the boil.

What to Expect at the Doctor's Office

If there is fever or a facial boil, the doctor will usually prescribe an antibiotic. Otherwise, antibiotics may not be used; they are of limited help in abscesslike infections. If the boil feels as though fluid is contained in a pocket but has not yet drained, the physician may lance the boil. In this procedure, a small incision is made to allow the pus to drain. After drainage the pain is reduced and healing is quite prompt. While "incision and drainage" is not a complicated procedure, it is tricky enough that you should not attempt it yourself.

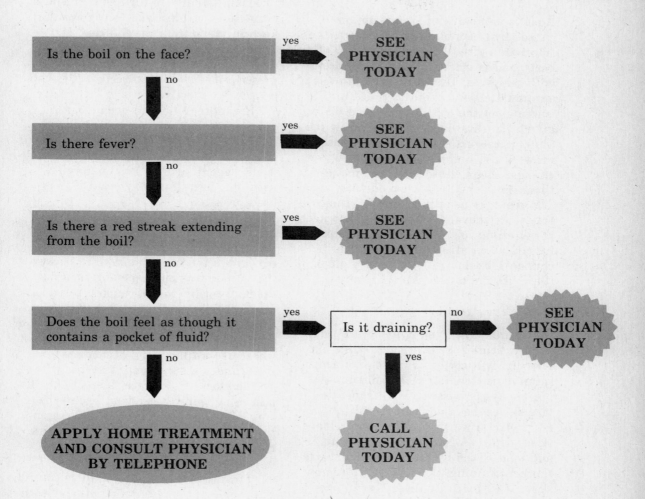

Is the boil on the face? — yes → SEE PHYSICIAN TODAY

no ↓

Is there fever? — yes → SEE PHYSICIAN TODAY

no ↓

Is there a red streak extending from the boil? — yes → SEE PHYSICIAN TODAY

no ↓

Does the boil feel as though it contains a pocket of fluid? — yes → Is it draining? — no → SEE PHYSICIAN TODAY

no ↓

APPLY HOME TREATMENT AND CONSULT PHYSICIAN BY TELEPHONE

Is it draining? — yes ↓ CALL PHYSICIAN TODAY

44 Acne

Acne is a superficial skin eruption caused by a combination of factors. It is triggered by the hormonal changes of puberty and is most common in children with oily skin. The increased skin oils accumulate below keratin plugs in the openings of the hair follicles and oil glands. In this stagnant area below the plug, secretions accumulate and bacteria grow. These normal bacteria cause changes in the secretions that make them irritating to the surrounding skin. The result is usually a pimple but sometimes may develop into a larger pocket of secretions, or cyst. Blackheads are formed when air causes a chemical change—"oxidation"—of keratin plugs; the irritation of the skin is minimal.

Home Treatment

Cleanliness and good hygiene are important principles for everyone. While excessive dirt will certainly aggravate acne, scrupulous cleaning will unfortunately not always prevent it. With acne, the face should be scrubbed several times daily with a warm washcloth to remove skin oils and keratin plugs. The rubbing and heat of the washcloth help dislodge the keratin plug. Soap will help remove skin oil and will decrease the number of bacteria living on the skin. If there are pimples on the back, a backbrush or washcloth should be used there. Greases and creams on the skin may aggravate the problem. The various patent medicines available over the counter appear to help some people; they are disappointing to others. Diet is not an important factor in most cases, but if certain foods tend to aggravate the problem, avoid them. There is scant evidence that chocolate aggravates acne, despite popular belief.

Several further steps may be taken at home. An abrasive soap, such as Pernox or Brasivol, may be used from one to three times daily to further reduce the oiliness of the skin and to remove the keratin plugs from the follicles.

Medications containing benzoyl peroxide are now widely available without prescription. Used as directed, these appear to be effective.

Steam may help to open clogged pores. Hot compresses are sometimes helpful. Some dermatologists recommend Vlem-Dome as a hot drying compress. A drying agent such as Fostex may be used, but irritation may occur if it is used too often.

Finally, natural sunlight or a sunlamp is effective if used conscientiously. We prefer natural sunlight and do not encourage the use of sunlamps. However, if a sunlamp is used, place it at a distance of twelve inches, expose three sides of the face in succession (left, center, right), wear goggles or place damp cotton over the eyes, treat two or three times a week, use a timer, and do not read or sleep under a sunlamp. Start at thirty seconds for each surface. Increase the exposure by thirty seconds at each exposure. Should a mild burn occur, discontinue for one week. Restart at one-half the previous time. Do not exceed ten minutes under the sunlamp.

Should these measures fail to control the problem, make an appointment with the physician.

What to Expect at the Doctor's Office

The physician will advise about hygiene and the use of medications. Several new topical preparations such as retinoic acid (Retin-A) and benzoyl peroxide have been found helpful; they act by fostering skin peeling, which prevents plugging of

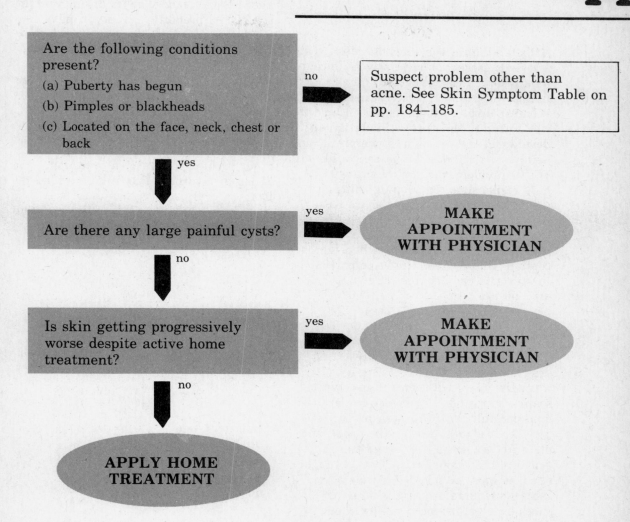

Are the following conditions present?
(a) Puberty has begun
(b) Pimples or blackheads
(c) Located on the face, neck, chest or back

no → Suspect problem other than acne. See Skin Symptom Table on pp. 184–185.

yes ↓

Are there any large painful cysts? — yes → **MAKE APPOINTMENT WITH PHYSICIAN**

no ↓

Is skin getting progressively worse despite active home treatment? — yes → **MAKE APPOINTMENT WITH PHYSICIAN**

no ↓

APPLY HOME TREATMENT

the hair follicles. This peeling is not noticeable if the medication is used properly.

In resistant cases an antibiotic (tetracycline or occasionally erythromycin) may be prescribed to be taken by mouth. Some physicians prescribe these antibiotics for application to the skin as well.

"Acne surgery" is a term generally applied to the physician's removal of blackheads with a suction device and an eyedropper. Large developing cysts are sometimes arrested with injection of steroids. Such procedures should be required only in severe cases and are more usually performed on the back than on the face.

45 Athlete's Foot

Athlete's foot is very common during and after adolescence, and relatively uncommon before. It is the most common of the fungal infections and is often persistent. When it involves toenails, it can be difficult to treat. Moisture is important in developing the problem. Some physicians believe bacteria and moisture cause most of this problem and that the fungus is only responsible for keeping things going. When many people share locker room and shower facilities, exposure to this fungus is impossible to prevent; and infection is the rule, rather than the exception. But you don't have to participate in sports to contact this fungus; it's all around.

Home Treatment

Scrupulous hygiene, without resorting to drugs, is often effective. *Twice a day* wash the space between the toes with soap, water, and a cloth; dry the entire area carefully with a towel, particularly between the toes (despite the pain); and put on clean socks. Use shoes that allow evaporation of moisture. Plastic linings of shoes must be avoided. Sandals or canvas sneakers are best. Changing shoes every other day to allow them to dry out is a good idea. Keeping the feet dry with the use of a powder is helpful in preventing reinfection. In difficult cases, over-the-counter drugs such as Desenex powder or cream may be used. The powder has the virtue of helping keep the toes dry. If these are not effective, a more expensive over-the-counter medication, tolnaftate (Tinactin), is available in either cream or lotion. Tin-

actin powder is better as a preventive preparation rather than a curative one. Recently, the twice-daily application of a 30% aluminum chloride solution has been recommended for its drying and antibacterial properties. You will have to ask your pharmacist to make up the solution, but it is inexpensive.

What to Expect at the Doctor's Office

Through history and physical examination, and possibly microscopic examination of a skin scraping, the physician will establish the diagnosis. Several other problems, notably a condition called dyshydrosis, may mimic athlete's foot. An oral drug, griseofulvin, may be used for fungal infections of the nails but is not recommended for athlete's foot.

Are both of the following conditions present?

(a) Redness and scaling between toes (may have cracks and small blisters)

(b) Itching

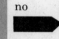 no → Suspect problem other than athlete's foot. Check Skin Symptom Table on pp. 184–185.

yes

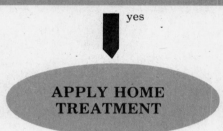

APPLY HOME TREATMENT

46 Jock Itch

We might wish for a less picturesque name for this condition, but *tinea cruris* is a term understood by relatively few. "Jock itch" is a fungus infection of the pubic region. It is aggravated by friction and moisture. It usually does not involve the scrotum or penis, nor does it spread beyond the groin area. For the most part, this is a male disease. Frequently the fungus grows in an athletic supporter turned old and moldy in a locker room far from a washing machine. The preventive measure for such a problem is obvious.

Home Treatment

The problem should be treated by removing the contributing factors—friction and moisture. This is done by wearing boxer-type shorts rather than closer-fitting shorts, by applying a powder to dry the area after bathing, and by frequently changing soiled or sweaty underclothes. It may take up to two weeks to completely clear this problem, and it may recur. The "powder-and-clean-shorts" treatment will usually be successful without any medication. Tolnaftate (Tinactin) will eliminate the fungus if the problem persists.

What to Expect at the Doctor's Office

Occasionally a yeast infection will mimic jock itch. By examination and history, the physician will attempt to establish the diagnosis and may also make a scraping in order to identify a yeast. Medicines for this problem are virtually always applied to the affected skin; oral drugs or injections are rarely used. Halo- prigin (Halotex) and Clotrimazole (Lotrimin) are prescription creams and lotions that are effective against both fungi and certain yeast infections.

Are all of the following conditions present?

(a) Involves only the groin and thighs

(b) Redness, oozing, or some peripheral scaling

(c) Itching

no →

Suspect problem other than jock itch. Check Skin Symptom Table on pp. 184–185.

yes

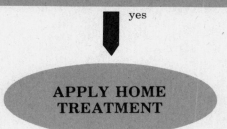

APPLY HOME TREATMENT

47 Sunburn

Sunburn is common, painful, and avoidable. Very rarely, persons with sunburn have difficulty with vision; if so, they should be seen by a physician. Otherwise, a visit to the doctor is unnecessary unless the pain is extraordinarily severe or extensive blistering (not peeling) has occurred. Blistering indicates a second-degree burn and rarely follows sun exposure. The pain of sunburn is worst between six and forty-eight hours after sun exposure. Peeling of injured layers of skin occurs later—between three and ten days after the burn.

Home Treatment

Cool compresses or cool baths with Aveeno (one cup to a tub full of water) may be useful. Ordinary baking soda (one-half cup to a tub) is nearly as effective. Lubricants such as Vaseline feel good to some people, but they retain heat and should not be used the first day. Avoid products that contain benzocaine. These may give temporary relief but can cause irritation of the skin and may actually prolong healing. Aspirin by mouth may ease pain and thus help sleep.

Sunburn is better prevented than treated. For protection, effective sunscreens are available. Protection is afforded by Block-out, Pabafilm, Pabonal, and Presun, among others.

What to Expect at the Doctor's Office

The physician will direct the history and physical examination toward determination of the extent of burn and the possibility of other heat-related injuries like sunstroke. If only first-degree burns are found, a prescription steroid lotion may be prescribed. This is not of particular benefit. The rare second-degree burns may be treated with antibiotics in addition to analgesics or sedation. There is no evidence that steroid lotions or antibiotic creams help at all in the *usual* case of sunburn; most physicians prescribe the same therapy that is available at home.

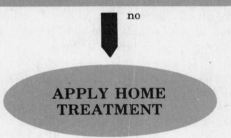

Are any of these conditions present following prolonged exposure to sun?

(a) Fever

(b) Fluid-filled blisters

(c) Dizziness

(d) Visual difficulties

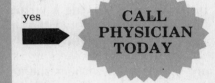

yes

CALL PHYSICIAN TODAY

no

APPLY HOME TREATMENT

48 Lice and Bedbugs

Lice and bedbugs are found in the best of families. Lack of prejudice with respect to social class is as close as these insects come to having a virtue. At best they are a nuisance and at worst they can cause real disability.

Lice themselves are very small and are seldom seen without the aid of a magnifying glass. Usually it is easier to find the "nits," which are clusters of louse eggs. Without magnification, nits will appear as tiny white lumps on hair strands. The louse bite leaves only a pinpoint red spot but scratching makes things worse. Itching and occasionally small, shallow sores at the base of hairs are clues to the disease. Pubic lice are not a "veneral disease" although they may be spread from person to person during sexual contact. Unlike syphilis and gonorrhea, lice may be spread by toilet seats, infected linen, and other sources. Pubic lice bear some resemblance to crabs; hence the use of the term "crabs" to indicate a lice infestation of the pubic hair. A different species of lice may inhabit the scalp or other body hair. Lice like to be close to a warm body all the time and will not stay for long periods of time in clothing that is not being worn, bedding, and other places.

Although related to lice, bedbugs present a considerably different picture. The adult is flat, wingless, oval in shape, reddish in color, and about one-quarter inch in length. Like lice, they stay alive by sucking blood. Unlike lice, they feed for only ten or fifteen minutes at a time and spend the rest of the time hiding in crevices and crannies. They feed almost entirely at night, both because that is when bodies are in bed and also because of a strong dislike of light. They have such a keen sense of the nearness of a warm body that the army has used them to detect the approach of an enemy at ranges of several hundred feet! Catching these pests out in the open is very difficult and may require some curious behavior. One technique is to dash into the bedroom at bedtime, flip on the lights and pull back the bedcovers in an effort to catch them in anticipation of their next meal.

The bite of the bedbug leaves a firm bump; usually there are two or three bumps clustered together. Occasionally, sensitivity is developed to these bites, in which case itching may be severe and blisters may form.

Home Treatment

Over-the-counter preparations are effective against lice; these include A200, Cuprex, and RID. RID has the advantage of supplying a fine tooth comb, a rare item these days. Instructions that come with these drugs must be followed carefully. Linen and clothing must be changed simultaneously. Sexual partners should be treated at the same time.

Since bedbugs don't hide on the body or in clothes, it is the bed and the room that should be treated. A 1% solution of malathion may be used. (**Caution:** *This is a dangerous pesticide and must be kept away from children.*) If the infestation is a light one, spray only the bed. Wet the slats, springs, and frame. Change the mattress cover, but spray the mattress only if there are seams or tufts that could harbor the bugs and if the child is older than five years. Use only a very light spray on mattresses. If the mattress is damaged so that stuffing is exposed, a new mattress is necessary. Never spray a mattress to be used by an infant or

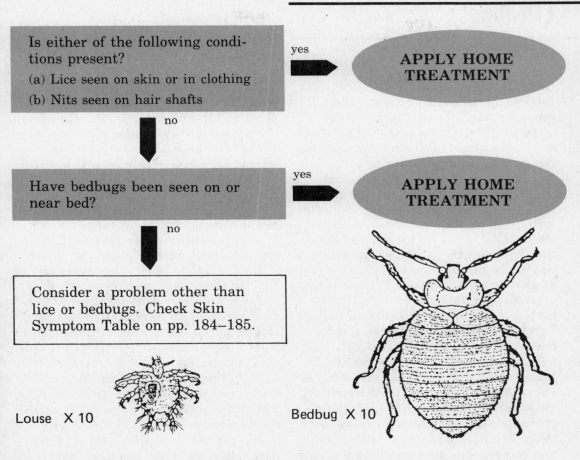

Is either of the following conditions present?
(a) Lice seen on skin or in clothing
(b) Nits seen on hair shafts

yes → APPLY HOME TREATMENT

no

Have bedbugs been seen on or near bed?

yes → APPLY HOME TREATMENT

no

Consider a problem other than lice or bedbugs. Check Skin Symptom Table on pp. 184–185.

Louse X 10

Bedbug X 10

young child. Malathion is dangerous if it contacts the skin. If the infestation is a heavy one, the furniture, walls, and floors of the bedroom should also be sprayed.

What to Expect at the Doctor's Office

If lice are the suspected problem, the doctor will make a careful inspection to find nits or the lice themselves. Doctors almost always use gamma benzene hexachloride (Kwell) for lice. It may be somewhat more effective than the over-the-counter preparations. It is more expensive and has more side effects.

The doctor will be hard-pressed to make a certain diagnosis of bedbug bites without information from you that bedbugs have been seen in the house. However, the bumps may be suggestive, and initially it may be decided to assume that the problem is bedbugs. If this is the case, treatment with an insecticide as under Home Treatment will be recommended.

219

49 Ticks and Chiggers (Redbugs)

Outdoor living has its dangers. While bears, mountain lions, and vertical cliffs can usually be avoided, shrubs and tall grasses hide tiny insects eager for a blood meal from a passing animal or person. Ticks and chiggers are the most common of the small hazards.

Ticks are rather easily seen, and a tick bite usually has the obvious cause sticking out. Ticks are about one-quarter inch long and easy to see. The tick buries its head and crablike pincers beneath the skin, with the body and legs protruding. Ticks feed on passing animals such as dogs or deer or people. In some areas, especially the southeastern United States, they carry other diseases, such as Rocky Mountain spotted fever; if a fever, rash, or headache follow a tick bite by a few days or weeks, the doctor should be consulted. If a pregnant female tick is allowed to remain feeding for several days, under certain circumstances a peculiar condition called tick paralysis may develop. The female tick secretes a toxin that can cause temporary paralysis, clearing shortly after the tick is removed; this complication is quite rare and can only happen if the tick stays in place many days. In tick-infested areas it is helpful to check your child's hair several times a day. By checking after hikes, you may be able to catch the ticks before they become embedded. Also check your pets.

Chiggers are small red mites, sometimes called "redbugs." Their bite contains a chemical that eats away at the skin, causing a tremendous itch. Usually the small red sores are around the belt line or other openings in clothes. Careful inspection may reveal the tiny red larvae in the center of the itching sore. Chiggers also live on grasses and shrubs.

Home Treatment

Ticks should be removed, although they will eventually "fester out"; complications are unusual. The trick is to get the tick to "let go" and not to squeeze the tick before getting it out. If the mouth parts and the pincers remain under the skin, healing may require several weeks. Rocky Mountain spotted fever is somewhat more likely if mouth parts are left in or the tick is squeezed during removal. Make the tick uncomfortable; gentle heat from a heated paperclip, alcohol, acetone, or oil will cause the tick to wiggle its legs and begin to withdraw. Grasp the tick with a tissue and remove it quickly. If the head is inadvertently left under the skin, soak gently with warm water twice daily until healing is complete. Call the doctor at once if the patient gets a fever, rash, or headache within three weeks.

Chiggers are better avoided then treated. Use of insect repellents, the wearing of appropriate clothing, and bathing after exposure help to cut down on the frequency of bites. Once you get them, they itch, often for several weeks. Keep the sores clean, and soak them with warm water twice daily. Cuprex and A200 applied the first few days will help kill the larvae, but the itch will persist.

Steroid creams (Cortaid, Lanacourt) may be tried, but usually are not much help (see Chapter 9, "The Home Pharmacy").

What to Expect at the Doctor's Office

The doctor can remove the tick but cannot prevent any illness that might have been transmitted. You can do as well.

CHIGGERS

Are any of the following present?

(a) Itching red sores around the belt line or other opening in clothes

(b) Itching red sores following contact with grass or shrubs

(c) Small red mites seen on the skin or red spot in center of sore.

 no → Suspect problem other than chiggers. See Skin Symptom Table on pp. 184–185.

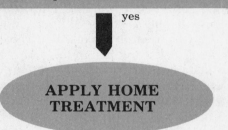

↓ yes

APPLY HOME TREATMENT

TICKS

Can tick be seen buried in skin, or is a swollen tick attached to skin?

 no → Suspect problem other than ticks. See Skin Symptom Table on pp. 184–185.

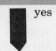

↓ yes

APPLY HOME TREATMENT

They are often removed from unusual places, such as armpits and belly buttons, but the scalp is the most common location. The technique is exactly the same, no matter where the tick is.

For chiggers, doctors will usually prescribe Kwell, which is perhaps slightly more effective than A200 or Cuprex but does not stop the itching either. Antihistamines make the patient drowsy and are not frequently used unless intense itching persists despite home treatment with aspirin, warm baths, oatmeal soaks, and calamine lotion.

50 Scabies

Scabies is an irritation of the skin caused by a tiny mite related to the chigger. No one knows why, but scabies seems to be on the rise in this country. As with lice, it is no longer true that scabies is related to hygiene. It occurs in the best of families and in the best of neighborhoods. The mite is easily spread from person to person or by contact with items that may harbor the mite such as clothing and bedding. Epidemics often spread through schools despite strict precautions against contacts with known cases.

The mite burrows into the skin to lay eggs; favorite locations for this burrowing are given in the decision chart. These burrows may be evident, especially at the beginning of the problem. However, the mite soon causes the skin to have a reaction to it so that redness, swelling, and blisters follow within a short period. Intense itching causes scratching so that there are plenty of scratch marks and these may become infected from the bacteria on the skin. Thus the telltale burrows are often obscured by scratch marks, blisters, and secondary infection. If you can locate something that looks like a burrow, you might be able to see the mite with the aid of a magnifying lens. This is the only way to be absolutely sure that the problem is scabies, but it is often not possible. The diagnosis is most often made on the basis of a problem that is consistent with scabies and the fact that scabies is known to be in the community.

Home Treatment

Benzyl benzoate (25% solution) is effective against scabies and does not require a prescription. Unfortunately, it is not widely available. If you are able to find it, apply it once to the entire body except for the face and around the urinary opening of the penis and the vaginal opening. Wash it off twenty-four hours later. This medicine does have an odor that some find unpleasant. If you cannot find benzyl benzoate, you'll have to get a prescription for Kwell from your doctor.

For itching, we recommend cool soaks, calamine lotion, or aspirin. Antihistamines may help but often cause drowsiness. Follow the directions that come with the package. As in the case of poison ivy, warmth makes the itching worse by releasing histamine, but if all the histamine is released, relief may be obtained for several hours. (See **Poison Ivy and Poison Oak**, Problem 39).

It will take some time before the skin becomes normal, even with effective treatment, but at least some improvement should be noted within seventy-two hours. If this is not the case, visit the doctor.

What to Expect at the Doctor's Office.

The doctor should examine the entire skin surface for signs of the problem and may examine the area with a magnifying lens in an attempt to identify the mite. A scraping of the lesion may be made for examination under the microscope. Most of the time the doctor will be forced to make a decision based on the probability of various kinds of diseases and then treat it much as you would at home. The proof will be whether or not the treatment is successful.

Kwell will often be prescribed. Because of the potency of this medication it should not be used more than two times, a week apart.

Are all of the following conditions present?

(a) Intense itching

(b) Raised red skin in a line (represents a burrow) and possibly blisters or pustules

(c) Located on the hands, especially between the fingers, elbow crease, armpit, groin crease, or behind the knees

(d) Exposure to scabies

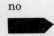 no

Consider a problem other than scabies. Check Skin Symptom Table on pp. 184–185.

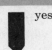 yes

APPLY HOME TREATMENT

51 Dandruff and Cradle Cap

Although they look somewhat different, cradle cap and dandruff are really part of the same problem; its medical term is *seborrhea*. It occures when the oil glands in the skin have been stimulated by adult hormones, leading to oiliness and flaking of the scalp. This occurs in the infant because of exposure to the mother's hormones and in older children when they begin to make their own adult hormones. However, it does occur between these two ages, and once a child has the problem, it tends to recur.

Seborrhea itself is a somewhat ugly but relatively harmless condition. However, it may make the skin more susceptible to infection with yeast or bacteria. Occasionally this condition is confused with problems such as ringworm of the scalp or psoriasis. Careful attention to the conditions listed in the decision chart will usually avoid this confusion. Remember also that ringworm would be unusual in the newborn and very young child. Psoriasis often stops at the hairline. Furthermore, the scales of psoriasis are on top of raised lesions called "plaques," which is not the case in seborrhea.

Children will frequently have redness and scaling of the eyebrows and behind the ears as well.

Home Treatment

The heavily advertised antidandruff shampoos are helpful in mild to moderate cases of dandruff. For severe and more stubborn cases, there are some less well-known over-the-counter shampoos that are effective. Selsun (available by prescription only) and Selsun Blue are brand names of shampoos that contain selenium sulfide; Selsun Blue is available over the counter and, while weaker, is just as good if you apply more of it more frequently. When using these shampoos, it is important that directions be followed carefully, since oiliness and yellowish discoloration of the hair may occur with their use. Sebulex, Sebucare, Ionil, and DHS are another series of antidandruff preparations that are very effective and also must be used strictly according to directions.

Cradle cap is best treated with a scrub brush. If the cradle cap is thick, then rub in warm baby oil, cover with a warm towel, and soak for fifteen minutes. Use a fine tooth comb or scrub brush to help remove the scale; then shampoo with Sebulex or other preparations listed above. Be careful to avoid getting shampoo in the eyes.

No matter what you do, the problem will often return, and you may have to repeat the treatment. If the problem gets worse despite home treatment over several weeks, see the doctor.

What to Expect at the Doctor's Office

Severe cases of seborrhea may require more than the medications given above; a cortisone cream is most often prescribed. Most often, a trip is made to the doctor in order to clear up some confusion concerning the diagnosis. The physician usually makes the diagnosis on the basis of the appearance of the rash. Occasionally, scrapings from the involved areas will be looked at under the microscope. Drugs by mouth or by injection are not indicated for seborrhea unless bacterial infection has complicated the problem.

In an infant, are all of the following conditions present?

(a) Thick, adherent, oily, yellowish scaling or crusting patches

(b) Located on the scalp, behind the ears, eyebrows, or (less frequently) in the skin creases of the groin

(c) Only mild redness in involved areas

 no → Suspect problem other than cradle cap. Check Skin Symptom Table on pp. 184–185.

In an older child (or adult), are all of the following conditions present?

(a) Fine, white, oily scales

(b) Confined to scalp and/or eyebrows

(c) Only mild redness in involved areas

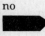 no → Suspect problem other than dandruff. Check Skin Symptom Table on pp. 184–185.

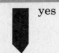 yes

APPLY HOME TREATMENT

52 Patchy Loss of Skin Color

Children are constantly getting minor cuts, scrapes, insect bites, and other minor skin infections. During the healing process it is common for the skin to lose some of its color. With time, the skin coloring generally returns.

Occasionally, ringworm, a fungal infection discussed in Problem 37, will begin as a small round area of scaling with associated loss of skin color.

In the summertime, many children have small round spots on their face in which there is little color. The white spots have probably been present for some time, but the tanning of the skin does not occur in these areas, thus making them visible. This condition is known as *pityriasis alba*; the cause is unknown, but it is a mild condition of cosmetic concern only. It may take many months to disappear and may recur, but there are virtually never any long-term effects.

If there are lightly scaled, tan, pink, or white patches on the neck or back, the problem is most likely due to a fungal infection known as *tinea versicolor*. This is a very minor and superficial fungal infection.

Home Treatment

Waiting is the most effective home treatment for loss of skin color. Tinea versicolor can be treated by applying Selsun Blue shampoo to the affected area, once every day or so until the lesions are gone.

Tolnaftate (Tinactin) lotion or cream is also effective. Unfortunately tinea versicolor almost always comes back no matter what type of treatment is used.

What to Expect at the Doctor's Office

A history of careful examination of the skin will be performed. Scrapings of the lesions may be taken, since tinea versicolor can be identified from these scrapings. Pityriasis alba should be distinguished from more severe fungal infections that may occur on the face. Again, scrapings will help to identify the fungus.

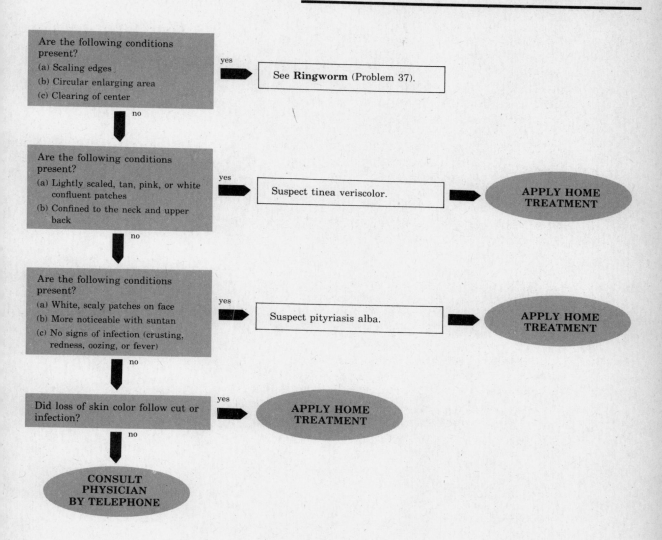

Are the following conditions present?
(a) Scaling edges
(b) Circular enlarging area
(c) Clearing of center

— yes → See **Ringworm** (Problem 37).

— no ↓

Are the following conditions present?
(a) Lightly scaled, tan, pink, or white confluent patches
(b) Confined to the neck and upper back

— yes → Suspect tinea veriscolor. → **APPLY HOME TREATMENT**

— no ↓

Are the following conditions present?
(a) White, scaly patches on face
(b) More noticeable with suntan
(c) No signs of infection (crusting, redness, oozing, or fever)

— yes → Suspect pityriasis alba. → **APPLY HOME TREATMENT**

— no ↓

Did loss of skin color follow cut or infection?

— yes → **APPLY HOME TREATMENT**

— no ↓

CONSULT PHYSICIAN BY TELEPHONE

I Childhood Diseases

229

53 Mumps

Mumps is a viral infection of the salivary glands. The major salivary glands are located directly below and in front of the ear. Before any swelling is noticeable, there may be a low fever, headache, earache, or weakness. Fever is variable; it may be only slightly above normal or as high as 104°F. After several days of these symptoms, one or both salivary glands (parotid glands) may swell. It is sometimes difficult to distinguish mumps from swollen lymph glands in the neck; in mumps you will not be able to feel the edge of the jaw that is located beneath the ear. Chewing and swallowing may produce pain behind the ear. Sour substances such as lemons and pickles may make the pain worse. When swelling occurs on both sides, people take on the appearance of chipmunks! Other salivary glands besides the parotid may be involved, including those under the jaw and tongue. The openings of these glands into the mouth may become red and puffy. Approximately one-third of all patients who have mumps do not demonstrate any swelling of glands whatsoever. Therefore, many persons who are concerned about exposure to mumps will already have had the disease without realizing it.

Mumps is quite contagious during the period from two days before the first symptoms to the complete disappearance of the parotid gland swelling (usually about a week after the swelling has begun). Mumps will develop in a susceptible exposed person approximately sixteen to eighteen days after exposure to the virus. In children, it is generally a mild illness. the chart is directed toward detection of the rare complications, which include encephalitis (viral infection of the brain), pancreatitis (viral infection of the pancreas), kidney disease, deafness, and involvement of the testicles or the ovaries. Complications are more frequent in adults than they are in children.

Home Treatment

The pain may be reduced with either aspirin or acetaminophen. There may be difficulty in eating, but adequate fluid intake is important. Sour foods should be avoided, including orange juice. Adults who have not had mumps should avoid exposure to the patient until complete disappearance of the swelling. Many adults who do not recall having mumps as a child may have had an extremely mild case and consequently are not at risk of developing mumps.

If swelling has not disappeared in three weeks, call the doctor.

What to Expect at the Doctor's Office

If a complication is suspected, a visit to the physician's office may be necessary. The history and physical examination will be directed at confirming the diagnosis or the presence of a complication. The rare complication of a right ovarian infection may be confused with appendicitis and blood tests may be required. Since mumps is a viral disease, there is no medicine that will directly kill the virus. Supportive measures may be necessary for some of the complications; fortunately these occur rarely and permanent damage to hearing or other functions is unusual. Mumps very rarely produces sterility in men or women even when the testes or ovaries are involved.

Is there lethargy, convulsions, or stiff neck?

yes → SEE PHYSICIAN NOW

no ↓

Are any of the following present?
(a) Pain and swelling of one or both testicles
(b) Abdominal pain and vomiting
(c) Dizziness and difficulty in hearing

yes → CALL PHYSICIAN TODAY

no ↓

APPLY HOME TREATMENT

54 Chicken Pox

How to recognize the chicken pox:

Before the rash: Usually there are no symptoms before the rash appears, but occasionally there is fatigue and some fever in the twenty-four hours before the rash is noted.

Rash: The typical rash goes through the following stages.

1. First it appears as flat red splotches.
2. They become raised and may resemble small pimples.
3. They develop into small blisters, called vesicles, which are very fragile. They may look like drops of water on a red base. The tops are easily scratched off.
4. As the vesicles break, the sores become "pustular" and form a crust. (The crust is made of dried serum, not true pus.) This stage may be reached within several hours of the first appearance of the rash. The crust falls away between the ninth and thirteenth day. Itching is often severe in the pustular stage.
5. The vesicles tend to appear in crops with two to four crops appearing within two to six days. All stages may be present in the same area. They often appear first on the scalp and in the mouth, and then spread to the rest of the body, but they may begin anywhere. They are most numerous over shoulders, chest, and back. They are seldom found on the palms of the hands or the soles of the feet. There may be only a few sores, or there may be hundreds.

Fever: After most of the sores have formed crusts, the fever usually subsides.

Chicken pox spreads very easily—over 90 percent of brothers and sisters catch it. It may be transmitted from twenty-four hours before the appearance of the rash up to about six days after. It is spread by droplets from the mouth or throat or by direct contact with contaminated articles of clothing. It is not spread by dry scabs. The incubation period is from fourteen to seventeen days. Chicken pox leads to lifelong immunity to recurrence with rare exceptions. However, the same virus that causes chicken pox also causes shingles and the individual who has had chicken pox may develop shingles (herpes zoster) later in life.

Most of the time, chicken pox should be treated at home. Complications are rare and far less common than with measles. The specific questions on the chart deal with two severe complications that may require more than home treatment: encephalitis (viral infection of the brain) and severe bacterial infection of the lesions. Encephalitis is rare.

Home Treatment

The major problem in dealing with chicken pox is control of the intense itching and reduction of the fever. Warm baths containing baking soda (one-half cup to a tubful of water) frequently help. Antihistamines may help; see Chapter 9, "The Home Pharmacy." Aspirin and acetaminophen are effective itch relievers.

Cut the fingernails or use gloves to prevent skin damage from intensive scratching. When lesions occur in the mouth, gargling with salt water (one-half teaspoon salt to an eight-ounce glass) may help give comfort. Hands should be washed three times a day and all of the skin should be kept gently but scrupulously clean in order to prevent a compli-

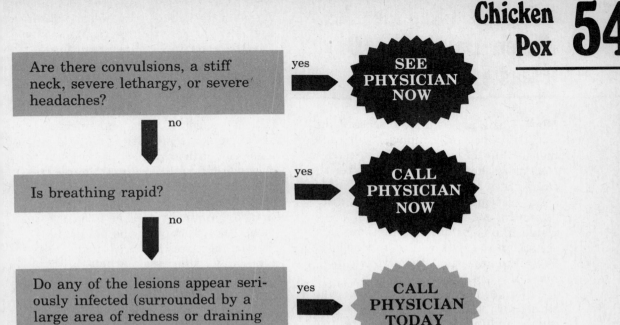

Are there convulsions, a stiff neck, severe lethargy, or severe headaches? — **yes** → SEE PHYSICIAN NOW

no

Is breathing rapid? — **yes** → CALL PHYSICIAN NOW

no

Do any of the lesions appear seriously infected (surrounded by a large area of redness or draining pus)? — **yes** → CALL PHYSICIAN TODAY

no

APPLY HOME TREATMENT

cating bacterial infection. Minor bacterial infection will respond to soap and time; if it becomes severe and results in return of fever, then call the physician. Scratching and infection can result in permanent scars.

If itching is unable to be controlled or problem persists beyond three weeks, call the doctor. Using the phone for questions to the doctor will avoid exposing others to the disease.

What to Expect at the Doctor's Office

Do not be surprised if the physician is willing and even anxious to treat the case "over the phone." If it is necessary to go to the doctor's office, then attempts should be made to keep the patient separate from the other patients. In healthy children, chicken pox has few lasting ill effects, but in persons with other serious illnesses, it can be a devastating or even fatal disease. A visit to the physician's office may not be necessary unless a complication seems possible.

55 Measles (Red Measles, Seven-Day or Ten-Day Measles)

Measles is a preventable disease. Unlike some of the other "childhood" illnesses, measles can be quite severe. It is tragic that more than thirteen years after the licensing of the measles vaccine, thousands of people still contract this disease annually, and some of them die. We would like to be able to eliminate this section in the next edition of this book. Only immunization of everyone can make this possible.

Measles is a viral illness that begins with fever, weakness, a dry "brassy" cough, and inflamed eyes that are itchy, red, and sensitive to the light. These symptoms begin three to five days before the appearance of the rash. Another early sign of measles is the appearance of fine white spots on a red base inside the mouth opposite the molar teeth (Koplik's spots). These fade as the skin rash appears.

The rash begins on about the fifth day as a pink, blotchy, flat rash. The rash first appears around the hairline, on the face, on the neck, and behind the ears. The spots, which fade when pressure is applied (early in the illness), become somewhat darker and tend to merge into larger red patches as they mature. The rash spreads from head to chest to abdomen and finally to the arms and legs. It lasts from four to seven days and may be accompanied by mild itching. There may be some light brown coloring to the skin lesions as the illness progresses.

Measles is a highly contagious viral disease. It is spread by droplets from the mouth or throat and by direct contact with articles freshly soiled by nose and throat secretions. It may be spread during the period from three to six days before the appearance of the rash to several days after. Symptoms begin in a susceptible person approximately eight to twelve days after exposure to the virus.

There are a number of complications of measles; sore throats, ear infections, and pneumonia are all common. Many of these complicating infections are due to bacteria and will require antibiotic treatment. The pneumonias can be life-threatening. A very serious problem that can lead to permanent damage is measles encephalitis (infection of the brain); life-support measures and treatment of seizures may be necessary when this rare complication occurs.

Home Treatment

Symptomatic measures are all that is needed for uncomplicated measles. Aspirin or acetaminophen should be used to keep the fever down, and a vaporizer can be used for the cough. Dim lighting in the room is often more comfortable because of the eyes' sensitivity to light. In general, the person feels "measley." The patient should be isolated until the end of the contagious period. All unimmunized people in contact with the patient should be immunized immediately. (People who have had the measles are considered to be immunized.)

What to Expect at the Doctor's Office

The history and physical examination will be directed at determining the diagnosis of measles and the nature of any complications. Bacterial complications, such as ear infections and pneumonia, can usually be treated with antibiotics. The person with symptoms suggestive of encephalitis (lethargy, stiff neck, convulsions) will be hospitalized and a spinal tap will be performed. Very rarely, there

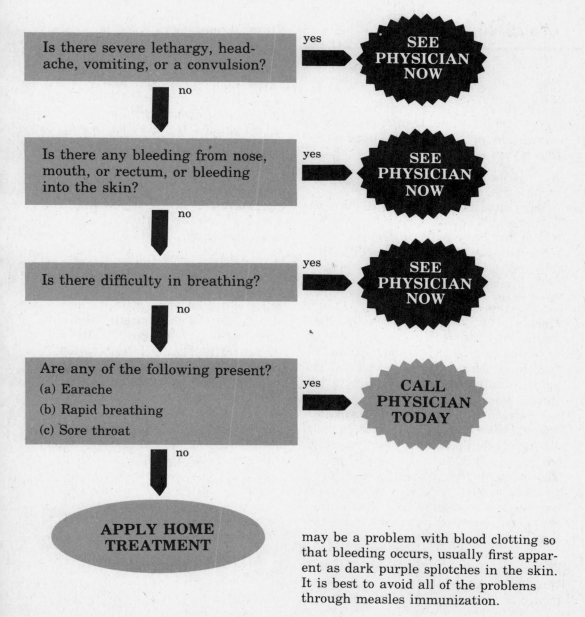

Is there severe lethargy, headache, vomiting, or a convulsion? — yes → **SEE PHYSICIAN NOW**

no ↓

Is there any bleeding from nose, mouth, or rectum, or bleeding into the skin? — yes → **SEE PHYSICIAN NOW**

no ↓

Is there difficulty in breathing? — yes → **SEE PHYSICIAN NOW**

no ↓

Are any of the following present?
(a) Earache
(b) Rapid breathing
(c) Sore throat
— yes → **CALL PHYSICIAN TODAY**

no ↓

APPLY HOME TREATMENT

may be a problem with blood clotting so that bleeding occurs, usually first apparent as dark purple splotches in the skin. It is best to avoid all of the problems through measles immunization.

235

56 German Measles (Rubella, Three-day Measles)

How to recognize the German measles:

Before the rash: There may be a few days of mild fatigue. Lymph nodes at the back of the neck may be enlarged and tender.

Rash: The rash first appears on the face as flat or slightly raised red spots. It quickly spreads to the trunk and the extremities and the discrete spots tend to merge into large patches. The rash of rubella is highly variable and is difficult for even the most experienced parents and physicians to recognize. Often, there is *no* rash.

Fever: The fever rarely goes above 101°F and usually lasts less than two days.

Joint pains occur in about 10 to 15 percent of older children and adults. The pains usually begin on the third day of illness.

German measles is a mild virus infection that is not as contagious as measles or chicken pox. It is usually spread by droplets from the mouth or throat. The incubation period is from twelve to twenty-one days, with an average of sixteen days. The specific questions on the chart are addressed to possible complications, which are extremely rare.

The main concern with German measles is an infection in an unborn child. If three-day measles occurs during the first month of pregnancy, there is a 50 percent chance that the fetus will develop an abnormality such as cataracts, heart disease, deafness, or mental deficiency. By the third month of pregnancy, this risk decreases to less than 10 percent and it continues to decrease throughout the pregnancy. Because of the problem of congenital defects, a vaccine for German measles has been developed.

Home Treatment

Usually no therapy is required. Occasionally, fever will require the use of aspirin or acetaminophen. Isolation is usually not imposed. Women who could possibly be pregnant should avoid any exposure to the patient. If a question of such exposure arises, the pregnant woman should discuss the risk with her physician. Blood tests are available that will indicate whether a pregnant woman has had rubella in the past and is immune, or whether problems with the pregnancy might be encountered.

What to Expect at the Doctor's Office

Visits to the physician's office are seldom required for uncomplicated German measles. Questions about possible infection of pregnant women are more easily and economically discussed over the telephone. The question of immunization is complex and it is discussed in detail in *Taking Care of Your Child.* (Robert Pantell, M.D., James Fries, M.D., and Donald Vickery, M.D., *Taking Care of Your Child* [Reading, Mass.: Addison-Wesley Publishing Co., 1977]).

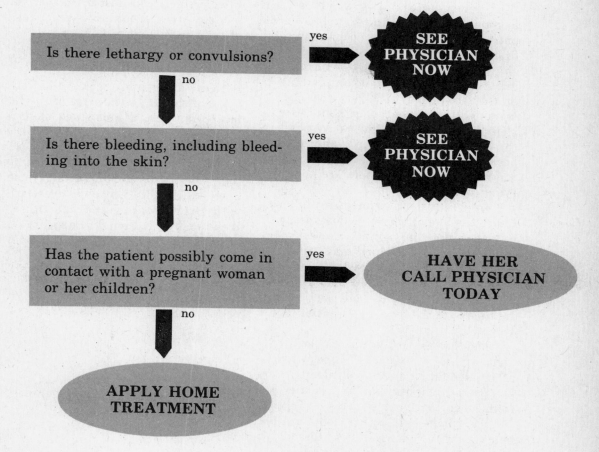

Is there lethargy or convulsions? — yes → **SEE PHYSICIAN NOW**

no ↓

Is there bleeding, including bleeding into the skin? — yes → **SEE PHYSICIAN NOW**

no ↓

Has the patient possibly come in contact with a pregnant woman or her children? — yes → **HAVE HER CALL PHYSICIAN TODAY**

no ↓

APPLY HOME TREATMENT

57 Roseola

How to recognize roseola: Before the rash appears there are usually several days of sustained high fever; sometimes this fever can trigger a convulsion or seizure in a susceptible child. Otherwise, the patient appears well. The rash appears as the fever is decreasing or shortly after it is gone. It consists of pink, well-defined patches that turn white on pressure and first appear on the trunk. It may be slightly bumpy. It spreads to involve the arms and neck but is seldom prominent on the face or legs. The rash usually lasts less than twenty-four hours. Occasionally, there is a slight runny nose, throat redness, or swollen glands at the back of the head, behind the ears, or in the neck. Most often, there are no other symptoms.

Roseola is most common in children under the age of three but may occur at any age. Its main significance lies in the sudden high fever, which may cause a convulsion. Such a convulsion is due to the high temperature and does not indicate that the child has epilepsy. Prompt treatment of the fever is essential (see **Fever,** Problem 17).

This disease is probably caused by a virus and is contagious. Contact with others should be avoided until the fever has passed. The incubation period is from seven to seventeen days.

Encephalitis (infection of the brain) is a very rare complication of roseola; roseola is basically a mild disease.

Home Treatment

Home treatment is based on two principles. The first is effective treatment of the fever, discussed in Problem 17. The second is careful watching and waiting. This depends on the fact that the patient should appear reasonably well and have no other significant symptoms when the fever is controlled. Especially watch for symptoms of ear infection (a complaint of pain or tugging at the ear), cough (see Problem 24), or lethargy. If these occur, then the appropriate sections of this book should be consulted. If the problem is still not clear, a phone call to the physician may be necessary. Remember that roseola should not last more than four or five days; you should call your physician about a persistent problem.

What to Expect at the Doctor's Office

Patients are usually seen soon after the onset of the illness because of the high fever. As noted, at this stage there is little else to be found in roseola. The ears, nose, throat, and chest should be examined. If the fever remains the only finding, then the physician will recommend home treatment (control of the fever with careful waiting and watching to see if the rash of roseola will appear). There is no medical treatment for roseola other than that available at home.

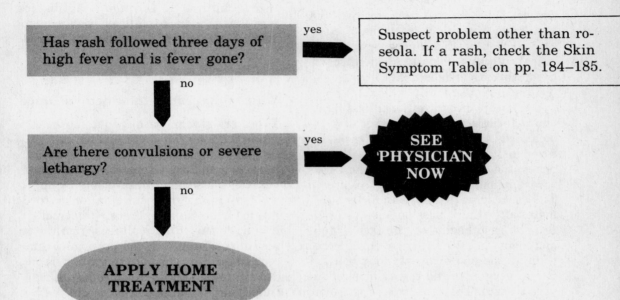

Has rash followed three days of high fever and is fever gone?

yes → Suspect problem other than roseola. If a rash, check the Skin Symptom Table on pp. 184–185.

no ↓

Are there convulsions or severe lethargy?

yes → SEE PHYSICIAN NOW

no ↓

APPLY HOME TREATMENT

58 Scarlet Fever

Scarlet fever derived its name over 300 years ago from its characteristic red rash. The illness is caused by a streptococcal infection, usually of the throat. Strep throats are discussed in **Sore Throat**, (Problem 19).

You can recognize the illness by its characteristic features. A fever and weakness usually precede the rash. The fever is often accompanied by a headache, stomachache, and vomiting. A sore throat is usually but not always present. The rash appears twelve to forty-eight hours after the illness begins.

The rash begins on the face, trunk, and arms and generally covers the entire body by the end of twenty-four hours. It is red, very fine, and covers most of the skin surface. The area around the mouth is pale. With your eyes closed, it has the feeling of fine sandpaper. Skin creases, such as in front of the elbow and the armpit, are more deeply red. Pressing on the rash will produce a white spot lasting several seconds. The intense redness of the rash lasts for about five days, although peeling of skin can go on for weeks. It is not unusual for peeling, especially of the palms, to last for more than a month.

Examination often reveals a red throat, spots on the roof of the mouth (soft palate), and a fuzzy white tongue, later becoming swollen and red. There may be swollen glands in the neck.

As with other streptoccal infections, the significance of scarlet fever is its connection with rheumatic fever (see **Sore Throat**, Problem 19).

Home Treatment

Since scarlet fever is due to a streptococcal infection, a medical visit is required for antibiotic treatment. Streptococcal infections are quite contagious, and other members of the family should also have throat cultures. In addition to antibiotics you should reduce the fever with aspirin or acetaminophen, keep up with fluid requirements, and give plenty of cold liquids to help soothe the throat.

What to Expect at the Doctor's Office

There are several rashes that can be confused with scarlet fever, including those of measles and drug reactions. If the rash is sufficiently typical of scarlet fever, the physician will probably begin antibiotics, usually penicillin (or erythromycin if the child is allergic to penicillin), and take throat cultures from the rest of the family. If the physician is uncertain of the cause of the rash, a throat culture may be taken before beginning treatment. Treatment that is delayed by a day or two while waiting for culture results will still prevent the complication about which we are most concerned: rheumatic fever.

Are both of the following present?

(a) Fever

(b) Fine, red rash on trunk and extremities which feels like sandpaper

no

Suspect problem other than scarlet fever. If there is a skin rash, check the Skin Symptom Table on pp. 184–185.

yes

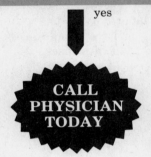

CALL PHYSICIAN TODAY

59 Fifth Disease

Consider the strange case of the fifth disease, whose only claim to fame is that it might be mistaken for another disease. It is so named because it is always listed last (and least) among the five very common contagious rashes of childhood. Its medical name, *erythema infectiosum*, is easily forgotten.

It comes very close to not being a disease at all. It has no symptoms other than rash, has no complications, and needs no treatment. It can be recognized because it causes a characteristic "slapped cheek" appearance in children. The rash often begins on the cheeks and is later found on the backs of the arms and legs. It often has a very fine, lacy, pink appearance. It tends to come and go and may be present one moment and absent the next. It is prone to recur for days or even weeks, especially as a response to heat (warm bath or shower) or irritation. In general, however, the rash around the face will fade within four days of its appearance, and the rash on the rest of the body will fade within three to seven days of its appearance. Its only significance is that it could worry you or cause you to make an avoidable trip to the doctor's office. It is very contagious; epidemics of fifth disease have resulted in unnecessary school closings. The agent responsible for this "nondisease" is not known; a virus is suspected. The incubation period is thought to be from six to fourteen days.

Home Treatment

There is no treatment. Just watch and wait to make sure you are dealing with fifth disease. Check that there is no fever; fever is very unusual with fifth disease. No restrictions on activities are necessary.

What to Expect at the Doctor's Office

The physician may be able to distinguish fifth disease from other rashes. If the rash fits the description given in this section, the physician is going to make the same diagnosis that you might have. Checking patients temperature and looking at the rash can be expected. Since there are no tests for the unknown cause, laboratory tests are unlikely. Waiting and watching are the means of dealing with fifth disease.

Are all of the following conditions present?

(a) No fever

(b) Rash is the first and only symptom

(c) Palms and soles are not involved

 no ⟶ Suspect problem other than fifth disease. If a rash, check the Skin Symptom Table on pp. 184–185.

yes

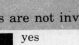

APPLY HOME TREATMENT

J Bones, Muscles, and Joints

60 Arthritis

Most "arthritis" is not arthritis at all! Misunderstanding comes from a different use of the term by doctors and by patients. The "arth" part of the word means "joint"—*not* muscle, tendon, ligament, or bone. The "itis" means "inflamed." Thus, true arthritis affects the joints, and the joints are red, warm, swollen, and painful to move. Pains in the muscles or ligaments are discussed in Problem 61.

There are over one hundred types of arthritis. The four most common types are "osteoarthritis," "rheumatoid arthritis," "gout," and "ankylosing spondylitis." Osteoarthritis is usually not serious, occurs in later life, and frequently causes knobby swelling at the most distant joints of the fingers. Rheumatoid arthritis usually starts in middle life and may cause you to feel sick and stiff all over, in addition to the joint problems. Gout occurs mostly in men, with sudden, severe attacks of pain and swelling in one joint at a time—frequently the big toe, the ankle, or the knee. Ankylosing spondylitis affects the back and joints of the lower back and may be suspected if your back is sore for a long time, particularly stiff in the morning, and you are unable to touch your toes.

Only rarely does a patient with arthritis need to be seen by a physician immediately. Home treatment and patience will usually resolve the problem. The relative emergencies are (1) infection, (2) nerve damage, (3) fractures near a joint, and (4) gout. In the first three, serious damage may result if the joint is neglected; in the fourth, the pain is so intense that immediate help is needed.

The complications of arthritis and treatment for arthritis occur very slowly and are more easily prevented than corrected. Arthritis results in more lost workdays and sickness than any other disease category—it must be managed correctly and with care.

Home Treatment

Aspirin is more powerful than prescription drugs for most patients with arthritis but only when used in high doses continued for a long period. Aspirin can reduce the swelling in the joints as well as the pain. For adult patients the usual dose is two to four tablets (10 to 20 grains), every four hours, for a total of sixteen tablets daily. **If the dose causes stomach pain, ringing in both the ears, dizziness, or affects hearing, it is too high and should be reduced**. Continued use of a high dose of aspirin may contribute to bleeding from the stomach or ulcers. Upset stomach usually can be avoided by taking the aspirin after meals, after an antacid (Maalox or Gelusil), or by using coated aspirin tablets (Ecotrin, A.S.A. Enseals). While aspirin has fewer side effects than most drugs, a physician should monitor treatment with these doses if it is maintained for more than a week. Note that aspirin substitutes (acetaminophen) do not have the anti-inflammatory property of aspirin. See Chapter 9, "The Home Pharmacy," for more information on aspirin and aspirin substitutes.

Resting an inflamed joint can speed healing. Heat may help. Usually, a painful joint should be worked through its entire range of motion twice daily to prevent later stiffness or contracture.

If arthritis persists more than six weeks, see a physician. For more information, consult James Fries, M.D., *Arthritis: A Comprehensive Guide* and Kate Lorig, R.N., and James Fries, M.D., *The*

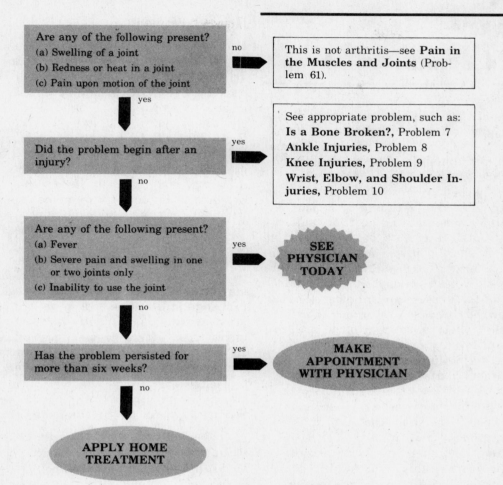

Are any of the following present?
(a) Swelling of a joint
(b) Redness or heat in a joint
(c) Pain upon motion of the joint

no → This is not arthritis—see **Pain in the Muscles and Joints** (Problem 61).

yes ↓

Did the problem begin after an injury?

yes → See appropriate problem, such as:
Is a Bone Broken?, Problem 7
Ankle Injuries, Problem 8
Knee Injuries, Problem 9
Wrist, Elbow, and Shoulder Injuries, Problem 10

no ↓

Are any of the following present?
(a) Fever
(b) Severe pain and swelling in one or two joints only
(c) Inability to use the joint

yes → **SEE PHYSICIAN TODAY**

no ↓

Has the problem persisted for more than six weeks?

yes → **MAKE APPOINTMENT WITH PHYSICIAN**

no ↓

APPLY HOME TREATMENT

Arthritis Helpbook—listed at the end of this volume.

What to Expect at the Doctor's Office

The physician will examine the joints, take several blood tests, and often will X-ray the involved joint areas. If a joint contains fluid, the fluid may also be removed and tested. A cortisone like drug may be injected (not more than three times) into a painful joint. Beware of the long-term oral use of such drugs—their side effects may be worse than the arthritis. If such drugs as prednisone are to be continued for more than a few weeks, we recommend that a consultant concur in their use. The good physician will invariably use aspirin or one of the "nonsteroidal anti-inflammatory agents" (such as indomethacin) before resorting to long-term use of cortisone or its derivatives.

61 Pain in the Muscles and Joints

Here are two new medical terms: "arthralgia" means pain (without inflammation) in the joints, and "myalgia" means pain in the muscles. These pains are not "arthritis" but can be very bothersome. Usually they are not serious, and will go away. They can be caused by tension, virus infections, unusual exertion, automobile or other accidents, or can be without obvious cause. Only seldom do they indicate a serious disease. Rarely, thyroid disease, cancer, polymyositis (inflammation of the muscles), or, in older patients, a newly-known disease termed "polymyalgia rheumatica" may cause arthralgias. If fever, weight loss, or severe fatigue are not present, give home treatment a trial of several weeks or even months before seeing a physician. If pain is pronounced at the upper neck and base of the skull, the problem is almost certainly minor.

Doctors often do not agree on diagnostic terms in this area, and two doctors may give different names to your problem. Some terms frequently used are: "fibrositis," "nonarticular rheumatism," "chronic muscle-contraction syndrome," "psychogenic rheumatism," and "psycho-physiological musculo-skeletal pain." These all mean about the same. Medical treatment is often not very helpful. Tranquilizers, muscle relaxants, and pain relievers may be prescribed, but the side effects are often more spectacular than the relief provided. The doctor is frequently unsure whether the problem is physical or emotional in origin. These problems are "diseases of civilization" and are rarely seen in underdeveloped societies.

Home Treatment

Both rest and exercise are important. Try to relax and gently stretch the involved areas. Warm baths, massage, and stretching exercises should be used as frequently as possible. Sponge-soled shoes may help if you work on hard floors. Better light or a better chair may help if you work at a desk. Regular exercise (slowly increased from very gentle to more vigorous) may help restore the proper muscle tone. We recommend walking, bicycling, and swimming. Aspirin, two tablets (10 grains) four times daily may help—higher doses usually are of no additional benefit. If aspirin is poorly tolerated, acetaminophen (Tylenol) may be substituted in the same dosage. A change in life style or a move to a different location is frequently followed by improvement. If the problem goes away on vacation, you can be relatively certain that everyday stress accounts for the problem.

What to Expect at the Doctor's Office

A physical examination. Often, some blood tests. Rarely, X-rays. Advice similar to that above. In general, pain relievers containing narcotics or codeine are not useful. Oral corticosteroids such as prednisone should almost never be used unless a specific diagnosis can be made. If a particular spot in the body is causing the pain, a corticosteroid injection into that area may help greatly; such injections should not be repeated if they do not help and should be repeated only two or three times even if they do give prolonged relief.

Are any of the following present?

(a) Swelling of a joint

(b) Redness or heat in a joint

(c) Pain on motion of the joint

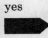 yes

See **Arthritis,** Problem 60.

 no

Are any of the following present?

(a) Fever not associated with "flu" symptoms

(b) Weight loss of ten or more pounds

 yes

MAKE APPOINTMENT WITH PHYSICIAN

 no

APPLY HOME TREATMENT

62 Low-back Pain

Few problems can frustrate patient and physician alike as much as "low-back pain." The pain is slow to resolve and apt to recur. The frustration then becomes a part of the problem and may also require treatment.

Low-back pain usually involves spasm of the large supportive muscles alongside the spine. Any injury to the back may produce such spasms; pain (often severe) and stiffness result. The onset of pain may be immediate or may occur some hours after the exertion or injury. Often the cause is not clear.

Most muscular problems in the back are linked to some exertion or lifting and must heal naturally; give them time. Back pain that results from a severe blow or fall may require immediate attention. As a practical matter, if back pain is caused by an injury received at work, examination by a physician is required by the workman's compensation laws.

The most common location of pain due to muscular strain is in the low back. Although many other pains have a muscular origin, pain that extends beyond the low-back area suggests a need for concern. Pain that extends down the leg to below the knee is different than pain confined to the low back. Such pain suggests pressure on the nerves as they leave the spinal cord and requires the help of a physician. If backache occurs with other symptoms (such as difficult menstrual periods), refer to the appropriate chart for that symptom.

Home Treatment

The low-back-pain syndrome is a vicious cycle in which injury causes muscle spasm, the spasm induces pain, and the pain results in additional muscle spasm. Therapy helps disrupt this cycle. Muscle spasm is intended to immobilize an injured part; sometimes it increases the problem.

Resting the muscles is of primary importance. When the pain first appears, rest, flat on your back, for at least twenty-four hours. Follow the period of complete bed rest by a gradual increase in activity, carefully avoiding reinjury. Severe muscle-spasm pain usually lasts for forty-eight to seventy-two hours and is followed by days or weeks of less severe pain. Strenuous activity during the next six weeks can bring the problem back and delay complete recovery. After healing, an exercise program will help prevent reinjury. *No* drug will hasten healing; they only reduce symptoms.

The patient should sleep, pillowless, on a very firm mattress, with a bedboard under the mattress, on a waterbed, or even on the floor. A folded towel beneath the low back and a pillow under the knees may increase comfort.

Heat applied to the affected area will provide some relief. Two to three aspirin every three hours should be continued as long as there is significant pain. To avoid upset stomach, take the medication with milk or food, or use buffered aspirin (such as Ascriptin and Bufferin).

There is little sound medical information of this subject. The advice given here is standard. If there is no nerve damage, hospitalization and the physician have little to offer. If significant pain persists beyond a week, call the doctor.

What to Expect at the Doctor's Office

Expect questions similar to those on the chart. The examination will center on the back, the abdomen, and the extremities, with special attention to testing the nerve function of the legs. If the injury

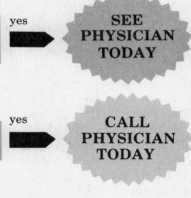

Is pain associated with any of the following?

(a) Abdominal pain

(b) Nausea or vomiting or diarrhea

(c) Pain, bleeding or frequency of urination

(d) Menstrual period

(e) Flu-like symptoms.

yes → See Problems 18, 82, 83, 85, 88, or 92

no ↓

Is there fever or does pain travel down the legs below the knee?

yes → **SEE PHYSICIAN TODAY**

no ↓

Is this due to a blow or fall?

yes → **CALL PHYSICIAN TODAY**

no ↓

APPLY HOME TREATMENT

is the result of a fall or a blow to the back, X-rays are indicated; otherwise, they usually are not. X-rays reveal injury only to bones, not to muscles. If the history and the physical examination are consistent with lower-back strain, the physician's advice will be similar to that described above. A muscle relaxant may be prescribed. If the history and physical examination indicate damage to the nerves leaving the spinal cord, a special X-ray may be necessary. Only if nerve damage is present or the condition fails to heal for a prolonged period should hospitalization, traction, or surgery be required.

63 Neck Pain

Most neck pain is due to strain and spasm of the neck muscles. The common "crick in the neck" upon arising is one example of neck muscle strain. This type of neck pain can be adequately treated at home. Neck pains that require the attention of the physician include those due to meningitis or a pinched nerve.

With fever and headache there is a possibility of meningitis. More commonly, neck pain is part of a "flu" syndrome with fever, muscle aches, and a headache. When generalized aching throughout the muscles is present, a visit to a physician will seldom be useful. Meningitis may cause intense spasm of the neck muscles and a very stiff neck. When stiff neck is due to one of the more common causes of muscle spasm, the patient usually can touch the chin to the chest, even if with difficulty. If in doubt, it is better to see the physician for an ordinary muscle spasm than to attempt to treat meningitis at home.

Arthritis or injury to the neck can result in a pinched nerve. When this is the cause of neck pain, the pain may extend down the arm, or there may be numbness or tingling sensations in the arm or hand. This pain is only on one side, and neck stiffness is not prominent.

Home Treatment

Neck pain in the morning may be due to sleeping habits. Sleep on a firm surface and discontinue use of a pillow. A firm mattress is best. If this is not possible, a bed board will make the present mattress firmer. Warmth may be of benefit in relieving spasms and pain. Heat may be applied with hot showers, hot compresses, or a heating pad. Heat may be used as often as practical, but don't burn the skin. Aspirin or acetaminophen (Tylenol, Tempra), two tablets every four hours, will help relieve pain and inflammation. Neck pain, like back pain, is slow to improve and may take several weeks to resolve. If an ordinary bath towel is folded lengthwise to a long four-inch wide strip, wrapped around the neck at bedtime and secured with tape or a safety pin, relief obtained overnight is often striking.

If pain does not lessen in a week, call the doctor.

What to Expect at the Doctor's Office

If meningitis is suspected, the physician will perform a spinal tap as well as several blood tests. If a pinched nerve is likely, X-rays of the neck will be done. A muscle relaxant may be prescribed and perhaps a more powerful pain reliever. Valium is a frequently prescribed muscle relaxant. Prescription drugs are not necessarily better than aspirin; usually you are just as well off with home therapy if no infection or nerve damage is present.

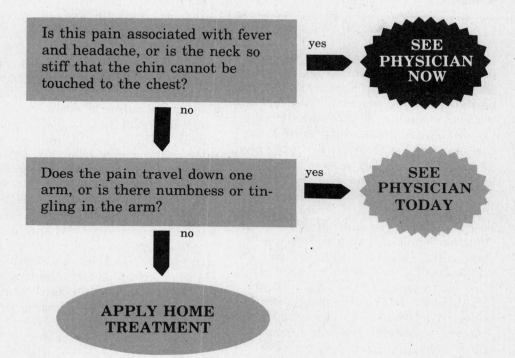

Is this pain associated with fever and headache, or is the neck so stiff that the chin cannot be touched to the chest?

yes → **SEE PHYSICIAN NOW**

no

Does the pain travel down one arm, or is there numbness or tingling in the arm?

yes → **SEE PHYSICIAN TODAY**

no

APPLY HOME TREATMENT

64 Elbow, and Shoulder Pain

Pain located around the elbow or shoulder is common and almost never poses a serious threat to life. Nonetheless, it can persist for a long time and cause discomfort and disability. Most of the time the pain comes from the "soft tissues" near the joint and not from the bones or the joint itself. These soft tissues include the ligaments, the tendons, and the "bursae" —small pockets of special tissue that separate and lubricate the cartilage and bones that form the joint. Medical terms for these conditions include "bursitis," "tendonitis," "calcific tendonitis," and the self-descriptive "tennis elbow" (Problem 65) and "frozen shoulder." If the hand and shoulder, but not the elbow, are involved, the "shoulder-hand syndrome" (a rather unusual problem) may be present and the physician should be consulted.

Therapy for these conditions is not very advanced. The physician usually recommends home treatment and reserves injection and surgery for only the very worst and long-lasting problems. Prescriptive medications are *not* predictably effective. The physician should be seen if the condition is very severe, if a fracture or dislocation is suspected, or if home treatment fails to relieve the problem. Unfortunately, you may be just as unhappy with the results of your physician's remedies.

Home Treatment

Irritation and inflammation of these soft tissues subsides with rest and time and becomes worse with active use of the involved part. Usually, about six weeks is required for the tissues to fully heal. If the part is too rigidly immobilized, two tissues may stick together (adhesion) during healing, resulting in permanent loss of a portion of the normal range of motion. Thus, treatment is designed to rest the part, and to exercise it enough to prevent adhesions.

The activity that caused the problem should be discontinued. An arm sling may be used to rest the shoulder or elbow. Gentle heat may help. Carefully work the shoulder or elbow through its range of motion twice daily to preserve mobility. This is best done immediately after application of heat or a warm bath or shower. Aspirin or acetaminophen (Tylenol), two tablets (10 grains) every four hours, may be taken as needed.

Some authorities in sports medicine feel that problems related specifically to tennis or golf swings are treated more appropriately with lessons from the local pro than with pills from the local doctor. Poor sports technique results in most of these sprains. This approach is well worth considering. The pro should be less expensive than the doctor and at least you can expect some help with your game.

The physician should be called if the condition persists beyond three weeks.

What to Expect at the Doctor's Office

The physician will examine the affected area and will give general suggestions similar to those above. If pressure at a particular place reproduces most of your pain, injection of a corticosteroid medication into that area sometimes gives relief. Even if they work, two or three injections are plenty; many prominent athletes, particularly baseball pitchers, have had joints damaged by a combination of continuing the irritating activity and using steroid injections to keep the

65 "Tennis" Elbow

Tennis elbow m[...]
cases of tenni[...]
tor's office[...]
sociated [...]
usual[...]
scv[...]

Is this due to an injury?

no

Are any of the following present?
(a) Fever
(b) Swelling and redness
(c) Inability to use the joint

no

Is this elbow pain associated with tennis or twisting motions of the forearm?

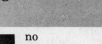

yes → See **"Tennis" Elbow** (Problem 65).

no

APPLY HOME TREATMENT

inflammation down. Oral cortisone-like drugs or narcotic pain relievers are generally *not* indicated. Common sense and good medical practice both require that local problems be treated with local therapies if possible.

...y be a misnomer. Of the ... s elbow that reach the doc- ... less than half are actually as- ... with playing tennis. The rest ... y result from work such as using a ...ewdriver.

Whether from use of a racket or screwdriver, tennis elbow seldom should be cause for a visit to a doctor. The doctor's help is needed only for prolonged cases of tennis elbow that don't get better; perhaps one person in a thousand needs such help.

One reason you may feel confident about tennis elbow is that you can diagnose it as well as your doctor can. The diagnosis does not depend on tests or special examinations. Tennis elbow is simply defined as pain in the lateral (outer) portion of the elbow and upper forearm, which occurs after repeatedly using a rolling or twisting motion of the forearm, wrist, and hand. A large number of medical disorders have been offered as the explanation for tennis elbow, including arthritis, tendonitis, and bursitis. But there is still no agreement among doctors as to exactly what the problem is, so you're not likely to get a precise diagnosis beyond "tennis elbow."

Professional tennis players get a different kind of tennis elbow from the rest of us. They have more problems with the inside portion of the elbow and forearm than the outside portion, probably due to the very hard serve which is such an important part of the professional game.

For amateurs, the cause of tennis elbow seems to be the tremendous impact transmitted to the forearm when the tennis ball is hit with the backhand motion.

When you realize that the tennis racket may be traveling at 300 to 350 miles per hour before it contacts the ball and is immediately slowed to perhaps 150 miles an hour at contact, it is easy to see that tremendous force is involved. Tennis players seem to raise the risk that this force will create tennis elbow by:

1. Hitting the ball with the elbow bent rather than locked in a position of strength.
2. Attempting to put top spin on the ball by rolling the wrist on contact.
3. Holding the thumb behind the racket.
4. Using a racket which is head-heavy, especially a wood racket.
5. Switching from a slower to a faster court surface.
6. Using heavier balls such as those of foreign manufacture and the pressureless type.
7. Using a very stiff racket.

If your "tennis" elbow comes from using a screwdriver, there may be similar types of practices that contribute to the problem.

According to the experts, the single most important preventive measure for tennis players is to employ a two-handed backhand stroke.

Home Treatment

The preventive measures, of course, are the things you should do at the first sign of tennis elbow. But suppose that you have already adopted a two-handed backhand, switched to a light and supple metal racket, stopped trying to put top spin on the ball by rolling your wrist, bought some lighter balls, switched to a slower surface, adjusted your grip so that the thumb is no longer behind the racket, and made a point of hitting every stroke with the elbow locked in a position of strength. Or suppose your job or favorite hobby requires repeated use of screwdrivers or other tools that aggravate the problem. What now? Well, rest-

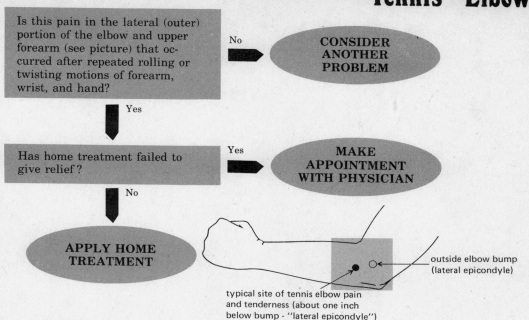

Is this pain in the lateral (outer) portion of the elbow and upper forearm (see picture) that occurred after repeated rolling or twisting motions of forearm, wrist, and hand?

No → **CONSIDER ANOTHER PROBLEM**

Yes ↓

Has home treatment failed to give relief?

Yes → **MAKE APPOINTMENT WITH PHYSICIAN**

No ↓

APPLY HOME TREATMENT

outside elbow bump (lateral epicondyle)

typical site of tennis elbow pain and tenderness (about one inch below bump - "lateral epicondyle")

ing the arm will surely make it hurt less, but most likely taking two weeks off will not cure it forever. Interestingly enough, most authorities now think that you can "play with pain" and not cause disastrous permanent injury.

We advocate a common sense approach: if you are having pain, cut down on your playing time, take it easy, and give your elbow a rest. When you do play, warm up slowly and do some stretching exercises of the wrist and elbow before you begin to hit the ball. Taking aspirin immediately before and after playing may help decrease the amount and duration of the discomfort.

What to Expect at the Doctor's Office

What can you expect if you are the one person in a thousand with tennis elbow who has persistent pain that is so severe that it interferes with your daily activities? If you really have employed all the measures above, the next step is for the doctor to inject a pain-reliever and corticosteroid (cortisone-like drug) into the painful area. Doctors usually give such an injection with a recommendation to rest the arm for two weeks. In most cases the combination of rest and injection will relieve the problem, but unfortunately the pain is likely to come back when you use the arm again. In this event the doctor may try another injection. But these injections cannot go on forever, and it is generally agreed that three or four injections into the same place should be the limit. And what if the problem continues? Yes, it can be operated on and the surgeons who operate say it seems to help in most cases. Unfortunately we can find no scientific study of the results of such operations. It appears to us that surgery should be a last resort—an act of desperation. If you get to this point, perhaps it's time to take up another game.

K Problems of Stress and Strain

66 Stress, Tension and Anxiety

Stress is a normal part of our lives. It is not necessarily good or bad. It is not a disease. But reactions to stress can vary enormously, and some of these reactions are undesirable. The most frequent undesirable reaction is anxiety. The degree of anxiety is much more a function of the individual than the degree of stress. A person who reacts with excessive anxiety to everyday stress has a personal rather than a medical problem. The person who does not recognize anxiety as the problem will have difficulty in solving the problem.

Some common symptoms of anxiety are insomnia and an inability to concentrate; these symptoms can lead to a vicious cycle that aggravates the situation. But the symptoms are effects, not causes, and the person who focuses on the insomnia or the lack of concentration as the cause of the problem is far from a solution.

Most communities have several resources that can help with problems of anxiety. Ministers, social workers, friends, neighbors, and family may each play a beneficial role. The physician is an additional resource but is not necessarily the first or the best place to seek help for these problems.

Grief is an appropriate reaction to certain situations, such as death of a loved one or loss of a job. In such cases, time is the healer although significant help may be gained from various family and community resources. Working through grief is an important part of getting over a loss. If the reaction persists several months, seek outside help.

The limitations of drugs such as tranquilizers or alcohol in this situation must be understood. While they may provide short-term symptomatic relief, they are brain depressants which do not enhance mental processes or solve problems. They are a crutch. In this instance, the long-term use of a crutch insures that the person using it will become a cripple. The underlying problem must be confronted.

Home Treatment

An honest attempt to identify the cause of the anxiety is a necessary first step in resolving the problem. When physical symptoms are due to job pressures, marital woes, wayward children, or dominating parents, the situation must be accurately identified, admitted, and confronted. When anxiety or depression is reactive, the cause is often obvious, and simply talking about it with friends or counselors will help. In other instances, identifying the source of the anxiety will be difficult, painful, time-consuming, and may eventually require the help of a professional counselor or psychiatrist. Unfortunately, no scientific studies have been able to show better results with any particular type of therapy. So pay your money and take your choice.

Additionally, sometimes these symptoms are simply an overdose of one of the minor poisons of everyday life—caffeine. Watch out for coffee if you drink more than four cups a day, and remember that No-Doz, APCs, and a variety of cold and headache remedies contain caffeine.

What to Expect at the Doctor's Office

The family physician will attempt to identify the problem and determine if

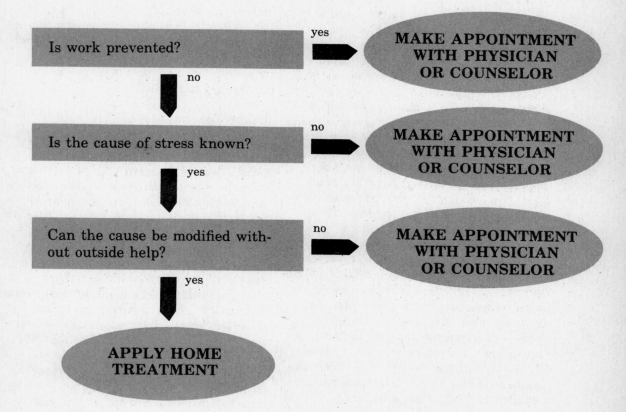

Is work prevented? — **yes** → MAKE APPOINTMENT WITH PHYSICIAN OR COUNSELOR

no ↓

Is the cause of stress known? — **no** → MAKE APPOINTMENT WITH PHYSICIAN OR COUNSELOR

yes ↓

Can the cause be modified without outside help? — **no** → MAKE APPOINTMENT WITH PHYSICIAN OR COUNSELOR

yes ↓

APPLY HOME TREATMENT

the help of a psychiatrist or psychiatric social worker is required. Personal questions may be asked, and frank, honest answers must be given. Try to report the underlying problems and avoid emphasis on the effects, such as insomnia, muscle aches, headache, or inability to concentrate.

67 Headache

Headache is the most frequent single complaint of modern times. Most commonly, the causes are tension and muscle spasms in the neck, scalp, and jaw. For this reason, massaging or otherwise relaxing neck muscles can help relieve headaches. Most tension headaches will respond to the simple measures outlined below. Headache *without any other associated symptoms* is almost always caused by tension. Fever and a neck so stiff that the chin cannot be touched to the chest suggest the possibility of meningitis rather than an ordinary tension headache. But even with these symptoms, meningitis is rare. Flu is much more likely. Muscle aches and pains are seldom seen in meningitis.

Most so-called "migraine" headaches are really severe tension headaches. True migraine headaches are often associated with nausea or vomiting and preceded by visual phenomena such as seeing "stars." They are caused by constriction and then relaxation of blood vessels in the head. True migraine headaches occur *only* on one side of the head during any particular attack. Drugs that constrict the blood vessels, such as Cafergot, will help migraine but not tension headaches.

Increased internal pressure due to head injury can cause headache and may also cause vomiting and difficulties with vision. See **Head Injuries**, Problem 11.

Headache is not a reliable indicator of blood pressure. A high-blood-pressure headache usually occurs in the morning; tension headaches are more common later in the day. When headaches increase in severity or frequency, involve the back or top of the head, or are worse in the morning, check the blood pressure. Headache patients frequently worry about brain tumors. In the absence of paralysis or personality change, the possibility that an intermittent headache is caused by a brain tumor is exceedingly remote. Although constant and slowly increasing headaches are frequently noted in patients with brain tumors, it is usually some other symptom that leads the physician to institute an investigation for tumor. Headache patients should not be routinely investigated for possible brain tumor, since the tests are both costly and hazardous.

Home Treatment

Aspirin is the superdrug. Use it or another pain-reliever such as acetaminophen (Tylenol, Tempra). All of the usual over-the-counter drugs are quite effective in relieving headache. Aspirin may be taken with milk or some food in order to prevent stomach irritation. Headache may frequently be relieved by massage or heat applied to the back of the upper neck or by simply resting with eyes closed and the head supported. Persistent headaches that do not respond to such measures should be brought to the attention of a physician. Headaches that are associated with difficulty in using the arms or legs, or with slurring of speech, as well as those which are rapidly increasing in frequency and severity, also require a visit to the doctor.

What to Expect at the Doctor's Office

The physician will examine the head, eyes, ears, nose, throat, and neck, and will also test nerve function. The temperature will be taken. Abnormalities are rarely found. The diagnosis of a headache is usually based on the history given by the patient. If the physician feels that the headache may be "migraine," an ergot preparation (Cafergot)

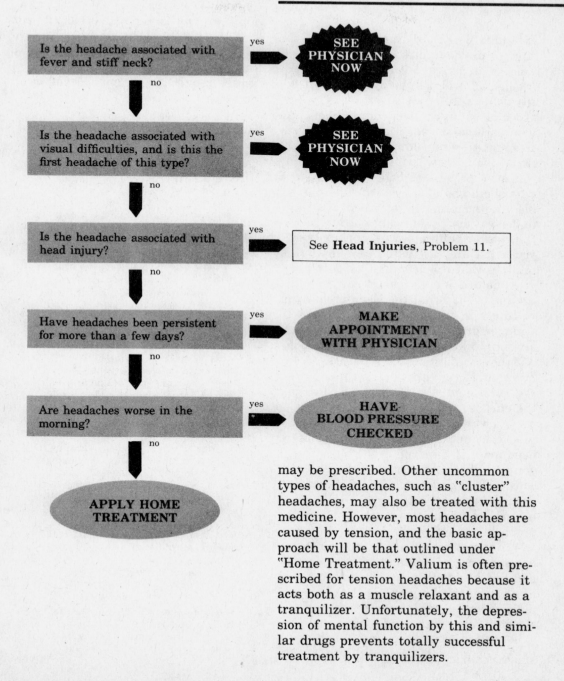

Is the headache associated with fever and stiff neck?

yes → **SEE PHYSICIAN NOW**

no ↓

Is the headache associated with visual difficulties, and is this the first headache of this type?

yes → **SEE PHYSICIAN NOW**

no ↓

Is the headache associated with head injury?

yes → See **Head Injuries**, Problem 11.

no ↓

Have headaches been persistent for more than a few days?

yes → **MAKE APPOINTMENT WITH PHYSICIAN**

no ↓

Are headaches worse in the morning?

yes → **HAVE BLOOD PRESSURE CHECKED**

no ↓

APPLY HOME TREATMENT

may be prescribed. Other uncommon types of headaches, such as "cluster" headaches, may also be treated with this medicine. However, most headaches are caused by tension, and the basic approach will be that outlined under "Home Treatment." Valium is often prescribed for tension headaches because it acts both as a muscle relaxant and as a tranquilizer. Unfortunately, the depression of mental function by this and similar drugs prevents totally successful treatment by tranquilizers.

68 Insomnia

Insomnia is not a disease, but it is a continuing problem for some 15 to 20 million Americans and causes occasional problems for almost everyone else. It is a frequent cause of physician visits, many of which could be avoided. Many of these visits are made specifically to obtain sleeping pills that are "better" than those available without a prescription. Yet most physicians believe that sleeping pills should be avoided whenever possible. The nonprescription sleep aids seem to depend mostly on what doctors call the "placebo effect"—they work only if you think they are going to. The antihistamines that they contain can increase daytime drowsiness and actually create the impression that the sleep problem is getting worse rather than better. The stronger drugs available by prescription are more likely to really knock you out, but they do not produce a natural sleep. They interfere with what is called rapid eye movement (REM) sleep, and this has the effect of making the sleep less restful. As a result, you feel more fatigued than ever and may conclude that you need more of the drug. The more drug you use, the more disturbed your sleep. This vicious cycle is called drug-dependent insomnia, is well recognized, and has become an unnecessary national health problem.

For most people, occasional insomnia is a response to excitement. Both good and bad events in your life can keep you awake and thinking at night. Other people develop "poor sleeping schedules"—sleeping late or napping during the day makes sleep at night more difficult. Finally, some people don't realize that they actually need less sleep as they get older. When they can't sleep the usual number of hours, they believe they have a sleeping problem.

A disease is rarely the cause of insomnia. Problems that wake you up at night are not insomnia; you should consult the sections of this book that deal with your particular complaints. Problems such as chest pain or shortness of breath require the prompt attention of a physician.

Home Treatment

Here are some suggestions for developing a successful approach to your insomnia:

1. Avoid using alcohol in the evening. Although one small after-dinner drink may do no harm, larger quantities of alcohol interfere with REM sleep and can cause you to feel agitated the next day.

2. Avoid caffeine for at least two hours before bedtime.

3. Establish a regular bedtime, but don't go to bed if you feel wide awake.

4. Use the bedroom for bedroom activities only. If the bedroom is used for activities such as paying bills, studying, having discussions or arguments, watching the late night news, and so on, entering the bedroom can be a signal to become more active rather than to go to sleep.

5. Break your chain of thought before retiring. Relax by reading, watching television, taking a bath, or listening to soothing music—something that helps to keep your mind from working overtime on life's more serious activities. The *National Geographic* is highly recommended as pleasant and distracting evening reading. Medical journals put many physicians asleep; it has been suggested that reading something that you feel you should but really don't want to is sure to put you to sleep.

6. A snack seems to help many people. In fact, some foods such as milk, meat, and lettuce have a natural sleep inducer called L-tryptophan. A

Has faithfully applied home treatment been unsuccessful for three weeks or more?

yes → **MAKE APPOINTMENT WITH PHYSICIAN**

no ↓

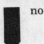

APPLY HOME TREATMENT

single glass of milk probably does not have enough tryptophan to induce sleep by itself, but the tradition of drinking a glass of warm milk seems to work well for many people. However, don't eat a big meal before going to bed since this seems to cause problems with sleep.

7. Exercise regularly, but not in the last two hours before going to bed. Exercise dispels tension and gives you what has been called "that good tired feeling."

8. Give up smoking. At least one study indicates that smokers have more difficulty in getting to sleep than nonsmokers.

9. Once you get into bed, the use of creative imagery and relaxation techniques to keep your mind off unrestful thoughts can be useful. "Counting sheep" is the oldest kind of creative imagery. Another technique is to progressively concentrate on relaxing each part of your body. Imagine that your toes weigh a thousand pounds and couldn't move if you wanted them to. Let them go completely limp. Work your way up to the top of your head by relaxing the muscles in each part of your body. Don't neglect the facial muscles—tension often centers in the forehead or jaw and keeps you from relaxing. An alternative is to imagine that your breath is coming in through the toes of your right foot, all the way up to your lungs, and back out through the same foot. Do this three times; repeat the procedure for the left foot and then for each of your arms. Another image technique is to concentrate on a pleasant scene that relaxes you, such as walking along a beach and hearing the sounds of the ocean.

10. Finally, many researchers believe that the most effective natural sleep inducer is—you guessed it—sex.

It may take several weeks or more to establish a new, natural sleeping routine. If you are unable to make progress after giving these methods an honest try, a visit to the physician may be necessary.

What to Expect at the Doctor's Office

The physician will focus on your sleeping schedule, factors that could be causing stress and anxiety, and other factors related to sleep such as the use of drugs. The physical examination is less important than the history and may be brief. In some instances, the physician may want to obtain further studies such as an electroencephalogram during sleep. On rare occasions it may be necessary to refer you to a center for the study of sleep disturbances where complex studies of your sleep pattern may be conducted.

69 The Hyperventilation Syndrome

Anxiety, especially unrecognized anxiety, can lead to physical symptoms. The hyperventilation syndrome is such a problem. In this syndrome a nervous or anxious person begins to be concerned by his or her breathing and rapidly develops a feeling of inability to get enough air into the lungs. This is often associated with a feeling of chest pain or constriction. The sensation of being out-of-breath leads to further overbreathing and a lowering of the carbon dioxide level in the blood; carbon dioxide is present in exhaled air. The lower level of carbon dioxide gives symptoms of numbness, tingling of the hands, and dizziness. The numbness and tingling may extend to the feet and also may be noted around the mouth. Occasionally, spasms of the muscles of the hands may occur.

This syndrome is almost always a disease of young adults. While it is more common in women it is also frequently seen in men. Usually this syndrome occurs in people who recognize themselves as being nervous and tense. It often occurs when such people are subjected to additional stress, to alcohol, or to situations where there is an advantage for the patient to have a sudden dramatic illness. A classical example is the occurrence of the hyperventilation syndrome during separation or divorce proceedings, so that a call for help is sent out to the estranged spouse.

Hyperventilation may also be a response to severe pain, particularly severe abdominal pain. A person with abdominal pain or severe pain of any type is not a candidate for home treatment. When in doubt, take a person who is hyperventilating due to anxiety to the physician's office rather than discount a potentially serious problem because it is associated with hyperventilation.

Home Treatment

The symptoms of the hyperventilation syndrome are due to the loss of carbon dioxide into the atmosphere as a result of the overbreathing. If the patient breathes into a paper bag, so that the carbon dioxide is taken back into the lungs rather than being lost into the atmosphere, the symptoms will be alleviated. This usually requires five to fifteen minutes with a small paper bag held loosely over both the nose and the mouth. This is not always as easy as it sounds, since a major feature of the hyperventilation syndrome is panic and a feeling of impending suffocation. Approaching such a person with a paper bag for their mouth and nose may prove to be difficult, so be sure first to reassure the patient.

Repeated attacks may occur. Once the patient has honestly recognized that the problem is anxiety rather than an organic disease, the attacks will stop because the panic component will not occur. Convincing the patient is the problem. Having the patient voluntarily hyperventilate (fifty deep breaths while lying on a couch) and demonstrating that this reproduces the symptoms of the previous episode is frequently helpful. Patients are usually afraid that they are having a heart attack or are on the verge of a nervous breakdown. Neither is true, and when fear is dissipated, hyperventilation usually ceases.

What to Expect at the Doctor's Office

The physician will obtain a history and direct attention primarily to the examination of the heart and lungs. In the young person with a typical syndrome,

266

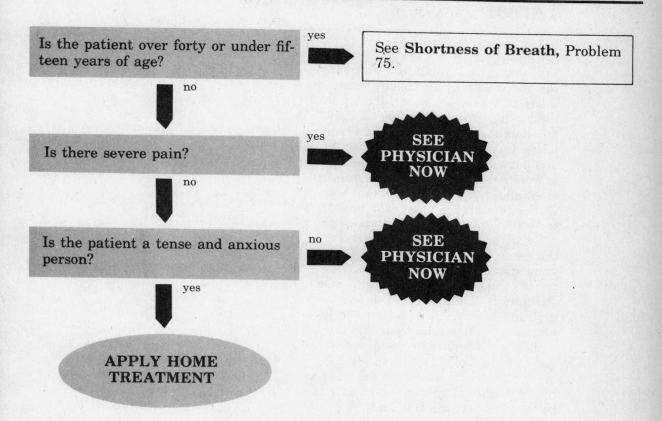

Is the patient over forty or under fifteen years of age?

yes → See **Shortness of Breath**, Problem 75.

no ↓

Is there severe pain?

yes → SEE PHYSICIAN NOW

no ↓

Is the patient a tense and anxious person?

no → SEE PHYSICIAN NOW

yes ↓

APPLY HOME TREATMENT

without abdominal pain and with a normal physical examination, the diagnosis of hyperventilation is easily made. Electrocardiograms and chest X-rays are seldom needed. These procedures may occasionally be necessary in less clear-cut cases. If the diagnosis of hyperventilation syndrome is made, the physician will usually provide a paper bag and the instructions given above. A tranquilizer may be administered; we prefer merely to reassure the patient. It is seldom possible to deal effectively with the cause of the anxiety during the hyperventilation episode. The patient should not assume that the underlying problem is solved simply because the hyperventilation has been controlled.

70 Lump in the Throat

The feeling of a "lump in the throat" is the best known of all anxiety symptoms. There may even be some difficulty in swallowing, although eating is possible if an effort is made. The sensation is intermittent and is made worse by tension and anxiety. The difficulty in swallowing is worst when the patient concentrates on swallowing and on the sensations within the throat. As an experiment, try to swallow rapidly several times without any food or liquid, and concentrate on the resulting sensation. You will then understand this symptom.

Several serious diseases can cause difficulty in swallowing. In these cases, difficulty in swallowing begins slowly, is noticed first with solid foods and then with liquids, results in loss of weight, and is more likely to be found in those over forty. "Lump in the throat," like the hyperventilation syndrome, is likely to be found in young adults, most frequently women.

Home Treatment

The central problem is not the symptom but, rather, the underlying cause of the anxiety state. See **Stress, Tension, and Anxiety**, Problem 66. Recognition that the symptom is minor is crucial to its disappearance.

What to Expect at the Doctor's Office

After taking a medical history and examining the throat and chest, a physician occasionally may feel that X-rays of the esophagus are necessary. If an abnormality of the esophagus is found, further studies may be performed. Reassurance will probably be the treatment that is given.

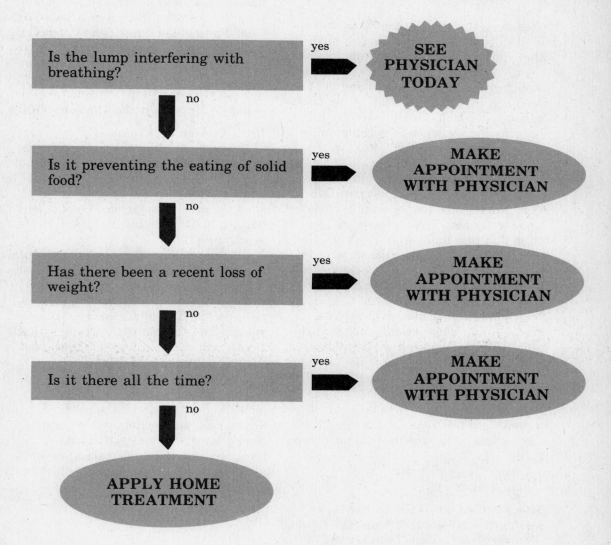

Is the lump interfering with breathing? — yes → **SEE PHYSICIAN TODAY**

no

Is it preventing the eating of solid food? — yes → **MAKE APPOINTMENT WITH PHYSICIAN**

no

Has there been a recent loss of weight? — yes → **MAKE APPOINTMENT WITH PHYSICIAN**

no

Is it there all the time? — yes → **MAKE APPOINTMENT WITH PHYSICIAN**

no

APPLY HOME TREATMENT

71 Weakness and Fatigue

Weakness and fatigue are often considered to be similar terms, but in medicine they have distinct and separate meanings. Weakness refers to lack of strength. Fatigue is tiredness, lack of energy, or lethargy. Weakness is usually the more serious condition. Weakness is particularly important when it is confined to one area of the body, as occurs in a stroke.

Lack of energy, on the other hand, is typically associated with a virus infection or with a feeling of anxiety, depression, or tension. Weakness in one area is often due to a problem in the muscular or nervous system, whereas general fatigue is caused by a large variety of illnesses, especially those that create anxiety or depression.

Hypoglycemia means "low blood sugar," and many patients fear that this problem is the cause of their tiredness. A few individuals do in fact feel shaky and tremulous several hours after a meal because their blood sugar level drops at that point. However, they do *not* feel fatigued. Low blood sugar throughout the day can cause fatigue, but this is a rare condition.

Home Treatment

There is time and need for careful reflection on the causes of fatigue. The most common situation has been termed "the tired housewife syndrome." This outdated slang is still sometimes used to describe the large number of young and middle-aged women who come to the physician's office complaining of fatigue and requesting tests for anemia or thyroid problems. Many adult women are mildly iron deficient, and thyroid problems may cause fatigue, but it is very unusual for one of these conditions to be the cause of fatigue. In most cases, fatigue is more closely related to boredom, unhappiness, disappointment, or just plain hard work. The patient should consider these possibilities before consulting the physician.

Vitamins are rarely helpful, but in moderation they do not hurt.

What to Expect at the Doctor's Office

If the problem is weakness of only part of the body, the physician will concentrate the examination on the nerve and muscle functions. A typical stroke will be identified by such an examination, whereas more uncommon ailments may require further testing and special procedures.

If the problem is fatigue, the medical history is the most important part of the encounter. Physical examination of heart, lungs, and the thyroid gland can be expected. The physician may test for anemia and thyroid dysfunction, as well as other problems. Inquiry into the patient's life-style and feelings is important. There are no direct cures for the most common fatigue syndromes. "Pep pills" do not work, and the rebound usually makes the problem worse. Tranquilizers generally intensify fatigue. Vacations, job changes, undertaking new activities, or making marital adjustments are far more helpful.

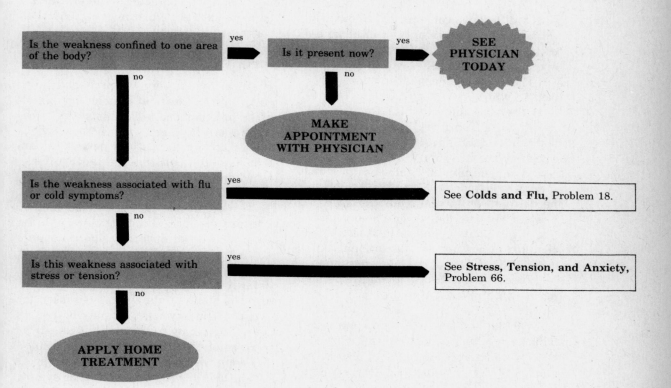

Is the weakness confined to one area of the body? — **yes** → Is it present now? — **yes** → **SEE PHYSICIAN TODAY**

no ↓

Is it present now? — **no** ↓ → **MAKE APPOINTMENT WITH PHYSICIAN**

Is the weakness associated with flu or cold symptoms? — **yes** → See **Colds and Flu,** Problem 18.

no ↓

Is this weakness associated with stress or tension? — **yes** → See **Stress, Tension, and Anxiety,** Problem 66.

no ↓

APPLY HOME TREATMENT

72 Dizziness and Fainting

Three different problems are frequently introduced by the complaint of dizziness or fainting: loss of consciousness, vertigo, and lightheadedness.

True unconsciousness includes a period in which the patient has no control over the body and of which there is no recollection. Therefore, if consciousness is lost while standing, the patient will fall and may sustain injury in doing so. The common symptom of "blackout" in which the patient finds it difficult to see and needs to sit or lie down but can still hear is not true loss of consciousness. Such "blackouts" may be related to changes in posture or to emotional experiences. True loss of consciousness may be caused by a number of conditions and needs to be investigated promptly by a physician.

Vertigo is caused by a problem in the balance mechanism of the inner ear. Since this balance mechanism also helps to control eye movements, there is loss of balance and the room seems to be spinning around. Walls and floors may seem to lurch in crazy motions. Most vertigo has no definite cause and is thought to be due to a viral infection of the inner ear. A physician should be seen since further studies may be needed, and the vertigo itself may be totally disabling.

"Lightheadedness" is by far the most common of these problems. It is that woozy feeling that is such a common part of flu or cold syndromes. If such a feeling is associated with other flu or cold symptoms, refer to Problem 18. Lightheadedness that is not associated with other symptoms is usually not serious either. Many such patients are tense or anxious. Others have low blood pressure and regularly feel lightheaded when suddenly standing up. This is called "postural hypotension" and does not require treatment. If lightheadedness is associated with the use of drugs, the physician should be contacted to determine if the drug should be discontinued. Alcohol is a frequent cause.

Home Treatment

"Postural hypotension" is probably the most common cause of momentary blackout or light-headedness. This problem becomes more frequent with increasing age. Typically, the patient notices a transient loss of vision or a lightheaded feeling when going suddenly from a reclining or sitting position to upright posture. The symptoms are caused by a momentary lack of blood flow to the brain. Most people will experience this phenomenon at one time or another. The therapy is to avoid sudden changes in posture. Unless postural hypotension suddenly becomes worse, it alone is not sufficient reason for a visit to the physician. It may be reported on the next routine visit unless it is extremely frequent and troublesome.

People who experience a persistent light-headed feeling without other symptoms should be reassured that this is not an indication of brain tumor or other hidden disease. This type of lightheadedness often disappears when anxiety is resolved. Not infrequently it is a problem with which the patient must learn to live.

What to Expect at the Doctor's Office

The physician will obtain a history with emphasis on making the distinctions outlined above. If loss of consciousness is the problem, the heart and lungs will be examined and the nerve function will be

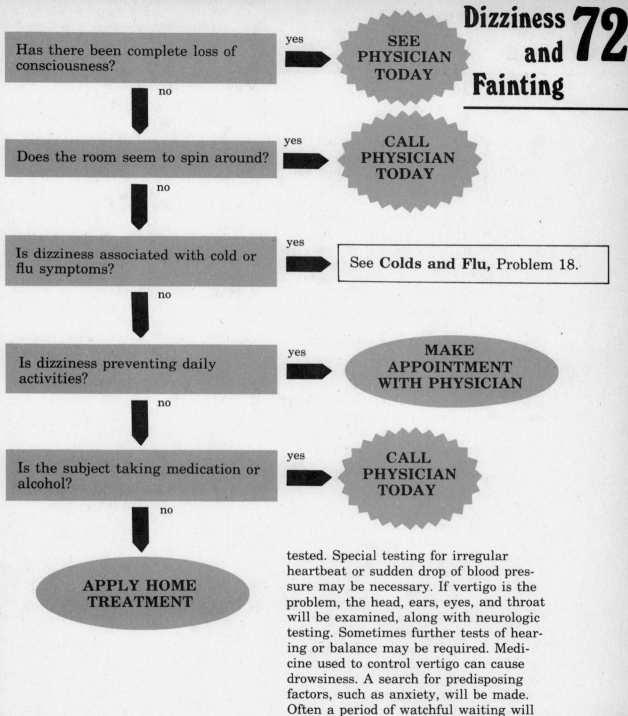

Has there been complete loss of consciousness?

yes → **SEE PHYSICIAN TODAY**

no ↓

Does the room seem to spin around?

yes → **CALL PHYSICIAN TODAY**

no ↓

Is dizziness associated with cold or flu symptoms?

yes → See **Colds and Flu,** Problem 18.

no ↓

Is dizziness preventing daily activities?

yes → **MAKE APPOINTMENT WITH PHYSICIAN**

no ↓

Is the subject taking medication or alcohol?

yes → **CALL PHYSICIAN TODAY**

no ↓

APPLY HOME TREATMENT

tested. Special testing for irregular heartbeat or sudden drop of blood pressure may be necessary. If vertigo is the problem, the head, ears, eyes, and throat will be examined, along with neurologic testing. Sometimes further tests of hearing or balance may be required. Medicine used to control vertigo can cause drowsiness. A search for predisposing factors, such as anxiety, will be made. Often a period of watchful waiting will be advised.

73 Depression

The blues and the blahs—everybody gets them sometime. There is no more common problem. It can range from a feeling of no energy all the way to such an overwhelming sense of unhappiness and defeat that ending it all seems the only way out.

Depression may seem to be simple fatigue or a general feeling of ill health. You just don't feel good, and you may not know the reason why. The future may seem to hold no promise. There is a sense of loss—a feeling of defeat or of having lost something—or someone—important.

In medical terms, most depression is "reactive," meaning that it is a reaction to an unhappy event. It is natural to have some depression after a loss such as a death of a friend or relative, or after a substantial disappointment at home or work.

Time and activity take care of most depressions. After all, life has its ups as well as its downs; happiness also is inevitable. But if the depression is so great as to disrupt your work or family life for a substantial period of time, put a time limit on it by making an appointment with your doctor.

If the problem is so severe that suicide has been considered, do not hesitate to call the physician immediately and let the doctor help. If you have no physician or you prefer to get help elsewhere, many communities have telephone "hotlines" for such situations. If there is no such service near you, call the nearest emergency room or health care facility. They will get help for you.

Home Treatment

Activity, both mental and physical, has long been recognized as the natural antidote for depression. Recently it has been shown that regular exercise is as effective in mild depression as the drugs usually prescribed by doctors. Make a plan for activity and include regular exercise in it. Stay involved with others and let them help.

Make a point to tell someone about your problems. Getting it out helps, and there may be some suggestions that the listener can make to ease the burden.

What to Expect at the Doctor's Office

The physician will explore the issues and events associated with depression. Listening and responding are the most important things; the physician will make some suggestions about activities and exercise. The use of drugs will be avoided if possible; hospitalization is best if suicide is a possibility.

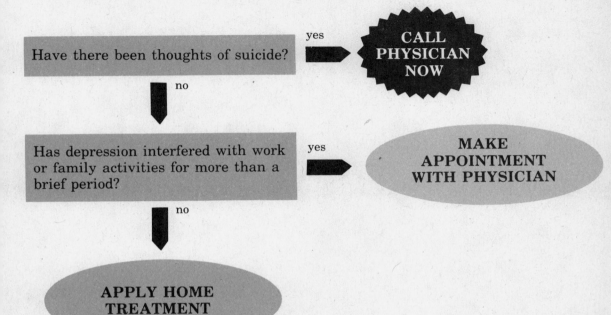

Have there been thoughts of suicide? — yes → **CALL PHYSICIAN NOW**

no ↓

Has depression interfered with work or family activities for more than a brief period? — yes → **MAKE APPOINTMENT WITH PHYSICIAN**

no ↓

APPLY HOME TREATMENT

L Chest Pain, Shortness of Breath, and Palpitations

74 Chest Pain

Chest pain is a serious symptom meaning "heart attack" to most people. Serious chest discomfort should usually be evaluated by a physician.

However, pain can *also* come from the chest wall (including muscles, ligaments, ribs, and rib cartilage), the lungs, the outside covering of the lungs (pleurisy), the outside covering of the heart (pericarditis), the gullet, the diaphragm, the spine, the skin, and the organs in the upper part of the abdomen. Often it is difficult even for a physician to determine the precise origin of the pain. Therefore, there can be no absolute rules that enable you to determine which pains may be treated at home. The following guidelines usually work and are used by doctors, but there are occasional exceptions.

A shooting pain lasting a few seconds is common in healthy young people and means nothing. A sensation of a "catch" at the end of a deep breath is also trivial and does not need attention. Heart pain almost never occurs in previously healthy men under thirty years of age or women under forty and is uncommon for the next ten years in each sex. Chest-wall pain can be demonstrated by pressing a finger on the chest at the spot of discomfort and reproducing or aggravating the pain. Heart and chest-wall pain are rarely present at the same time. The hyperventilation syndrome (Problem 69) is a frequent cause of chest pain, particularly in young people. If you are dizzy or have tingling in your fingers, suspect this syndrome.

Pleurisy gets worse with a deep breath or cough; heart pain does not. When inflammation of the outside covering of the heart is present, the pain may throb with each heartbeat. Ulcer pain burns with an empty stomach and gets better with food; gallbladder pain often becomes more intense after a meal. Each of these four conditions, when suspected, should be evaluated by a physician.

While heart pain may be mild, it is usually intense. Sometimes a feeling of pressure or squeezing on the chest is more prominent than actual pain. Almost always, the pain or discomfort will be beneath (inside) the breastbone. It may also be felt in the jaw or down the inner part of either arm. There may be nausea, sweating, dizziness, or shortness of breath. When shortness of breath or irregularity of the pulse is present, it is particulary important that a physician be seen immediately. Heart pains may occur with exertion and go away with rest—in this case they are not an actual "heart attack" but are termed "angina pectoris" or "angina."

Home Treatment

You should be able to deal effectively with pain arising from the chest wall. Pain medicines such as aspirin or acetaminophen, topical treatments such as Ben-Gay or Vicks Vaporub, and general measures such as heat and rest should help. If symptoms persist for more than five days, see the physician.

What to Expect at the Doctor's Office.

The physician will thoroughly examine the chest wall, lungs, and heart and will frequently order an electrocardiogram and blood tests. A chest X-ray is usually not helpful and may not be ordered. If the pain remains mysterious, a whole battery of expensive and complex tests may be recommended or required. Pain relief, by injection or by mouth, will sometimes be needed. Hospitalization will be required in instances when the heart is involved or the cause of the pain is not clear.

Do any of these conditions exist?

(a) Chest pain associated with short-ness of breath

(b) Irregular pulse

(c) Sweat or dizziness

(d) Severe pain

yes **SEE PHYSICIAN NOW**

no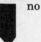

Is chest tender to touch in area of pain?

no ⮞ **MAKE APPOINTMENT WITH PHYSICIAN**

yes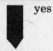

APPLY HOME TREATMENT

75 Shortness of Breath

This symptom is normal under circumstances of strenuous activity. The medical use of "shortness of breath" does not include shortness of breath after heavy exertion, "breathless" with excitement, or having clogged nasal passages. These instances are not cause for alarm.

When you get "winded" after slight exertion or at rest, or wake up in the night out of breath, or have to sleep propped up on several pillows to avoid becoming short of breath, you have a serious symptom that should be promptly evaluated by your physician. If wheezing is present, the problem is probably not as serious, but attention is needed just as promptly. In this instance, you may have asthma or early emphysema.

The hyperventilation syndrome (Problem 69) is a common cause of shortness of breath in previously healthy young people and is almost always the problem if the complaint of tingling fingers is present. In this syndrome the patient is actually overbreathing but has the sensation of shortness of breath. A second emotional problem that may present the complaint of difficult breathing is mental depression; deep sighing respirations are a frequent symptom in depressed individuals.

Home Treatment

Rest, relax, use the treatment described for the hyperventilation syndrome (Problem 69) if indicated. If the problem persists, see the physician. There isn't much that you can do for this problem at home.

What to Expect at the Doctor's Office

The physician will thoroughly examine the lungs, heart, and upper airway passages. Sometimes, electrocardiograms (EKG), chest X-rays, and blood tests will be necessary. Depending upon the cause and the severity of the problem, hospitalization, fluid pills, heart pills, or asthma medications may be needed. Oxygen is less frequently helpful than commonly imagined and can be very hazardous for patients with emphysema.

Is there shortness of breath at rest, or is shortness of breath associated with wheezing?

yes → **SEE PHYSICIAN NOW**

no ↓

Is there tingling in the fingers?

yes → See **The Hyperventilation Syndrome** (Problem 69).

no ↓

MAKE APPOINTMENT WITH PHYSICIAN

76 Palpitations

Everyone experiences palpitations. Pounding of the heart is brought on by strenuous exercise or intense emotion and is seldom associated with serious disease. Most of us have experienced the "bent-bumper syndrome"; after a near collision with another car, the heart seems to almost stop, then pounds with such force that you feel like you're being punched in the chest. Simultaneously, the knees become wobbly and the palms become sweaty. These events are due to a large discharge of adrenalin from the adrenal glands. Almost no one is concerned by such pounding of the heart. But if there is no obvious exertion or frightening event, many people become worried.

Most people who complain of palpitations do not have heart disease but are overly concerned about the possibility of such disease and thus overly sensitive to normal heart actions. Often this is because of heart disease in parents, other relatives, or friends.

An irregular or very fast pulse may be more serious. There is a normal variation in the pulse with respiration (faster when breathing in, slower when breathing out). Even though the pulse may speed or slow, the normal pulse has a regular rhythm. Occasional extra heartbeats occur in nearly everyone. Consistently irregular pulses, however, are usually abnormal. The pulse can be felt on the inside of the wrist, in the neck, or over the heart itself. Ask the nurse to check your method of taking pulses on your next visit. Take your own pulse and those of your family, noting the variation with respiration.

The most common time for palpita-

tions to occur is just before going to sleep. If the pulse rate is under 120, relax.

Hyperventilation may also cause pounding and chest pain, but the heart rate remains less than 120 beats per minute (see Problem 69).

In adults, a heart rate greater than 120 beats per minute (without exercise) is cause to check with your physician. Young children may have normal heart rates in that range, but they rarely complain of the heart pounding. If one does, check the situation with your physician. Keep in mind that the most frequent causes of rapid heart beat (other than exercise) are anxiety and fever. The presence of shortness of breath (Problem 75) or chest pain (Problem 74) increases the chances of a significant problem.

Home Treatment

If a patient seems stressed or anxious, focus on this rather than upon the possibilities of heart disease. If anxiety does not seem likely and the patient has none of the other symptoms on the chart, discuss it with the physician by phone. If the problem persists, see the physician.

What to Expect at the Doctor's Office

Tell the doctor the exact rate of the pulse and whether or not the rhythm was regular. Usually, the symptoms will disappear by the time you see the doctor, so the accuracy of your story becomes crucial. The doctor will examine your heart and lungs. An electrocardiogram (EKG) is unlikely to help if the problem is not present when it's being done. A chest X-ray is seldom needed. Do not expect reassurance from a physician that your heart will be sound for the next month, year, or decade. Your doctor has no crystal ball nor can he or she perform an annual tune-up or oil change. You, not the doctor, are in charge of preventive maintenance of your heart (see Chapters 1 and 2).

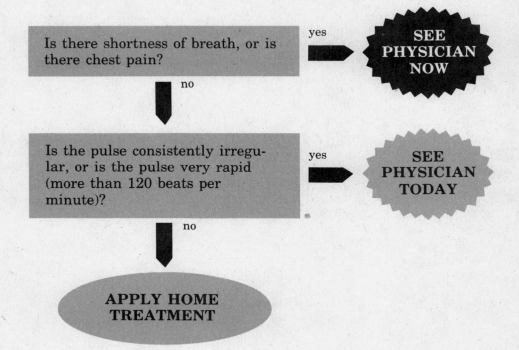

Is there shortness of breath, or is there chest pain?

yes → SEE PHYSICIAN NOW

no

Is the pulse consistently irregular, or is the pulse very rapid (more than 120 beats per minute)?

yes → SEE PHYSICIAN TODAY

no

APPLY HOME TREATMENT

M Eye Problems

285

77 Foreign Body in Eye

Eye injuries must be taken seriously. If there is any question, a visit to the physician is indicated.

A foreign body must be removed to avoid the threat of infection and loss of sight in that eye. Be particularly careful if the foreign body was caused by the striking of metal on metal; this can cause a small metal particle to strike the eye with great force and penetrate the eyeball.

Under a few circumstances, you may treat at home. If the foreign body was minor, such as sand, and did not strike the eye with great velocity, it may feel like it is still in the eye even when it is not. Small round particles like sand rarely stick behind the upper lid for long.

If it feels like a foreign body is present but it is not, then the cornea has been scraped or cut. A minor corneal injury will usually heal quickly without problems; a major one requires medical attention.

Even if you think the injury is minor, run through the decision chart daily. If any symptoms at all are present after forty-eight hours and are not clearly resolving, see the physician. Minor problems will heal within forty-eight hours—the eye repairs injury quickly.

Home Treatment

Be gentle. Wash the eye out. Water is good; a weak solution of boric acid is even better if readily available. Inspect the eye yourself and have someone else check it as well. Use a good light and shine it from both the front and the side. Pay particular attention to the cornea—the clear membrane that covers the colored portion of the eye. Do not rub the eye; if a foreign body is present, you will abrade or scratch the cornea. An eye patch will relieve pain; take it off each day for recheck—it is usually needed for twenty-four hours or less. Make the patch with several layers of gauze and tape firmly in place—you want some gentle pressure on the eye. Check vision each day; compare the two eyes, one at a time, by reading different sizes of newspaper type from across the room. If you are not sure that all is going well, see the doctor.

What to Expect at the Doctor's Office

The physician will check your vision and inspect the eye, including inspection under the upper lid—this is not painful. Usually, a fluorescent stain will be eye-dropped into the eye and the eye will then be examined under ultraviolet light—this is not painful or hazardous. An ophthalmologist (surgeon specializing in diseases of the eye) will examine the eye with a slit lamp. A foreign body, if found, will be removed. In the office, this may be done with a cotton swab, an eye-wash solution, or a small needle or "eye spud." An antibiotic ointment is sometimes applied, and an eye patch may be provided. Eye drops that dilate the pupil may be employed. X-rays may be taken if it is possible that a foreign body is inside the eye globe.

Are any of the following present:

(a) Can the foreign body be seen and does it remain after gentle washing?

(b) Could the injury have penetrated the globe of the eye?

(c) Can you see blood in the eye?

yes →

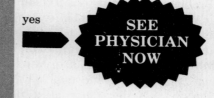

SEE PHYSICIAN NOW

no

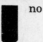

Is there any problem with vision, or does it feel like a foreign body might be trapped behind the upper lid?

yes →

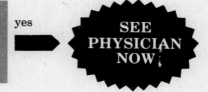

SEE PHYSICIAN NOW

no

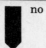

APPLY HOME TREATMENT

78 Eye Pain

Pain in the eye can be an important symptom and cannot be safely ignored for long. Fortunately, it is an unusual complaint. Itching and burning (see Problem 80) are more common. Eye pain may be due to injury, infection, or to an underlying disease. An important disease that can cause eye pain is "glaucoma," which may slowly lead to blindness if not treated. In glaucoma, the fluid inside the eye is under abnormally high pressure, and the globe is tense, causing discomfort. Lateral vision is the first to be lost. Gradually and almost imperceptibly, the field of vision is constricted until the patient has "tunnel vision." In addition, a patient often will see "halos" around lights. Unfortunately, this sequence can occur even when there is no associated pain.

Eye pain is a nonspecific complaint, and questions relating to the pain are often better answered under the more specific headings of **Foreign Body in Eye** (Problem 77), **Decreased Vision** (Problem 79), **Eye Burning, Itching, and Discharge** (Problem 80), and **Styes and Blocked Tear Ducts** (Problem 81). A feeling of tiredness in the eyes, or some discomfort after a long period of fine work (eye strain) is generally a minor problem and does not really qualify as eye pain. Severe pain behind the eye may result from migraine headaches and pain either over or below the eye may suggest sinus problems. Pain in both eyes, particularly upon exposure to bright light (photophobia), is common with many viral infections such as flu and will go away as the infection improves. More severe photophobia, particularly when only one eye is involved, may indicate inflammation of the deeper layers of the eye and requires a physician.

Home Treatment

Except for eye pain associated with a viral illness or eyestrain, or minor discomfort that is more tiredness than pain, we do not recommend home treatment. In these instances, resting the eyes, taking a few aspirin, and avoiding bright light may be of help. Follow the chart to the discussion of other problems where appropriate. When symptoms persist check them out in a routine appointment with your physician.

What to Expect at the Doctor's Office

The physician will check vision, eye movements, and the back of the eye with an ophthalmoscope. An ophthalmologist (surgeon specializing in diseases of the eye) may perform a slit lamp examination. If glaucoma is possible, the doctor may check the pressure of the globe. This is simple, quick, and painless. (Many physicians feel uncomfortable with eye symptoms, and referral to an ophthalmologist is common; you may wish to go directly to an ophthalmologist if you have major concern).

Is the pain related to a significant injury, or is a foreign body present?

yes → See **Foreign Body in Eye** (Problem 77).

no ↓

Is the pain an itching or burning sensation, or are the eyes runny?

yes → See **Eye Burning, Itching, and Discharge** (Problem 80).

no ↓

Is there any decrease in vision?

yes → See **Decreased Vision** (Problem 79).

no ↓

Is the pain severe or prolonged beyond forty-eight hours?

yes → **SEE PHYSICIAN TODAY**

no ↓

Is the pain more of a feeling of tiredness in the eyes or are flu-like symptoms present?

no → **MAKE APPOINTMENT WITH PHYSICIAN**

yes ↓

APPLY HOME TREATMENT

79 Decreased Vision

Few people need urging to protect their sight. Decrease in vision is a major threat to the quality of life. Usually, professional help is needed. A few syndromes do not require a visit to a health professional. When small, single "floaters" drift across the eye from time to time and do not affect vision, they are not a matter for concern. Slight, reversible blurring of vision may occur after outdoor exposure or with overall fatigue. In young people, sudden blindness in both eyes is commonly a hysterical reaction and is not a permanent threat to sight; such patients need a doctor but not an eye doctor. After a problem has disappeared, it is often impossible to tell what it was; if your problem has reversed itself, wait to see if it comes back before seeing the physician.

Usually, the question is not whether to see a health professional but, rather, which one to see. The choice is generally between the ophthalmologist, the optometrist, and the primary-care physician (generalist, internist, or pediatrician). An *optician* dispenses glasses and does not diagnose eye problems. The *optometrist* is not a physician but is capable of evaluating the need for glasses and determining what prescription lens gives the best vision. Conditions treated by the optometrist are myopia (nearsightedness), hyperopia (farsightedness), and astigmatism (crooked-sightedness). If another disease of the eye is suspected, the optometrist may refer you to an *ophthalmologist*, who is a highly trained physician and surgeon. The ophthalmologist is the final authority on diseases localized to the eye. Sometimes an eye problem is part of a general health problem; in these cases the primary physician is sometimes appropriate.

Try to find the right health professional on the first attempt; this will save you time and money. Eventually, you will be referred to the right person, but it is in your interest to make the process simpler. Following are some examples that usually work, although you may have to modify them for your particular situation. Depending upon the physician availability in your area, the choice will often be different.

- School nurse detects decreased vision in child: ophthalmologist or optometrist—possibly myopia (nearsightedness)
- Sudden blindness in one eye in an elderly person: ophthalmologist or internist—possible stroke or temporal arteritis
- Halos around lights and eye pain: ophthalmologist—possibly acute glaucoma (increased pressure in the eye)
- Gradual visual decrease in an adult who wears glasses: ophthalmologist or optometrist—change in refraction of the eye
- Sudden blindness in both eyes in a healthy young person: internist or ophthalmologist—possible hysterical reaction
- Gradual blurring of vision in an older person, not helped by moving closer or farther away: ophthalmologist—possible cataract (scar tissue forming in the lens of the eye)
- Older person who sees far objects best: optometrist or ophthalmologist—presbyopia or farsightedness
- Blurred vision, thirst, large urine output: internist—possible diabetes
- Visual change while taking a medi-

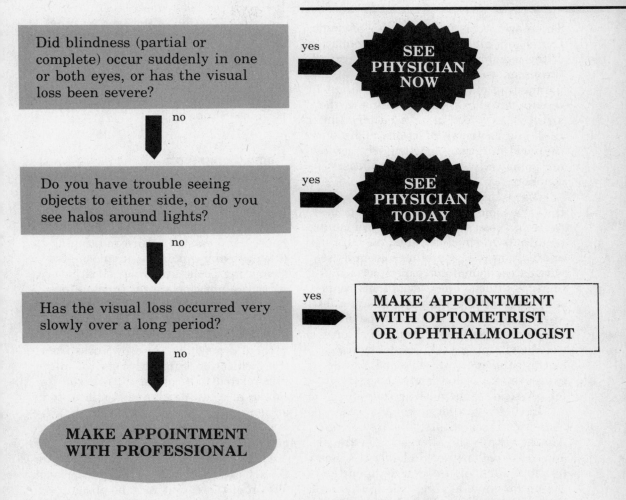

Did blindness (partial or complete) occur suddenly in one or both eyes, or has the visual loss been severe? — yes → **SEE PHYSICIAN NOW**

no

Do you have trouble seeing objects to either side, or do you see halos around lights? — yes → **SEE PHYSICIAN TODAY**

no

Has the visual loss occurred very slowly over a long period? — yes → **MAKE APPOINTMENT WITH OPTOMETRIST OR OPHTHALMOLOGIST**

no

MAKE APPOINTMENT WITH PROFESSIONAL

cine: call the prescribing physician—the drug may be responsible

• Decreased vision, one eye, with a "shadow" or "flap" in the visual field: ophthalmologist—possible retinal detachment

What to Expect at the Doctor's Office

The physician will check vision, eye movements, pupils, back of eye, and eye pressure when indicated; slit lamp examination will be done on occasion. A general medical evaluation will be done as required. Refraction to determine a proper corrective lens may be needed; busy ophthalmologists will sometimes refer this procedure to an optometrist. Surgery will be recommended for some conditions.

291

80 Eye Burning, Itching, and Discharge

These symptoms usually mean "conjunctivitis" or "pink eye," with inflammation of the membrane that lines the eye and the inner surface of the eyelids. The inflammation may be due to an irritant in the air, an allergy to something in the air, a virus infection, or a bacterial infection. The bacterial infections and some of the viral infections (particularly herpes) are potentially serious but are least common.

Many tourists have trouble reading the "Welcome to Los Angeles" sign because of these symptoms. Environmental pollutants in smog can produce burning and itching that sometimes seem as severe as the symptoms experienced in a tear-gas attack. These symptoms represent a chemical conjunctivitis and affect anyone exposed to enough of the chemical. The smoke-filled room, the chlorinated swimming pool, the desert sandstorm, sunglare on a ski slope, or exposure to a welder's arc can give similar physical or chemical irritation.

In contrast, allergic conjunctivitis affects only those people who are allergic. Almost always the allergen is in the air, and grass pollens are probably the most frequent offender. Depending upon the season for the offending pollen, this problem may occur in spring, summer, or fall and usually lasts two to three weeks.

A minor conjunctivitis frequently accompanies a viral cold, giving the well-known symptoms and lasting only a few days. Some viruses, such as herpes, cause deep ulcers in the cornea and interfere with vision. Bacterial infections cause pus to form, and a thick plentiful discharge runs from the eye. Often the eyelids are crusted over and "glued" shut upon wakening. These infections can cause ulceration of the cornea and are serious.

Some major diseases affect the deeper layers of the eye—those layers that control the operation of the lens and the size of the pupillary opening. This condition is termed "iritis" or "uveitis" and may cause irregularity of the pupil or pain when the pupil reacts to light. Medical attention is required. For true eye pain, see Problem 78.

Home Treatment

If a physical, chemical, or allergic exposure is the cause of the symptoms, there is nothing to do but avoid the exposure. Dark glasses, goggles at work, closed houses and cars with air-conditioning to filter the air, avoidance of chlorinated swimming pools, and other such measures are appropriate. Antihistamines, either over the counter or by prescription, may help slightly if the problem is an allergy—but don't expect total relief without a good deal of drowsiness from the medication. Similarly, a viral infection related to a cold or flu will run its course in a few days, and it is best to be patient.

If it doesn't clear up, if the discharge gets thicker, or if you have eye pain or a problem with vision, see your physician. Do not expect a fever with a bacterial infection of the eye; it may be absent. Since the infection is superficial, washing the eye gently will help remove some of the bacteria, but the physician should still be seen. Murine, Visine, and other eyedrops may soothe minor conjunctivitis but do not cure.

This is a complaint that should urge you to social action. If the smoking of others around you is annoying, say so. If an industrial plant in your area is polluting, get them to clean up their act.

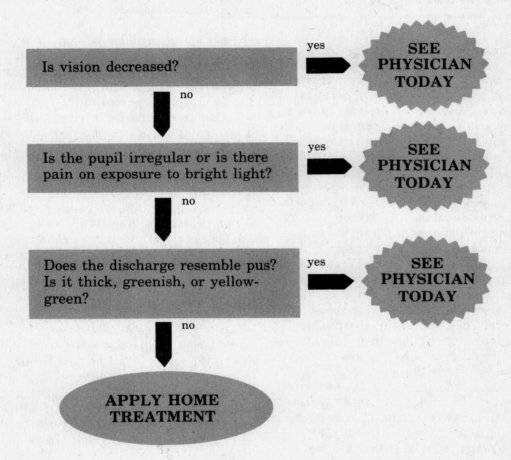

Is vision decreased? — **yes** → SEE PHYSICIAN TODAY

no ↓

Is the pupil irregular or is there pain on exposure to bright light? — **yes** → SEE PHYSICIAN TODAY

no ↓

Does the discharge resemble pus? Is it thick, greenish, or yellow-green? — **yes** → SEE PHYSICIAN TODAY

no ↓

APPLY HOME TREATMENT

What to Expect at the Doctor's Office

The physician will check vision, eye motion, eyelids, and the reaction of the pupil to light. An ophthalmologist (surgeon specializing in eye diseases) may perform a slit-lamp examination. Antihistamines may be prescribed and general advice may be given. Antibiotic eyedrops or ointments are frequently given. Cortisone-like eye ointments should be prescribed infrequently; certain infections (herpes) may get worse with these medicines. If herpes is diagnosed—usually by an ophthalmologist—special eyedrops and other medicines will be needed.

293

Styes and Blocked Tear Ducts

We might have called this problem "bumps around the eyes," since that is how they appear. Styes are infections (usually with staphylococcal bacteria) of the tiny glands in the eyelids. They are really small abscesses and the bumps are red and tender. They grow to full size over a day or so. Another type of bump in the eyelid, called a chalazion, appears more slowly over many days or even weeks and is not red or tender. A chalazion often requires drainage by a doctor, whereas most styes will respond to home treatment alone. However, there is no urgency in the treatment of a chalazion, and home treatment will not cause any harm.

Tears are the lubricating system of the eye. They are continually produced by the tear glands and then drained away into the nose by the tear ducts. These tear ducts are often incompletely developed at birth so that the drainage of tears is blocked. When this happens, the tears may collect in the tear duct and cause it to swell, appearing as a bump along the side of the nose just below the inner corner of the eye (see figure). This bump is not red or tender unless it has become infected. Most blocked tear ducts will open by themselves in the first month of life and most of the remainder will respond to home treatment. Tears running down the cheek are seldom noted in the first month of life because the infant produces only a small volume of tears.

The eyeball itself is *not* involved in a stye or a blocked tear duct. Problems with the eyeball, and especially with vision, should not be attributed to these two relatively minor problems.

Home Treatment

Stye: Apply warm, moist compresses for ten to fifteen minutes at least three times a day. As with all abscesses, the objective is to drain the abscess. The compresses help the abscess to "point," which means that the tissue over the abscess becomes quite thin and the pus in the abscess is very close to the surface. After an abscess points, it often will drain spontaneously. If this does not happen, the abscess may need to be lanced by the physician. Most styes will drain spontaneously; they may drain inwardly toward the eye or outwardly onto the skin. Sometimes the stye goes away without coming to a point and draining. Chalazions usually do not respond to warm compresses but they will not be harmed by them. If no improvement is noted with home treatment after forty-eight hours, see the doctor.

Blockage of the tear ducts: Simply massage the bump downward with warm, moist compresses several times a day. If the bump is not red and tender (indicating infection), this may be continued for up to several months. If the problem exists for this long, discuss it with your physician. If the bump becomes red and swollen, antibiotic drops will be needed.

What to Expect at the Doctor's Office

If the stye is pointing and ready to be drained, the physician will open it with a small needle. If it is not pointing, compresses will usually be advised and antibiotic eyedrops sometimes will be added. Attempting to drain a stye that is not pointing is usually not very satisfactory. If the physician feels that the problem is a chalazion, it may be removed with mi-

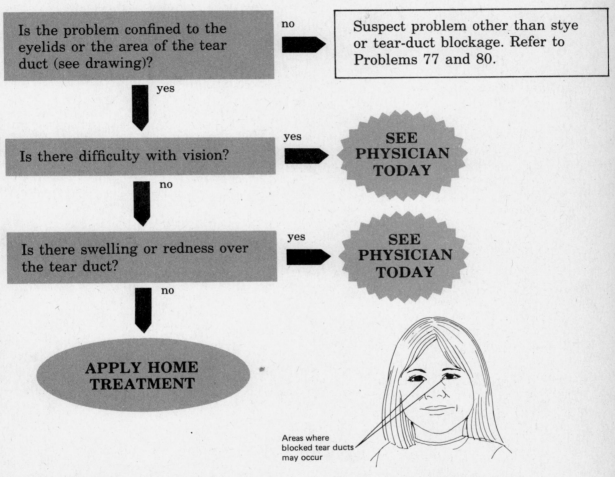

Is the problem confined to the eyelids or the area of the tear duct (see drawing)?

no → Suspect problem other than stye or tear-duct blockage. Refer to Problems 77 and 80.

yes ↓

Is there difficulty with vision?

yes → **SEE PHYSICIAN TODAY**

no ↓

Is there swelling or redness over the tear duct?

yes → **SEE PHYSICIAN TODAY**

no ↓

APPLY HOME TREATMENT

Areas where blocked tear ducts may occur

nor surgery. Whether to have the surgery will be up to you; chalazions are not dangerous and usually do not require removal.

If a child is over six months of age and is still having problems with blocked tear ducts, they can be opened in almost all cases with a very fine probe. This probing is successful on the first try in about 75 percent of all cases and on subsequent attempts in the remainder. Only rarely is a surgical procedure necessary to establish an open tear duct. For red and swollen ducts, antibiotic drops as well as warm compresses will usually be recommended.

N The Digestive Tract

82 Nausea and Vomiting

Viral infections are the most common cause of nausea and vomiting. When viruses are to blame, diarrhea is usually present as well. These illnesses will cure themselves with time; antibiotics do not help. There are drugs that may decrease the frequency of vomiting while waiting for the body to cure itself, but the results are often unimpressive. Many physicians believe that in most cases the risks of these drugs outweigh their benefits, especially in children.

The real threat in most vomiting is that of dehydration. The speed with which dehydration develops is dependent upon the size of the individual and the frequency of the vomiting. Therefore, infants who are vomiting very frequently are at the greatest risk. Signs of dehydration are:

- Marked thirst
- Infrequent urination or dark yellow urine.
- Dry mouth or eyes that appear sunken.
- Skin that has lost its normal elasticity. To determine this, gently pinch the skin on the stomach using all five fingers. When you release it, it should spring back immediately; compare with another person's skin if necessary. When the skin remains tented up and does not spring back normally, dehydration is indicated.

In addition to dehydration, evidence of bleeding (bloody or black vomitus), or severe abdominal pain require the physician's attention immediately. Some abdominal discomfort accompanies almost every case of vomiting, but severe pain is unusual.

Head injuries may be associated with vomiting. Careful observation as indicated in the discussion of **Head Injuries** (Problem 11) is necessary in order to correctly interpret the importance of vomiting in this situation.

Pregnancy, diabetes, or medications may all cause vomiting; when these are present, the doctor's advice over the phone is usually sufficient to determine the approach you should take. Headache and stiff neck along with vomiting are sometimes seen in meningitis so that an early call to the doctor's office for further advice is wise. Lethargy or marked irritability in a young child has a similar implication.

Home Treatment

The objective of home treatment is to provide as much fluid as possible without upsetting the stomach any further. Sip clear fluids such as water or ginger ale. Suck on ice chips if nothing else will stay down. Don't drink much at any one time, and avoid solid foods. Vomiting, diarrhea, and fever will increase your need for fluid, so take in as much as possible. As your condition improves, add soups, bouillon, jello, and applesauce. Milk products may help but sometimes aggravate the situation. Work up slowly to a normal diet. Popsicles® or iced fruit bars often work well with children. If symptoms persist for more than seventy-two hours, or if hydration is not adequate, call your physician.

What to Expect at the Doctor's Office

The history and physical examination will be focused on determining the degree of dehydration as well as the possible causes. Blood tests and a urinalysis may be ordered but are not always necessary. Plain X-rays of the abdomen are

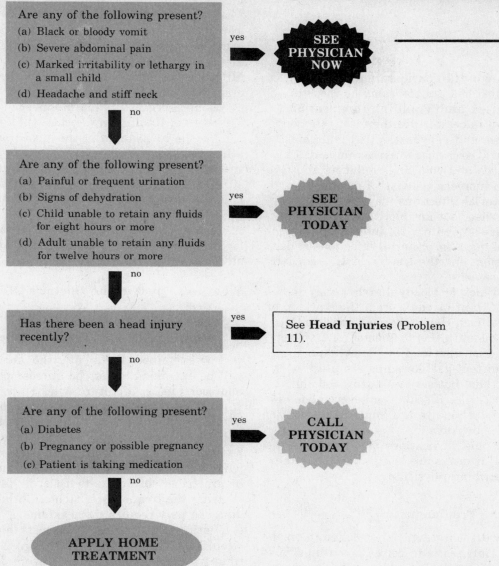

Are any of the following present?

(a) Black or bloody vomit

(b) Severe abdominal pain

(c) Marked irritability or lethargy in a small child

(d) Headache and stiff neck

yes → **SEE PHYSICIAN NOW**

no ↓

Are any of the following present?

(a) Painful or frequent urination

(b) Signs of dehydration

(c) Child unable to retain any fluids for eight hours or more

(d) Adult unable to retain any fluids for twelve hours or more

yes → **SEE PHYSICIAN TODAY**

no ↓

Has there been a head injury recently?

yes → See **Head Injuries** (Problem 11).

no ↓

Are any of the following present?

(a) Diabetes

(b) Pregnancy or possible pregnancy

(c) Patient is taking medication

yes → **CALL PHYSICIAN TODAY**

no ↓

APPLY HOME TREATMENT

usually not very helpful, but special X-ray procedures may be necessary in some cases. If dehydration is severe, intravenous fluids may be given. This may require hospitalization although this can often be done in the doctor's office. The use of antivomiting drugs is controversial, and they should be used only in severe cases. In addition to side effects involving the nervous system, there has been speculation that these drugs may contribute to the development of a serious illness known as Reyes syndrome in children.

83 Diarrhea

Many of the considerations with respect to diarrhea are the same as those in **Nausea and Vomiting** (Problem 82). Viral infections are the most common cause, and dehydration is the greatest risk. Diarrhea is often accompanied by nausea and vomiting; vomiting and fever both increase the risk of dehydration. Bacterial infections may also produce diarrhea, but antibiotics are seldom necessary. As with viral infections, the major danger in bacterial infections is dehydration, and the treatment is essentially the same.

Black or bloody diarrhea may signal significant bleeding from the stomach or intestines. However, medicines containing bismuth (Pepto Bismol) or iron may also turn the stool black. Cramping, intermittent gaslike pains are usual with diarrhea, but severe, steady abdominal pain is not. Bleeding or severe abdominal pain require the immediate attention of the physician.

Some medications may cause diarrhea; if drugs are being taken, call the prescribing physician.

Home Treatment

As with vomiting, the objective in treating diarrhea is to get as much fluid in as possible without upsetting the intestinal tract any further. Sip clear fluids such as water or ginger ale. If nothing else will stay down, sucking on ice chips is usually tolerated and provides some fluids. Popsicles®, iced fruit bars, apple juice, or flat sodas often work well in children. Gatorade and Pedialyte are fine but offer little advantage over the more common sources of fluid. Bouillon and jello can be used as well. When clear fluids are tolerated, constipating foods such as bananas, rice, applesauce, and toast can be given. The first letter of each of these foods combine to spell "brat," and this "brat" diet is often suggested by physicians. Milk and fats should be avoided for several days.

Nonprescription preparations such as Kaopectate, Kaolin, and Pectin will change the consistency of the stool from a liquid to a semisolid state, but they will not reduce the amount or frequency of the bowel movements. Adults may try narcotic preparations such as Parepectolin or Parelixir, but these should be avoided in children. If symptoms persist for more than ninety-six hours, call your physician.

What to Expect at the Doctor's Office

A thorough history and physical examination with special attention to assessing dehydration will be done. The abdomen will be examined. Frequently the stools will be examined under the microscope, and occasionally a culture will be taken. A urine specimen may be examined to assist in assessing dehydration. In cases of bacterial infection, an antibiotic may be used but this is uncommon. A narcoticlike preparation (such as Lomotil) may be prescribed for adults to assist in decreasing the frequency of stools. Chronic diarrhea may require more extensive evaluation of the stools, blood tests, and often, X-ray examinations of the intestinal tract. As with vomiting, severe dehydration will require intravenous fluids; this may be done in the doctor's office or may require hospitalization.

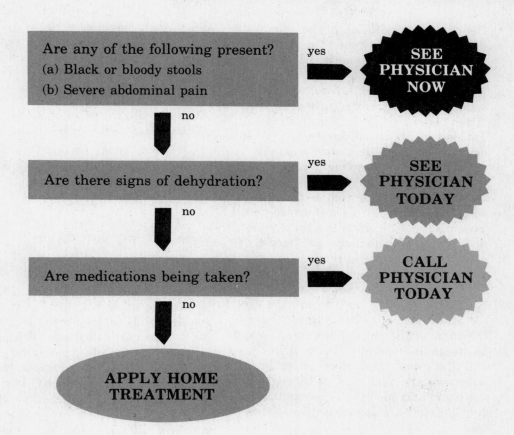

Are any of the following present?
(a) Black or bloody stools
(b) Severe abdominal pain

yes → **SEE PHYSICIAN NOW**

no

Are there signs of dehydration?

yes → **SEE PHYSICIAN TODAY**

no

Are medications being taken?

yes → **CALL PHYSICIAN TODAY**

no

APPLY HOME TREATMENT

84 Heartburn

Heartburn is irritation of the stomach or the esophagus, the tube that leads from the mouth to the stomach. The stomach lining is usually protected from the effects of its own acid; but certain factors, such as smoking, caffeine, aspirin, and stress cause this protection to be lost. The esophagus is not protected against acid, and a backflow of acid from the stomach into the esophagus causes irritation.

Ulcers of the stomach or the upper bowel (duodenum) may also cause pain. Treatment for ulcers is the same as for uncomplicated heartburn, provided that pain is not severe and there is no evidence of bleeding. Vomiting of black, "coffee ground" material or of bright red blood indicates the need to call the doctor. Black stools, rather like tar, have the same significance; however, iron supplements and bismuth (Pepto Bismol) will also cause black stools. Heartburn pain ordinarily does not go through to the back, and such pain may signal involvement of the pancreas or a severe ulcer.

Home Treatment

Avoid substances that aggravate the problem. The most common irritants are coffee, tea, alcohol, and aspirin. The contribution of smoking or stress must be considered in every patient. Relief is often obtained with the frequent (every one to two hours) use of nonabsorbable antacids like Maalox, Mylanta, or Gelusil (see Chapter 9, "The Home Pharmacy"). Antacids should be used with caution by people with heart disease or high blood pressure because of their high salt content. Sodium bicarbonate or Alka-Seltzer may provide quick relief but are not suitable for repeated use. Milk may be substituted for antacid but adds calories.

If the pain is worse when lying down, the esophagus is probably the problem. Measures that help prevent the backflow of acid from the stomach into the esophagus should be employed:

- Avoid reclining after eating.
- Elevate the head of the bed with four-inch to six-inch blocks.
- Discontinue wearing tight-fitting clothes (girdles, etc.), if applicable.
- Avoid eating or drinking for two hours prior to retiring.

If the problem lasts for more than three days, call your doctor.

What to Expect at the Doctor's Office

The physician will determine if the problem is due to stomach acid (a peptic acid syndrome). If so, treatment will be similar to that outlined above. Medications to reduce secretion of acid may be prescribed. X-rays of the stomach after swallowing barium (upper G.I.) may be done to determine the presence of ulcers and to note if backflow of acid from the stomach into the esophagus ("hiatal hernia") is present. Since the treatment for any acid syndrome is essentially the same, an X-ray is usually not done on the first visit. Any indication of bleeding will require a more vigorous approach to therapy.

Is there vomiting of black or bloody material, or is the patient passing tar-like black stools?

→ **yes** → **SEE PHYSICIAN NOW**

↓ **no**

Does the pain go through to the back?

→ **yes** → **SEE PHYSICIAN TODAY**

↓ **no**

Are all of these present?
(a) Burning pain just below breast bone or ribs.
(b) Some relief obtained with milk or bland food.
(c) Aggravated by coffee or tea, or alcohol.

→ **no** → **MAKE APPOINTMENT WITH PHYSICIAN**

↓ **yes**

APPLY HOME TREATMENT

85 Abdominal Pain

Abdominal pain can be a sign of a serious condition. Fortunately, minor causes for these symptoms are much more frequent.

Although abdominal pain can come from the esophagus, the stomach, the bowel, the female organs, the rectum, the gallbladder, an outpouching of the bowel, or other organs, such pain frequently raises immediate concern about possible appendicitis. Appendix pain usually occurs in the right lower quarter; kidney pain involves the back; the gallbladder—the right upper quarter; the stomach—the upper abdomen; and the bladder or female organs—the lower areas. Exceptions to these rules do occur. Pain from hollow organs (such as the bowel or gallbladder) tends to be intermittent and resembles gas pains (colic). Pain from solid organs (kidneys, spleen, liver) tends to be more constant. There are exceptions to these rules also.

If the pain is very severe or if bleeding from the bowel occurs, see a physician. Similarly, if there has been a significant recent abdominal injury, see the doctor—a ruptured spleen or other major problem is possible. Pain during pregnancy is potentially serious and must be evaluated; an "ectopic pregnancy" (in the fallopian tube rather than the uterus) can occur before the patient is even aware she is pregnant. Pain localized to one area is more suggestive of a serious problem than generalized pain (again, there are exceptions).

The most constant signal of appendicitis is the *order* in which symptoms occur:

- Pain—usually first around the belly button or just below the breast bone; only later in the right lower quarter of the abdomen; then
- Nausea or vomiting, or at the very least, loss of appetite;
- Local tenderness in the right lower quarter of the abdomen; then
- Fever—in the range of 100° to 102°F.

Appendicitis is unlikely if: fever precedes or is present at the time of first pain; there is *no* fever or a *high* fever (greater than 102°F) in the first twenty-four hours; vomiting accompanies or precedes the first bout of pain.

Rupture of the appendix, which is the complication we try to prevent by surgery, is unlikely within the first twelve to eighteen hours of pain. Many pains that may be confused with appendicitis will disappear in six to eight hours.

Of course, there are major problems other than appendicitis that cause abdominal pain. Gas pains and minor viral infections are the most common of the various causes. Use the chart to deal with abdominal pain logically.

Home Treatment

If the pain eventually proves to be due to a serious problem, the stomach should be emptied to allow prompt surgery or diagnostic tests. Sips of water or other clear fluids may be taken, but avoid solid foods. A bowel movement, passage of gas through the rectum, or a good belch may give relief—don't hold back. A warm bath helps some patients. The key to home treatment is periodic reevaluation; any persistent pain should be evaluated at the emergency room or the physician's office. Home treatment should be reserved for mild pains that resolve within

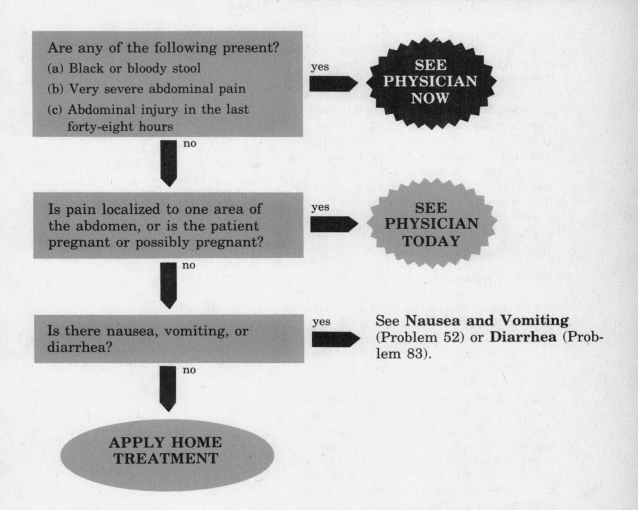

Are any of the following present?

(a) Black or bloody stool

(b) Very severe abdominal pain

(c) Abdominal injury in the last forty-eight hours

yes → **SEE PHYSICIAN NOW**

no ↓

Is pain localized to one area of the abdomen, or is the patient pregnant or possibly pregnant?

yes → **SEE PHYSICIAN TODAY**

no ↓

Is there nausea, vomiting, or diarrhea?

yes → See **Nausea and Vomiting** (Problem 52) or **Diarrhea** (Problem 83).

no ↓

APPLY HOME TREATMENT

twenty-four hours or are clearly identifiable as viral gastroenteritis, heartburn, or another minor problem.

What to Expect at the Doctor's Office

The physician will give a thorough examination, particularly of the abdomen. Usually, a white blood count and urinalysis and often other laboratory tests will be done. X-rays are often not important with pain of short duration but are sometimes needed. Observation in the hospital may be required. If the initial evaluation was negative but pain persists, reevaluation is necessary.

86 Constipation

Many patients are preoccupied with constipation. Concern about the shape of the stool, its consistency, its color, and the frequency of bowel movements is often reported to physicians. Such complaints are medically trivial. Only rarely (and then usually in older patients) does a change in bowel habits signal a serious problem. Weight loss and thin pencil-like stools suggest a tumor of the lower bowel. Abdominal pain and a swollen abdomen suggest a possible bowel obstruction.

Home Treatment

We like to encourage a healthy diet for the bowel, followed by a healthy disinterest in the details of the stool elimination process. The diet should contain fresh fruits and vegetables for their natural laxative action and adequate fiber residue. Fiber is present in brans, celery, and whole wheat breads and is absent in foods that have been too completely processed. Fiber draws water into the stool and adds bulk, thus it decreases the transit time from mouth to bowel movement and softens the stool.

Bowel movements may occur three times daily or once each three days and still be normal. The stools may change in color, texture, consistency, or bulk without need for concern. They may be regular or irregular. Don't worry about them unless there is a major deviation.

If laxatives are required, we prefer Metamucil, which is a fiber and bulk laxative. Milk of magnesia is satisfactory, but it and stronger traditional laxatives should not be used over a long period. For an acute problem, an enema may help. Fleet's enemas are handy and disposable. If such remedies are needed more than occasionally, ask your doctor about the problem on your next routine visit.

What to Expect at the Doctor's Office

If you have had a major change in bowel habits, expect a rectal examination and, usually, inspection of the lower bowel through a long (and sometimes cold) metal tube called a sigmoidoscope. An X-ray of the lower bowel (barium enema) is often needed. These procedures are generally safe and only mildly uncomfortable. If you have only a minor problem, you may receive advice similar to that under "Home Treatment," without examination or procedures.

Is constipation associated with the following?

(a) Very thin, pencil-like stools

(b) Abdominal pain and bloating

(c) Weight loss

no ↓

APPLY HOME TREATMENT

87 Rectal Pain, Itching, or Bleedi

Seld
th

...m is a rectal problem major, but ...e discomfort it can cause may materially interfere with the quality of life, and, unlike most other medical problems, rectal pain does not yield the dividend of a good topic for social conversation.

Hemorrhoids, or "piles," are the most common cause of these symptoms. There is a network of veins around the anus, and they tend to enlarge with age, particularly in individuals who sit a great deal during the day. Straining to have a bowel movement and the passage of hard, compacted stools tends to irritate these veins and they may become inflamed, tender, or clogged. The veins themselves are the "hemorrhoids." They may be external to the anal opening and visible, or they may be inside and invisible. Pain and inflammation usually disappear within a few days or a few weeks, but this interval can be extremely uncomfortable. After healing, a small flap (or "tag") of vein and scar tissue often remains.

Bleeding from the digestive tract should be taken seriously. We are *not* talking here about the bright red, relatively light bleeding that originates from the hemorrhoids but blood from higher in the digestive tract, which will be burgundy or black. Blood from hemorrhoids may be on the outside of the stool but will not be mixed into the stool substance and frequently will be seen on the toilet paper after wiping. Such bleeding

is not medically significant unless it persists for several weeks.

Often a child will suddenly awake screaming in the early evening with rectal pain. This almost always means pinworms. Though these small worms are seldom seen, they are quite common. They live in the rectum, and the female emerges at night and secretes a sticky and irritating substance around the anus into which she lays her eggs. Occasionally, the worms move into the vagina, causing pain and itching in that area. This is not a major problem; it may be treated at home *if* you have clearly identified the pinworms. The whole family should be treated to prevent reinfection.

If rectal pain persists more than a week, the physician should be consulted. In such cases, a fissure in the wall of the rectum may have developed, or an infection or other problem may be present.

Home Treatment

Hemorrhoids: Soften the stool by including more fresh fruits and fiber (bran, celery, whole wheat bread) in the diet, or by use of fiber bulk (Metamucil) or laxatives (milk of magnesia). Keep the area clean. Use the shower as an alternative to rubbing with toilet paper. After gently drying the painful area, apply zinc oxide paste or powder, which will protect against further irritation. The various proprietary hemorrhoid preparations are less satisfactory. We prefer not to use compounds with a local anesthetic agent, because these compounds may sensitize and irritate the area and may prolong healing. Such compounds have a "caine" in the brand name or in the list of ingredients. "Internal" hemorrhoids sometimes may be helped by using a soothing suppository in addition to stool-softening measures. If relief is not complete within a week, see the doctor. Even if the problem resolves quickly, mention it to your doctor on your next visit.

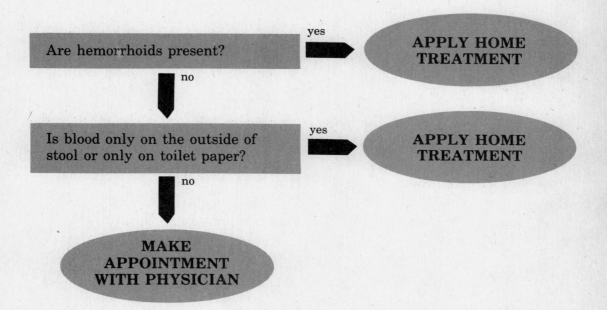

Are hemorrhoids present? — yes → **APPLY HOME TREATMENT**

no ↓

Is blood only on the outside of stool or only on toilet paper? — yes → **APPLY HOME TREATMENT**

no ↓

MAKE APPOINTMENT WITH PHYSICIAN

Pinworms: The Food and Drug Administration has indicated that pyrantel pamoate (Antiminth) will be available without prescription. Follow the directions supplied. If the problem persists, call your physician.

What to Expect at the Doctor's Office

Examination of the anus and rectum. If a clot has formed, the vein may be lanced and the clot removed. Major hemorrhoid surgery is seldom required and should be reserved for the most persistent problems. Usually, advice such as that given in "Home Treatment" will be given.

0 The Urinary Tract

88 Painful, Frequent, or Bloody Urination (Female)

The best-known symptoms of bladder infection are: (1) pain or burning upon urination, (2) frequent urgent urination, and (3) blood in the urine.

These symptoms are not always caused by infection due to bacteria. They can be due to a viral infection, excessive use of caffeine-containing beverages (coffee, tea, and cola drinks), bladder spasm, or they can have no known cause ("nerves"). When the cause is not bacteria, antibiotics will do no good.

Bladder infection is more common in women than it is in men (most women have it at one time or another) because the female urethra, the tube leading from the bladder to the outside of the body, is only about one-half inch long—a short distance for bacteria to travel to reach the bladder. Sometimes bladder infection is related to sexual activity; hence "honeymoon cystitis" has become a well-known medical syndrome.

Vomiting, back pain, or teeth-chattering, body-shaking chills are not typical of bladder infections but suggest kidney infection. This requires a more vigorous treatment and follow-up. A history of kidney disease (infections, inflammations, and kidney stones) also alters the treatment.

Bladder infections are common during pregnancy and may be more difficult to treat. Treatment must, of course, take the pregnancy into account.

Some physicians have developed procedures by which a patient with these symptoms may obtain a urinalysis without first seeing the physician. If the urinalysis indicates a possible bacterial infection, the patient is seen and appropriate therapy begun. If this is not the case, the patient is directed to use home treatment for twenty-four hours. If there is no relief during that time, the patient is then seen.

It is quite possible that many bacterial bladder infections will respond to home treatment alone. Still it makes good sense to use antibiotics when appropriate and this has become standard medical practice. Antibiotics may be especially important in recurrent bladder infections. Even if you are inclined toward doing without drugs, you should see the doctor unless the symptoms respond quickly and completely to home treatment.

Home Treatment

Definitive treatment of a urinary tract infection requires an antibiotic (which may not alter the symptoms for twenty-four hours). Quicker relief is afforded by home treatment, which should be started immediately.

- Drink a lot of fluids: Increase fluid intake to the maximum (up to several gallons of fluid in the first twenty-four hours). Bacteria are literally washed from the body during the resulting copious urination.
- Drink fruit juices: Putting more acid into the urine, while less important than the quantity of fluids, may help bring relief. Cranberry juice is the most effective, as it contains a natural antibiotic.

Begin home treatment as soon as symptoms are noted. For women with recurrent problems, an important preventive measure is to wipe the toilet tissue from front to back (*not* back to front) following urination. Most bacteria that cause bladder infections come from the rectum.

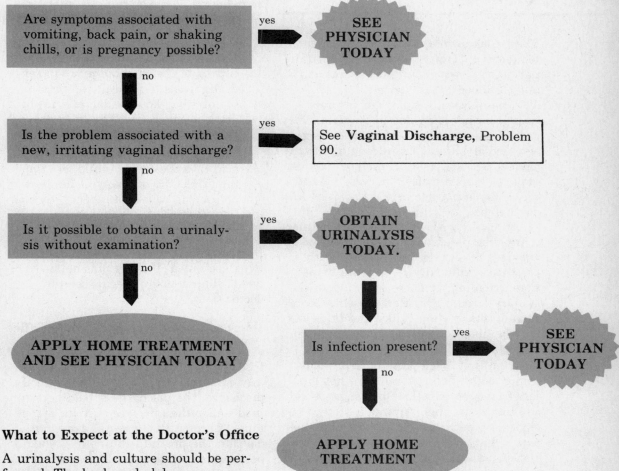

Are symptoms associated with vomiting, back pain, or shaking chills, or is pregnancy possible? — yes → **SEE PHYSICIAN TODAY**

no ↓

Is the problem associated with a new, irritating vaginal discharge? — yes → See **Vaginal Discharge**, Problem 90.

no ↓

Is it possible to obtain a urinalysis without examination? — yes → **OBTAIN URINALYSIS TODAY.**

no ↓

APPLY HOME TREATMENT AND SEE PHYSICIAN TODAY

Is infection present? — yes → **SEE PHYSICIAN TODAY**

no ↓

APPLY HOME TREATMENT

What to Expect at the Doctor's Office

A urinalysis and culture should be performed. The back and abdomen are usually examined. In women with a discharge, an examination of both the vagina and the discharge is often necessary. With preexisting kidney disease or symptoms of kidney infection, a more detailed history and physical are needed and extra laboratory studies may be necessary.

If urinary tract infection is proved, an antibiotic should be prescribed. Sulfa and ampicillin are the most commonly used, unless there is an allergy. Tetracycline is also used but should not be given to pregnant women or young children.

88 Painful, Frequent, or Bloody Urination (Male)

The best-known symptoms of bladder infection are: (1) pain or burning upon urination, (2) frequent urgent urination, and (3) blood in the urine.

These symptoms are not always caused by infection due to bacteria. They can be due to a viral infection or excessive use of caffeine-containing beverages (coffee, tea, and cola drinks), or they can have no known cause ("nerves"). When the cause is not bacteria, antibiotics will do no good.

In males with these symptoms, infection of the prostate gland (prostatitis) or venereal disease is quite likely. With prostatitis, difficulty in starting urination, dribbling, or decreased force of the urinary stream are often present. Gonorrhea discharges are milky and thick but may be noted only intermittently (refer to Problem 89).

Vomiting, back pain, or teeth-chattering, body-shaking chills are not typical of bladder infections but suggest kidney infection. This requires a more vigorous treatment and follow-up. A history of kidney disease (infections, inflammations, and kidney stones) also alters the treatment.

It is quite possible that many bacterial bladder infections will respond to home treatment alone. Still it makes good sense to use antibiotics when appropriate, and this has become standard medical practice. Antibiotics may be especially important in recurrent bladder infections. Even if you are inclined toward doing without drugs, you should see the doctor unless the symptoms respond quickly and completely to home treatment.

Home Treatment

Definitive treatment of a urinary tract infection requires an antibiotic (which may not alter the symptoms for twenty-four hours). Quicker relief is afforded by home treatment, which should be started immediately.

- Drink a lot of fluids: Increase fluid intake to the maximum (up to several gallons of fluid in the first twenty-four hours). Bacteria are literally washed from the body during the resulting copious urination.
- Drink fruit juices: Putting more acid into the urine, while less important than the quantity of fluids, may help bring relief. Cranberry juice is the most effective, as it contains a natural antibiotic.

Begin home treatment as soon as symptoms are noted. If symptoms persist for twenty-four hours or recur, see the doctor.

What to Expect at the Doctor's Office

A urinalysis and culture should be performed. The back and abdomen are usually examined. In males with urethral discharge, the discharge should be examined under the microscope. With symptoms of prostatitis, a rectal examination (so that the prostate can be felt) should be expected. With preexisting kidney disease or symptoms of kidney infection, a more detailed history and physical as well as extra laboratory studies may be needed.

If urinary tract infection is proved, an antibiotic should be prescribed. Tetracycline, erythromycin, and ampicillin are the most commonly used, unless there is an allergy. Tetracycline should not be given to young children.

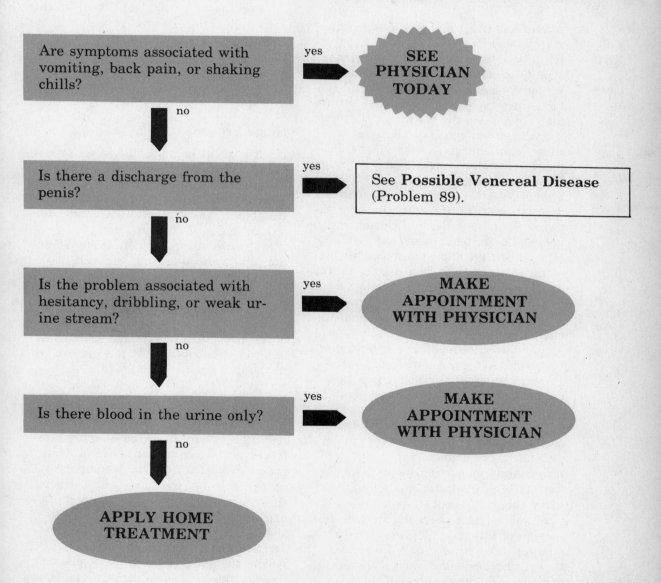

Are symptoms associated with vomiting, back pain, or shaking chills?

yes → **SEE PHYSICIAN TODAY**

no ↓

Is there a discharge from the penis?

yes → See **Possible Venereal Disease** (Problem 89).

no ↓

Is the problem associated with hesitancy, dribbling, or weak urine stream?

yes → **MAKE APPOINTMENT WITH PHYSICIAN**

no ↓

Is there blood in the urine only?

yes → **MAKE APPOINTMENT WITH PHYSICIAN**

no ↓

APPLY HOME TREATMENT

89 Discharge from the Penis or Possible Venereal Disease in Men

A venereal disease is any disease that is transmitted by sexual contact, but the term "VD" usually refers to gonorrhea or syphilis. Seldom are these diseases spread by means other than sexual contact, since the organisms do not survive for long outside the body.

Gonorrhea (the clap, the strain) causes a discharge from the penis. Primary symptoms—burning and pain upon urination and a thick, mucous discharge—start within two to fourteen days of exposure. If not treated, the patient may note difficulty in urinating, fever, and pain, tenderness, and swelling of the testicles. Repeated infections may result in sterility or in a scarred urethra which requires surgical dilatation, a most unpleasant procedure. Following possible exposure, symptoms such as discharge, sore throat, rash, or a hot, swollen joint require medical consultation.

Syphilis has three distinct phases. *Primary syphilis* may result in a small, painless ulcer (chancre) on the genitalia (occasionally on the mouth or hands) which appears ten to ninety days after sexual contact with an infected person. If untreated, the chancre will heal in approximately four to six weeks. The patient is highly infectious during the primary stage. In about 30 percent of all male cases, there is no chancre and thus no sign of this phase. *Secondary syphilis* occurs shortly after the first stage (although it occasionally occurs simultaneously with the chancre). This stage is a rash which may have small bumps, flat red lesions, or may, in fact, take almost any form except blisters. It is especially likely to involve the soles, palms, and face. The *tertiary stage* occurs years later. This is the stage in which people die or go insane. Tertiary syphilis may affect virtually any part of the body, but death usually comes from involvement of the heart or nervous system.

Persons who have had sexual contact with individuals infected with syphilis or gonorrhea must be contacted so that adequate therapy may be given. Public health departments often provide free care. Unnecessary consequences can be avoided.

Home Treatment

Don't treat at home with leftover or borrowed medicines. If you have venereal disease, think you might have it, or have been exposed to it, see the doctor. Home treatment can be used only in *preventing* VD.

The use of condoms offers some but not total protection from venereal disease. Urination immediately following intercourse appears effective in reducing the probability of gonorrhea (the problem of having intercourse when your bladder is full notwithstanding). The usefulness of antibiotics given prior to exposure (as in the military) is questionable.

What to Expect at the Doctor's Office

A diagnosis of gonorrhea is confirmed by testing a culture from the discharge (or from the infected throat or joints) for gonococcus bacteria. The gonococcus is seldom cultured from the genital tract if there is no discharge. Examination of the discharge under the microscope tentatively differentiates between gonorrhea and so-called "nonspecific urethritis," which, though it is probably a venereal disease, has no known serious long-term

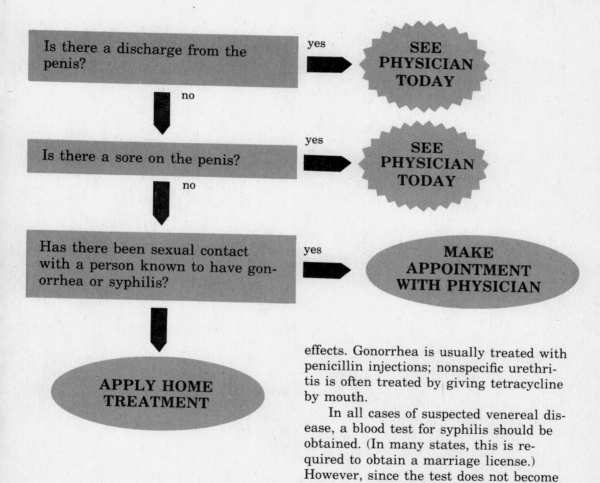

Is there a discharge from the penis?

yes → **SEE PHYSICIAN TODAY**

no

Is there a sore on the penis?

yes → **SEE PHYSICIAN TODAY**

no

Has there been sexual contact with a person known to have gonorrhea or syphilis?

yes → **MAKE APPOINTMENT WITH PHYSICIAN**

APPLY HOME TREATMENT

effects. Gonorrhea is usually treated with penicillin injections; nonspecific urethritis is often treated by giving tetracycline by mouth.

In all cases of suspected venereal disease, a blood test for syphilis should be obtained. (In many states, this is required to obtain a marriage license.) However, since the test does not become positive for from three weeks to three months after exposure, any negative test during that period must be repeated when the three months has elapsed.

P For Women Only

HOW TO DO A BREAST SELF-EXAMINATION

Most lumps in the breast are not cancer. Most women will have a lump in a breast at some time during their life. Many women's breasts are naturally lumpy (so-called "benign fibrocystic disease"). Obviously every lump or possible lump cannot and should not be subjected to surgery.

Cancer of the breast does occur, however, and is best treated early than late. Regular self-examination of your breasts gives you the best chance of avoiding serious consequences. Self-examination should be monthly, just after the menstrual period.

The technique is as follows:

- Examine your breasts in the mirror, first with your arms at your side and then with both arms over your head. The breasts should look the same. Watch for any change in shape or size, or for dimpling of the skin. Occasionally a lump that is difficult to feel will be quite obvious just by looking.

- Next, while lying flat, examine the left breast using the inner finger tips of the right hand and pressing the breast tissue against the chest wall. Do not "pinch" the tissue between the fingers; all breast tissue feels a bit lumpy when you do this. The left hand should be behind your head while you examine the inner half of the left breast and down at your side when you examine the outer half. Do not neglect the part of the breast underneath the nipples or that which extends outward from the breast toward the underarm. A small pillow under the left shoulder may help.

- Repeat this process on the opposite side.

Any lump detected should be brought to the attention of your physician. Regular self-examination will tell you how long it has been present and whether it has changed in size. This information is very helpful in deciding what to do about the lump; even the doctor often has difficulty with this decision. Self-examination is an absolute necessity for a woman with naturally lumpy breasts; she is the only one who can really know whether a lump is new, old, or has changed size. For all women, regular self-examination offers the best hope that surgery will be performed when, and only when, it is necessary.

THE GYNECOLOGICAL EXAMINATION

Examination of the female reproduction organs, usually called a "pelvic" examination, may be expected for complaints related to these organs and in conjunction with the annual "Pap" smear. This examination yields a great deal of information and often is absolutely essential for diagnosis. By understanding the phases of the examination and your role in them, you can make it possible for an adequate examination to be done quickly and with a minimum of discomfort.

Positioning: Lying on your back, put your heels in the stirrups (the nurse will often assist in this step). Move down to the very end of the examination table, with knees bent. Get as close to the edge as you can. Now let your knees fall out to the sides as far as they will go. Do not try to hold the knees closed with the inner muscles of the thigh. This will tire you and make the examination more difficult.

The key word during the examination is "relax"; you may hear it several times. The vagina is a muscular organ and if the muscles are tense, a difficult and uncomfortable examination is inevitable. You may be asked to take several deep breaths in an effort to obtain relaxation. We hope that understanding what is happening will also help you relax.

External examination: Inspection of the labia, the clitoris and vaginal opening is the first step in the examination. The most common findings are cysts in the labia, rashes, and so-called "venereal warts." These problems have effective treatments or may need no treatment at all.

Speculum examination: The speculum is the "duck-billed" instrument used to spread the walls of the vagina, so that the inside may be seen. It is *not* a clamp. It may be constructed of metal or plastic. The plastic ones will "click" open and closed, don't be alarmed. Contrary to popular opinion, the speculum is not stored in the refrigerator; it is usually warmed before use.

If a Pap smear or other test is to be made, the speculum examination usually will come before the finger (manual) examination and the speculum will be lubricated with water only. A lubricant or a manual examination may spoil the test. If these tests are not needed, the manual examination may come first. The speculum also opens the vagina so that insertion of an intrauterine device (IUD) or other procedures can be done.

Manual examination: By inserting two lubricated, gloved fingers into the vagina and pressing on the lower abdomen with the other hand, the physician can feel the shape of the ovaries and uterus as well as any lumps in the area. The accuracy of this examination depends on the degree of relaxation of the patient and the skill of the physician. Fat women cannot be examined as well; this is another good reason not to be overweight. Usually, the best pelvic examinations are done by those who do them most often. You do not need a gynecologist, but be sure that your internist or family practitioner does "pelvics" on a regular basis before you request a yearly gynecological exam. The nurse practitioner who does pelvic examinations regularly is usually expert also. The Pap smear alone does *not* require a great deal of experience and is the single most important part of the examination.

Many physicians will also perform a rectal or rectovaginal (one finger in rectum and one in vagina) examination. These examinations can provide additional information.

If you are nervous about the pelvic examination, ask the physician to explain what is going on during the examination. Usually there is a drape over your knees and the physician sits on a stool out of your line of sight. You can cooperate better if you understand the procedures, and you will feel less awkward during this examination if you and the physician are communicating effectively.

The "Pap" Smear

Since the Pap test is of unique importance to women, you should be familiar with the basics of this procedure. As explained above, a scraping of the cervix and a sample of the vaginal secretions is obtained with the aid of a speculum. This provides cells for study under the microscope. A trained technician (a cytologist) can then classify the cells according to their microscopic characteristics. There are five classes: Classes I and II are negative for tumor cells; Classes III and IV are suspicious but not definite for tumors; Class V is definite for tumors. If your smear is Classes III or IV, your physician will ask you to return for another pap test or a biopsy of the cervix. This does *not* mean that cancer is definite. If your smear is Class V, your physician will explain the approach to confirming the diagnosis and starting treatment.

The Pap smear is our most effective tumor-finding test for two reasons. First, a single test detects approximately 90 percent of the most common cancers of the womb and 70 to 80 percent of the second most common. Second, both of these common types of cancer grow slowly; current evidence indicates that it may take 10 years or more for a single focus of cancer of the cervix to spread. Thus there is an excellent chance that regular Pap smears will detect the cancer before it spreads. Although Pap smears are usually done annually, this is not magical, and an argument can be made for longer intervals. Cancer of the cervix is rare under the age of twenty-five. Pap smears are usually begun at that age. However, cancer of the cervix is more frequent with moderate-to-heavy sexual activity, especially if there are multiple partners, and regular Pap testing probably should begin when regular sexual activity begins. There is almost no evidence that the use of birth control pills requires more frequent Pap smears.

90 Vaginal Discharge

Abnormal discharge from the vagina is common, but should not be confused with the normal vaginal secretions. Some of the many possible causes require the physician. If the discharge is slight, doesn't hurt or itch, and is not cheesy, smelly, or bloody, and if there is no possibility of a venereal disease and the patient is past puberty, the problem may be treated at home— for a time.

Abdominal pain suggests the possibility of serious disease, ranging from gonorrhea to an ectopic pregnancy in the fallopian tube. Bloody discharge between periods, if recurrent or significant in amount, suggests much the same. Discharge in a girl before puberty is rare and should be evaluated.

If sexual contact in the past few weeks might possibly have resulted in a venereal disease, the physician *must* be seen. Do not be afraid to take this problem to the doctor; be frank in naming your sexual contacts, for their own benefit. Information will be kept confidential and you will not be embarrassed by the physician, who will have confronted this situation many times.

Monilia is a fungus that may infect the walls of the vagina and cause a white, cheesy discharge. Trichomonas is a common microorganism which can cause a white frothy discharge and intense itch. A mixture of bacteria may be responsible for a discharge, so-called non-specific vaginitis. These infections are not serious and do not spread to the rest of the body, but they are bothersome. They will sometimes but not always go away by themselves. If discharge persists beyond a few weeks, make an appointment with the physician.

In older women, lack of hormones can cause "atrophic" vaginitis. Prescription creams are sometimes needed if symptoms are bothersome. Foreign bodies, particularly a forgotten tampon, are a surprisingly frequent cause of vaginitis and discharge.

Home Treatment

Hygiene and patience are the home remedies. If you have a discharge, douche daily (and following intercourse) with a Betadine solution (2 tablespoons to a quart of water) or baking soda (one teaspoon to a quart). If you are taking an antibiotic such as tetracycline for some other condition, call your physician for advice on changing medication. If the discharge persists despite treatment for more than two weeks, or becomes worse, see the physician. Do not douche for twenty-four hours prior to seeing the physician. Some physicians will prescribe over the phone for a vaginitis. Multipurpose medications (AVC, Sultrin Creams) or those active against yeast (Mycostatin, Vanobid, Candeptin) are useful in this situation.

What to Expect at the Doctor's Office

Pelvic examination. If a venereal disease is suspected, a culture of the mouth of the womb (cervix) is mandatory. If not, examination of the discharge under the microscope or a culture of the discharge is sometimes but not always needed. Suppositories or creams are the usual treatment. If venereal disease is at all likely, antibiotics (usually penicillin) will be prescribed. Oral medication for fungus or trichomonas may be used in severe cases. The sexual partner(s) may require treatment as well.

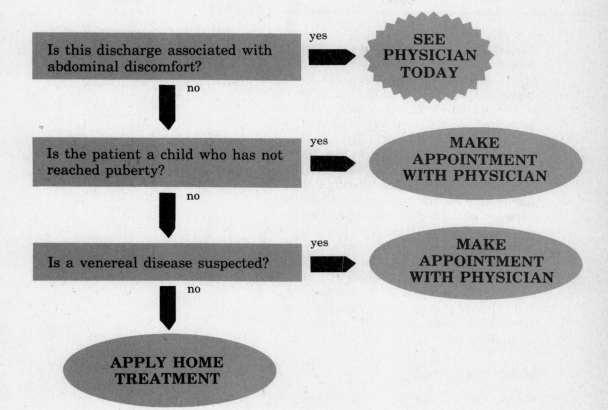

Is this discharge associated with abdominal discomfort?

yes → SEE PHYSICIAN TODAY

no ↓

Is the patient a child who has not reached puberty?

yes → MAKE APPOINTMENT WITH PHYSICIAN

no ↓

Is a venereal disease suspected?

yes → MAKE APPOINTMENT WITH PHYSICIAN

no ↓

APPLY HOME TREATMENT

91 Bleeding between Periods

Some personal questions, a pelvic examination, and a Pap smear should be expected. If bleeding is active, the pelvic examination and Pap smear may be postponed but should be performed within a few weeks.

Most often, the interval between two menstrual periods is free of bleeding or spotting. Many women experience such bleeding, however, even though no serious condition is present. Women with an intrauterine birth control device (IUD) are particularly likely to have occasional spotting. If bleeding is slight and occasional, it may be ignored. Serious conditions such as cancer and abnormal pregnancy may be first suggested by bleeding between periods. So if bleeding is severe or occurs three months in a row, a physician must be seen. Often a serious problem can be detected best when the bleeding is *not* active. The gynecologist or the family physician is a better resource than the emergency room. Any bleeding after the menopause should be evaluated by a physician.

Home Treatment

Relax, and use pads or tampons. Avoid use of aspirin if possible; in theory, it may prolong the bleeding. If in doubt about the effect of other medicines, call your doctor.

The relationship between tampons and the toxic shock syndrome is a subject of medical controversy, but many doctors believe that leaving tampons in place too long increases the risk of this problem. Change tampons regularly, at least twice daily. Be sure that tampons are removed: a surprising number of women occasionally forget about them. We do not think that tampons should be avoided but feel that they should be used with care.

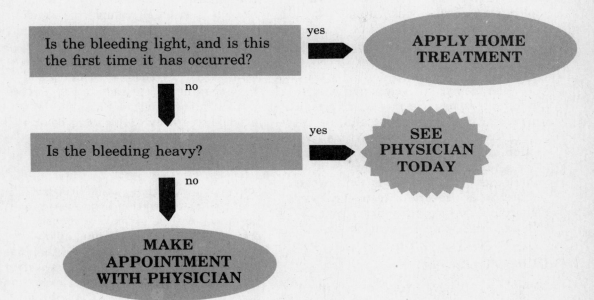

Is the bleeding light, and is this the first time it has occurred? — yes → **APPLY HOME TREATMENT**

no ↓

Is the bleeding heavy? — yes → **SEE PHYSICIAN TODAY**

no ↓

MAKE APPOINTMENT WITH PHYSICIAN

92 Difficult Periods

Adverse mood changes and fluid retention are very common in the several days prior to the menstrual period. Such problems are vexing and can be difficult to treat but are a result of normal hormonal variations during the menstrual cycle.

The menstrual cycle is different for different women. Periods may be regular, irregular, light, heavy, painful, pain-free, long, or short, and still be normal. Variation in the menstrual cycle is medically less significant than bleeding, pain, or discharge between periods. Only when problems are severe or recur for several months is medical attention required. Emergency treatment is seldom needed.

Home Treatment

We do not believe that diuretics (fluid pills) or hormones are frequently indicated. Perhaps this is callous. Still, as we have said in other sections of this book, we prefer the simple and natural to the complex and artificial. Following hormone treatment, all too frequently we have seen mood changes that are worse than the premenstrual tension, as well as potassium loss, gouty arthritis, and psychological drug dependency from diuretics.

Salt tends to hold fluid in the tissues and to cause edema. The most natural diuretic is to cut down on salt intake. In the United States the typical diet has ten times the required amount of salt; many authorities feel that this is one cause of high blood pressure and arteriosclerosis. No matter how hard you try to eliminate salt from your diet, you will still have more than enough. If you can eliminate some salt, you may have less edema and fluid retention. If food tastes flat without salt, try using lemon juice as a substitute. The commercial salt substitutes are also satisfactory. Products with the word "sodium" or the symbol "Na" anywhere in the list of ingredients contain salt.

For menstrual cramps, use aspirin. Products claimed to be designed for menstrual cramps (such as Midol) have aspirin as the main ingredient. Many patients swear by such compounds, and they are fine if you want to pay the premium. But we don't understand, on a scientific basis, why they should be any better than plain aspirin.

What to Expect at the Doctor's Office

The doctor will give you advice. Frequently, a prescription for diuretics or hormones will be given. For menstrual cramps, drugs known as prostaglondin inhibitors are now the accepted therapy. Pelvic examination is often unrewarding and sometimes may not be performed. In cases of heavy bleeding, a "D and C" may be required. Hysterectomy should not be performed for this complaint alone. If a tumor is found, surgery will sometimes be needed, but the common "fibroid" tumor will often stop growing by itself and surgery may not be needed. Such tumors often grow slowly and stop growth at the menopause, so an operation can be avoided by waiting. If the Pap smear is positive, however, surgery is often indicated.

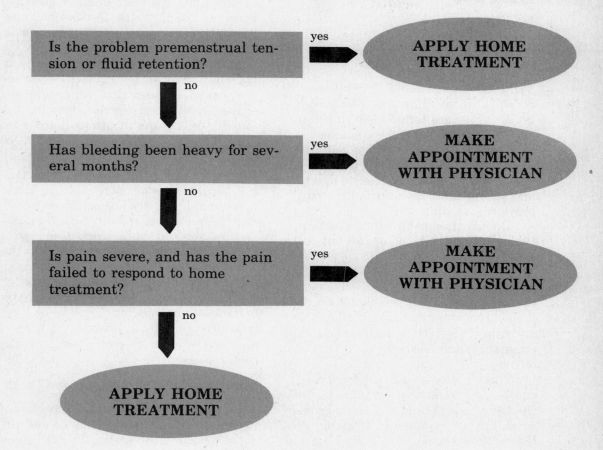

Is the problem premenstrual tension or fluid retention? — **yes** → APPLY HOME TREATMENT

↓ no

Has bleeding been heavy for several months? — **yes** → MAKE APPOINTMENT WITH PHYSICIAN

↓ no

Is pain severe, and has the pain failed to respond to home treatment? — **yes** → MAKE APPOINTMENT WITH PHYSICIAN

↓ no

APPLY HOME TREATMENT

93 Possible Venereal Disease in Women

VD. Clap. Gonorrhea. GC. Whites. Strain. PID. Syphilis. Lues. Chancre. Sores. These are terms for venereal disease. VD is not for home treatment, and if VD is suspected, you must contact a physician. These conditions require antibiotic treatment after accurate diagnosis, and sexual contacts must be treated to prevent spreading.

Do *not* attempt to use antibiotics that you have at home or can buy in the street for these serious infections. You do not know the potency, the dose, or the duration of treatment required, and we are not going to tell you. Tragedies from inadequate home treatment include sterility, heart infection, death from ectopic pregnancy, and needless infection of others.

There are two main venereal diseases—gonorrhea and syphilis—and of the two, gonorrhea is considerably more common than syphilis. In women, infection with either disease is often hard to determine, since it is "inside" rather than "outside." A vaginal discharge may be dismissed for several months until gonorrhea infection has moved to the fallopian tubes, the joints, or into the bloodstream. Gonorrhea is painful as well as dangerous. The male partner with gonorrhea may report "clap," "whites," or "strain"; all common names for gonorrhea or "GC." In syphilis, the male may report a "sore" on the penis (see Problem 89). The sore on the woman is often not noticed. An unexplained skin rash (on the body and including the palms and soles) occurs several weeks after the infection and indicates the secondary stage of the disease.

"Crabs," "lice," "trich," and several other conditions may be spread by sexual exposure but are more often transmitted by nonvenereal routes. Don't force any unreasonable accusations on your partner when one of these is found. Only syphilis and gonorrhea are invariably transmitted by sexual contact. When recent experience includes oral or anal sex, either syphilis or gonorrhea may be found infecting the mouth or the rectum.

Home Treatment

Hygiene after sexual contact is of potential benefit. Douche thoroughly after the encounter if you are suspicious or worried. Inspection of the penis during foreplay for sores or white thick discharge is useful for the uncertain situation. In the world's "oldest profession," such inspection is routinely practiced. A condom or "rubber" is a reasonably effective barrier to disease transmission. Thus home treatment consists of *prevention*. After infection, or after possible infection, you need a doctor.

What to Expect at the Doctor's Office

Pelvic examination and treatment. For gonorrhea, the doctor will take a culture of the mouth of the womb. The culture may be positive even if there is no abnormal discharge. For syphilis, a blood test and a scraping of the sore will be done. Venereal disease (VD) clinics are available in most large cities and provide high-quality service at little or no cost.

Your sexual contacts *must* be treated, even if they have no symptoms, for they can continue to spread the disease and can develop serious complications themselves. Do not withhold names. Treatment of contacts is discreetly performed.

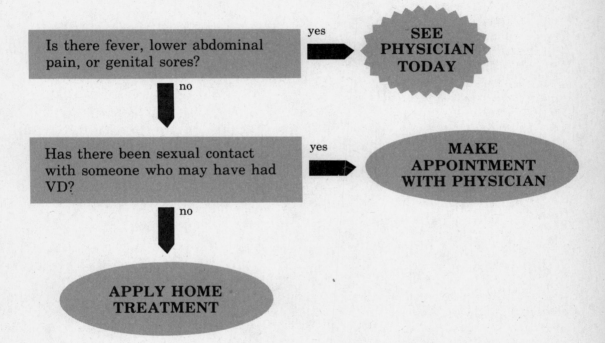

Is there fever, lower abdominal pain, or genital sores?

yes → **SEE PHYSICIAN TODAY**

no ↓

Has there been sexual contact with someone who may have had VD?

yes → **MAKE APPOINTMENT WITH PHYSICIAN**

no ↓

APPLY HOME TREATMENT

Treatment is with antibiotics, usually penicillin by injection. Be sure to tell the doctor if you have an allergy to penicillin. Treatment with the program recommended by the United States Public Health Service is almost always curative—but you can catch another dose of venereal disease a few days later. Be prepared.

Q Herpes Infections of the Genitalia

Herpes infections of the genitalia (herpes progenitalis) are well on their way to occupying a unique place in medicine as the first popular venereal disease. Certainly herpes progenitalis is the only venereal disease with its own membership organization, complete with newsletter and telephone service. With an estimated 20 million Americans having a recurrent problem with herpes, the prospects for building membership of this organization seem to be excellent.

There are two types of herpes simplex virus. Infections of the genitalia are usually caused by Type 2, but may be due to Type 1 viruses, especially in children. Herpes Type 1 is responsible for the all too frequent fever blisters and cold sores of the lips and mouth (see **Mouth Sores**, Problem 31). Whereas Type 1 infections are usually spread by kissing and other similar contact, Herpes Type 2 infections are almost always spread by sexual contact. The virus takes up a permanent home in about one-third of the people it infects and goes on to cause recurrent outbreaks of the painful, red blisters. These recurrences may be triggered by other illnesses, trauma, or emotional distress. The blisters usually last from five to ten days.

Herpes is most contagious during and just before the period when the blisters are present. Many people with recurrent herpes can tell a day or two before an outbreak actually occurs. They develop an itchy or tingling feeling called a *prodome*. The key to preventing transmission of herpes is to avoid sexual contact when the prodrome or blisters are present. Condoms probably give some protection against transmitting the disease but may be painful when sores are present and the protection is not complete.

There is no drug that cures herpes. Many things have been tried to decrease the frequency of attack or to make an attack go away more quickly. Application of cream containing an anticancer chemical (Stoxil) does not seem to help this problem although it works in herpes infections of the eye. Repeated smallpox vaccinations have been tried in an attempt to build up immunity to the virus but have not met with demonstrated success. "Photo inactivation" of the virus, using light and a dye applied directly to the lesions, may give some help but also creates a risk of skin

333

cancer. Ether and chloroform may speed resolution of the blisters in some, but the relief is not dramatic and these can be difficult to use. Some experts believe that emotional upset or anxiety makes these blisters even worse. They advocate relaxation techniques to reduce stress and anxiety. A *hot* tub bath for five to ten minutes can inactivate the virus and seems to speed healing.

The painful, reddened, grouped blisters of herpes are seldom mistaken for the painless shallow ulceration (chancre) which is the initial sign of syphilis. However, if you are unsure about the problem you are dealing with, you should not assume that it is herpes. A call or a visit to your physician may be necessary.

Several studies have indicated that herpes infections are associated with cancer of the cervix, but it is not known if herpes is involved in causing this cancer. If you have recurrent herpes infections, this is another reason for a Pap smear. However, you should be having Pap smears anyway, and it is not known if the presence of herpes indicates a need for more frequent Pap smears.

HOME TREATMENT

The painful truth is that the treatment of herpes primarily consists of "grin and bear it." Various salves such as calamine lotion, alcohol, and ether have been tried; they may provide some relief in individual cases, but none have been remarkably successful. The "hot tub" treatment mentioned above has the advantage of being readily available at low-cost and seems to work as well as anything. We think that a major concern should be to prevent the spread of herpes as indicated above.

As mentioned, some people believe that reducing stress and anxiety may be helpful. This is one of the approaches advocated by HELP, a program of the American Social Health Association that provides personal support for people with herpes. You may be interested in contacting this organization at P.O. Box 100, Palo Alto, California 94302.

If the problem lasts for more than two weeks or you are unsure of the diagnosis, a call or visit to the physician is indicated.

WHAT TO EXPECT AT THE DOCTOR'S OFFICE

The history will focus on recurrences, possible exposure to herpes and other venereal diseases, and how the blisters developed. On occasion a microscopic examination of material scraped from the bottom of a blister will be made, but this is usually not necessary. If herpes is diagnosed, treatment is essentially as outlined in "Home Treatment."

Is this a group of small, painful blisters on reddened skin?

no  **CONSIDER ANOTHER PROBLEM**

yes

APPLY HOME TREATMENT

R Contraception

Every woman must decide to abstain from sex, have babies, or use a contraceptive technique. Ideally the male partner participates in this decision, but through a peculiar quirk of nature, he does not participate in the most direct consequences. This chapter is concerned with the *medical* considerations involved in making decisions about contraception and childbearing. These decisions have a major effect on your health, both directly and indirectly, whether you are male or female. Directly, childbearing and every form of contraception has a definite risk. Indirectly, the threat to the health of an ever-increasing population is equally real.

Few women will pursue one course of action for all their childbearing years. Abstention will be a reasonable choice for only a few; for most it is neither a practical nor healthy suggestion. The majority of women employ some form of contraception except for specific periods when they are attempting to get pregnant or are not engaging in sexual intercourse. If you are sure that you do not want any more children, tubal ligation or vasectomy are the safest methods for ensuring this. Here are brief descriptions of the most popular forms of contraception:

- *Oral Contraceptives*. Birth-control pills use hormones to prevent pregnancy and must be taken on a daily basis. When used safely, they are very effective in preventing pregnancy. However, they may cause blood clots, and these clots have been fatal on occasion. They may also contribute to high blood pressure. There are also less dangerous but annoying side effects, such as weight gain, nausea, fluid retention, migraine headaches, vaginal bleeding, and yeast infections of the vagina.

- *Intrauterine Device (IUD)*. This device is inserted into the uterus by a physician and remains there until removed or expelled. If the IUD is expelled, it may not be noticed, and in such cases some pregnancies have resulted. The IUD may also cause bleeding and cramps. In rare instances they are associated with serious infections of the uterus, although the type with which this most frequently occurred (the Dalkon Shield) has been removed from the market.

- *Diaphragm*. A diaphragm is a rubber membrane that fits over the opening to the uterus in the vagina. It must be inserted before intercourse and retained in place for a number of hours thereafter. There are no side effects or complications from diaphragms. They are best used with a contraceptive foam or jelly.

• *Contraceptive Foams, Jellies, and Suppositories.* These contain chemicals that kill or immobilize the male's sperm. In the past they have been used by themselves but now are almost always used in conjunction with a diaphragm. Side effects are unusual and consist of some irritation to the walls of the vagina. Their effect will last for only about sixty minutes, and many people find these preparations inconvenient or just plain messy.

• *Condoms.* These are enjoying a resurgence of popularity. If used correctly, they are 90 percent effective in preventing pregnancy. There are no side effects, they are inexpensive and widely available, and they give some protection against venereal disease. However, remembering to use them seems to be a problem and they do result in decreased sensitivity for the male.

• *The Rhythm Method.* Intercourse is avoided during the time when ovulation is expected. This method requires fairly regular periods and a willingness to carefully take daily temperatures in order to predict the time of ovulation. Under the best of circumstances, it is only moderately effective.

• *Coitus Interruptus.* Here the male withdraws from the vagina just before ejaculation. Since there are sperm present in the secretions of the penis *before* ejaculation occurs, and since withdrawal at just the right time is a tricky business at best, this method reduces the chances of pregnancy by reducing the number of sperm deposited in the vagina.

• *Douche.* Douching after intercourse also decreases the number of sperm in the vagina and therefore decreases the chance of pregnancy somewhat.

Table 1 gives the relative risk of pregnancy for unprotected intercourse and for the most popular forms of contraception. Table 2 indicates the risk to life for pregnancy and contraceptives for any year on "average." Table 3 takes into account changing risks associated with age by totaling the risk for the period from age thirty to the end of the reproductive years.

A number of facts are clear from these tables:

• Unprotected intercourse is by far the most hazardous choice.

• The least hazardous techniques require the availability of abortions or involve sterilization.

• Except for oral contraceptives, the hazard of each contraceptive technique depends mostly on the probability of pregnancy.

• There is a substantial difference in risk between "used correctly" and "average experience." How well you use the method counts a great deal.

As far as your health is concerned, it would seem clear that you should consider "mechanical" forms of contraception (IUD, condom, diaphragm with foam) and assure yourself of access to facilities to interrupt an unwanted pregnancy. You may find that mechanical methods simply are not for you. You may have ethical or religious objections to abortion—or to contraception, for that matter. The objective here is not to promote any

TABLE 1

Expected Pregnancies

Number of pregnancies for 100 women using contraceptive methods in a year. (The "average experience" group includes women who were using the method inconsistently or incorrectly.)

	Used correctly	Average experience
Birth control pills	0.340	4 to 10
Condoms and foam	1	5
IUD	1 to 3	5
Condom	3	10
Diaphragm and foam	3	17
Foam	3	22
Coitus interruptus	9	20 to 25
Rhythm	13	21
No protection	90	90
Douche	?	40

Source: Robert A. Hatcher et al., *Contraceptive Technology, 1976–1977* (New York: Irvington, 1976), page 676. Reprinted by permission.

TABLE 2

Risks of Pregnancy versus Contraceptives

	Deaths per 100,000 women per year
Pregnancy	16
Diaphragm or condom (death resulting from 20 percent becoming pregnant)	3
Unprotected intercourse and abortion	2.6
Oral contraceptive users	0.3 to 3
IUD	1.0
Diaphragm or condom, and abortion for pregnancy	0.6

Source: Adapted from Robert A. Hatcher et al., *Contraceptive Technology, 1976–1977* page 676. Reprinted by permission.

particular method but to ensure that your decision is an informed one. To risk your health unknowingly is the truly tragic choice.

You may accept an increased risk to health for the best of reasons—your own reasons. Contraception is one of the most intensely personal decisions, and the rest of us should respect your right to make up your mind. Ideally, your choice depends only upon the feelings of you and your partner.

TABLE 3

Safety of Family Planning Alternatives for Women Beginning Birth Control at Age Thirty

Method of Fertility Control	Cumulative Reproduction—Related Deaths From Age Thirty to End of Reproductive Years
	(deaths per 100,000 women)
No contraception	245
Abortion only	92
Oral contraception to end of reproductive years*	188
Oral contraception to age forty, followed by diaphragm or condom use	80
Intrauterine device	22
Diaphragm or condom	55
Diaphragm or condom with legal abortion as backup	14
Tubal sterilization	10 to 20
Vasectomy (male risk)**	0

* Oral contraceptives usually are not recommended for women over forty.
** Recent animal studies suggest that vasectomy could contribute to arteriosclerosis ("hardening of the arteries"), but the importance of this in men, if any, is unknown.
C. Tietze, J. Bongaarts, B. Shearer, *Mortality Associated With the Control of Fertility* Family Planning Perspectives, Vol. 8, 1976) p. 6–14.

Unfortunately, the consequences of childbearing go far beyond the immediate family. Environment and the standard of living have a major influence on health, far outweighing the contribution of medical care. It is most likely that the demands of an ever-increasing population on an ever-decreasing supply of resources should not adversely affect the environment and the economy. It is most unlikely that advances in medical science will be able to counter these adverse effects. It is likely that economic and environmental factors can overwhelm the protective effects of a beneficial lifestyle.

In 1900, the population of the United States was 76 million. In 1950 it was 152 million. Today it is approximately 226 million. The Bureau of Census estimates that by the year 2000 it could be 287 million. The energy crisis may become just one of many crises—the job crisis, the housing crisis, the food crisis, and so on. Attempts to produce more jobs, housing, and food inevitably consume resources and produce waste. This brings us closer to what may well be the last crisis—too many people, too few resources, too much pollution. Unlike some developing nations, the United States has never been forced to formulate a national policy concerning population control. It seems obvious that it would be advantageous for each of us to consider this issue now before our options become limited and our crises become impossible to solve.

In curious contrast to population control, methods of contraception have always been a public issue. Not only have specific methods been illegal, but until recently even giving information about birth control was illegal in some states. Again, the purpose here is not to argue for or against any method, much less discuss the ethical or moral aspects of contraception. But from the point of view of public health, the banning of contraceptive methods or information must be regarded as a detrimental step. In the current debate on abortion, then, you must consider the fact that this procedure is a part of the safest approach to contraception. Even if you oppose abortion, a decision by you that every other woman must accept an increased risk to health must not be taken lightly.

S Sexual Problems

Sex is an area in which we all experience some insecurity. Every individual has anxieties and fears; everyone thinks that friends and colleagues are free from such problems. There are no personal experts in sex. No personal experience can constitute both a broad sampling of individual differences and probe the depths of a long-standing, profoundly intimate relationship. Since everyone knows his or her own activities, and for the most part imagines what others are doing, myths abound.

Each generation and most individuals discover anew the exhilaration of a good sexual experience. In a perverse game played between the generations, a variety of contradictory rules for the conduct of sexual relationships are dogmatically advocated. Accusations are formulated, anxieties created, and health disturbed.

Good feelings are what sex is all about. But the good feelings go beyond the pleasurable physical sensations of sexual arousal. Feeling good about yourself, your partner, intimacy—these are good feelings you need for sex to be its most satisfying and pleasurable. A number of factors may prevent these good feelings; only a minority of these are related to sexual function itself. Anxiety or depression from any cause may result in problems with sex. Attitudes toward sex create problems, usually unnecessarily. We are particularly concerned with an emerging view of the sexual partner as an orgasm machine, a preoccupation with technique rather than feeling, and with the resulting depersonalization of the sexual relationship.

Anxiety about sex, especially in the learning stage, must be counted as normal simply because it is a universal phenomenon. This anxiety has been compounded by both of the two dominant contemporary approaches toward sex. The first approach considers sex as an unspeakable subject. Moralistic fantasies develop. A feature of the human mind is that fantasies cannot be suppressed by thinking about them. If you avoid guilt about your fantasies, you promote your sexual health.

Virility is another major myth. We frequently encounter patients who have fears that their sexual activity is too frequent or too infrequent. Part of this problem stems from publication of average figures from large-scale sex surveys. People who find that their practices are distant from the averages often are concerned. Relax. It may be eight times a day or eight times a year. The only rule worth remembering is that in a stable relationship, the frequency of sexual activity should be a workable compromise between the desires of the partners.

Another area of anxiety concerns the *sexual equipment*. Men worry about the size of their penis. Women worry that their breasts are too big or too small, their legs too fat or too thin. Men worry about a pigeon-chest, no hair on their chest, or too much hair on their chest. Women are concerned that their hair does not properly frame their face, that they have hairs around the nipples, or that their total image is too dowdy, too awkward, or too cheap. There is little that is worthwhile in such concerns.

Some individuals are more attractive than others. In the dimension of sensuality, some are more sensual than others. However, the breadth of taste runs from thick to thin. Somebody likes you the way you are. Men may like large women or slender women who wear clothes well. Women may be excited by broad shoulders or by a thoughtful gesture. Whether this whole business is due to cultural indoctrination or to innate differences between the sexes, the point is the same. Usually, the sexual equipment is the least important part of the problem! If you fear that you were not created as the most attractive of creatures to the opposite sex, you will find that this difficulty can be reduced by warmth, affection, and humanity. In sex, how you feel *about* each other is more important than how you feel *to* each other.

The man frequently worries unnecessarily about penis size. In fact, there is little difference in size of the erect penis between different men, although there are significant differences in the resting state. Moreover, the vaginal canal, which accommodates birth, is potentially much larger than the thickest of penises. The size and rigidity of the penis will vary for the same man at different times. Some factors affecting erect penile size are physical—such as the length of time since previous intercourse—and some are psychological. Impotence is seldom due to disease of genitalia, nerves, or blood vessels. No male is equally potent at all times, and all males are, on some occasions, impotent. Chronic impotence implies chronic anxiety, at least partially compounded by worry over the impotence.

Premature ejaculation, while physically the opposite of impotence, has the same cause. Again, relaxation is usually a solution. There are some other potential aids. A firm pinch on the tip of the penis will delay ejaculation. A condom (rubber) usually will decrease sensation for the male so that ejaculation is delayed. Seldom are such measures necessary for more than a few occasions.

Female orgasm is the most written-about sexual phenomenon of recent years. This subject has been linked inseparably to aspects of the women's movement. It has been pointed out that some women are multiorgasmic and may climax several times during a single coupling. It has been held that equality of orgasm is a principal requirement for sexual equality. On the other hand, it has been observed that a large number of women do not have orgasms with regularity. The emerging sexual myth is that these women are in some way abnormal. In fact, many women relating a deep and satisfactory sexual experience over many years do not report frequent orgasms during that experience. If you let others tell you what you should be doing, and then allow guilt to develop when you don't meet false "norms," you are promoting these myths. Of all human activities, sexual activity, more than any other, should be directed by the individual, at his or her own pace and style.

A variety of sexual practices have been recently reemphasized. These include "swinging," group sex, sex with the aid of various appliances, and sex in a virtual infinity of positions. Such practices are recorded in all eras of human literature, but advocates of sexual variety were discouraged by legal and ethical barriers until recently. Medically, there is no reason either to encourage or discourage sexual variety and experimentation. The problems presently seen are a reaction to earlier attitudes. People now feel guilty that their sex life has insufficient variety. For example, the majority of heterosexual activity takes place in the "male-superior" position. This position is often the most satisfactory for both partners, since it allows the deepest penetration and the sensitivity value of being face to face. Recent derogation of this technique as the "missionary position" illustrates ignorance of history and anatomy; the accusatory tone of the phrase suggests an attempt to arouse guilt and anxiety about a normal practice.

Other individuals, for equally good reasons, prefer many different positions or find their greatest satisfactions with a particular alternative technique. There is no right way and no standard pattern for sexual expression. Averages are meaningless in a personal relationship between two individuals. Such relationships may be physically expressed in a wide variety of ways, none of which have any superiority to the others. You have personal freedom to be either ordinary or exotic—with pleasure, and without guilt.

Sex is not a competitive sport. Sexual health, for the great majority of individuals, reduces to common sense. If it feels good to both partners, do it. If it doesn't feel good, don't do it. Don't allow the fear of being "hung up" to become the major hang-up. Individuals should not allow other individuals, equally nonexpert, to define their satisfaction for them; there remain "different strokes for different folks."

T High Blood Pressure

Discussion of the major chronic diseases—heart disease, diabetes, arthritis, cancer, and so on— is beyond the scope of this book, but we think that it is important to make an exception in the case of high blood pressure. This is the most common of significant chronic problems and is the most treatable. It has been estimated that 30 to 40 million Americans have high blood pressure, more than 1 out of every 10.

Many of those who have high blood pressure do not know it. This is a uniquely silent disease. There are no symptoms until it is too late; the catastrophe of a heart attack or stroke is all too often the first indication of a problem. Do not wait for headaches or nosebleeds to give you fair warning; these are not reliable indicators of high blood pressure. Even if you have these symptoms, it is quite unlikely that they are due to high blood pressure.

Because high blood pressure is silent and can be treated effectively, early detection (screening) is important. Hypertension is unique in this regard; it is much more difficult to make the argument for routine screening than for any other major diseases. Therefore, we prefer to put our emphasis on early detection of high blood pressure. Put a blood pressure check first on your list.

It is true that you can have high blood pressure even though you are slim and exercising regularly. But it is also true that being overweight and out of shape increases the risk of high blood pressure. Most importantly, recent studies have confirmed that people with high blood pressure who are overweight and not exercising can lower their blood pressure by losing weight and exercising regularly. Many can control their blood pressure entirely without the use of drugs, and most others can reduce the amount of medication that they require. Drug treatment of high blood pressure is effective but is expensive and has risks and side effects. Getting off drugs is very desirable and is only surpassed by never needing the drugs in the first place. In both cases, exercise and weight control can be the keys for most hypertensive people.

Here is a summary of what you need to know about high blood pressure:

KNOW IF YOU HAVE IT

Once a year have your blood pressure checked. This is a reliable, cheap, painless test. Often the doctor's office is not the best place to have this done since just being in the doctor's office can raise the blood pressure. Blood pressure checks are available without charge through corporations, public health departments, and voluntary health agencies; a visit to the doctor's office is almost never necessary. The blood pressure machines available in many stores are reasonably accurate.

Don't be panicked by any one reading. Since your blood pressure varies up and down, you will need to have several readings if the first reading is elevated. At least one-third of the people whose first reading is high will be found to have normal readings on subsequent checks. The blood pressure reading has two numbers; the higher one is the *systolic pressure* and the lower is the *diastolic pressure*. Blood pressure is considered to be high if the higher number exceeds 140 or the lower number exceeds 90. Traditionally, "normal" is said to be 120/80, but this has been overemphasized. Generally, the lower the blood pressure, the better (unless the low reading is due to disease). A low reading due to disease is unusual; low readings are usually found in youngsters and in older people who are in excellent physical condition.

Do not buy a blood pressure cuff unless you actually have high blood pressure or unless you plan to do many blood pressures as a public service or for some other reason. You can obtain your reading once a year for nothing, so that the purchase of a kit is unnecessary. While taking a blood pressure is not difficult or mysterious, you do need some practice and doing it once or even several times a year is not enough.

IF YOU HAVE HIGH BLOOD PRESSURE, YOU MUST TAKE CARE OF IT

If you have high blood pressure, the most important thing to realize is that *you* must manage this problem yourself. It will be up to you to control your weight, your exercise, and to take your medicines. We think that it should be up to you to take your own blood pressure. Your physician should be your trusted advisor but cannot assume your responsibility. No matter how much the physician would like to take care of this for you, he or she cannot. You are in control, and good physicians will emphasize this point. After the initial investigation and when the blood pressure is controlled, you should be able to handle the management of this problem with relatively few visits to the physician.

If you have high blood pressure, you should buy a blood pressure kit. Blood pressure readings tell pretty much the whole story. If you are going to manage this problem, you need the blood presure readings so that you can report changes or difficulties to the physician.
Make exercise and weight control a part of your program.

In mild to moderate high blood pressure, drug treatment should be seen as a last resort. Even if drugs prove to be necessary, your attention to exercise and weight will enable you to use drugs less, which means less expense, risks, and side effects.
If you do take drugs, understand how to manage them.

Each drug has its own side effects and warning signs of which you should be aware. Chart the use of your drugs along with your blood pressure readings. This is essential; it is the only way that you and your physician can make rational decisions about your program.
Stick with it.

The management of high blood pressure is a lifelong undertaking. You cannot stop your program because you feel good or wait for signs or symptoms to tell you what you need to do. This is the silent disease. If you take care of your blood pressure, the odds are overwhelmingly against it causing you a major problem. If you ignore high blood pressure or hope that someone else will take care of it, you are needlessly endangering your life and well-being.

Section III FAMILY RECORDS

Immunizations

DPT = Diphtheria, Pertussis (Whooping Cough), and Tetanus (Lockjaw)

DT = Diphtheria and Tetanus (Lockjaw)

Polio = Oral Polio

Measles = Measles Vaccine

Mumps = Mumps

Rubella = German Measles (Three Day Measles)

Name: _____ _____ _____ _____ _____ _____

Recommended Age:	Date	Date	Date	Date	Date	Date
2 months						
DPT #1						
Polio #1						
4 months						
DPT #2						
Polio #2						
6 months						
DPT #3						
Polio #3						
12 months						
Measles						
Mumps						
Rubella						
18 months						
Polio Booster						
DPT Booster						
5 Years						
Polio Booster						
DPT Booster						

Others

_____ _____ _____ _____ _____ _____

_____ _____ _____ _____ _____ _____

_____ _____ _____ _____ _____ _____

_____ _____ _____ _____ _____ _____

Note: Diphtheria and Tetanus is recommended every 10 years for life, with an additional tetanus booster for contaminated wounds more than 5 years after the last booster.

Childhood Diseases

Whooping Cough

Name	Date	Place	Remarks

Chicken Pox

Measles

Mumps

German Measles (Rubella)

Other Diseases:

_____

_____   _____   _____   _____
_____   _____   _____   _____
_____   _____   _____   _____
_____   _____   _____   _____
_____   _____   _____   _____

_____

_____   _____   _____   _____
_____   _____   _____   _____
_____   _____   _____   _____
_____   _____   _____   _____
_____   _____   _____   _____

_____

_____   _____   _____   _____
_____   _____   _____   _____
_____   _____   _____   _____
_____   _____   _____   _____
_____   _____   _____   _____

_____

_____   _____   _____   _____
_____   _____   _____   _____
_____   _____   _____   _____
_____   _____   _____   _____
_____   _____   _____   _____

Family Medical Information

Name	Blood type	RH Factor	Allergies (including drug allergies)
_____	_____	_____	_____
_____	_____	_____	_____
_____	_____	_____	_____
_____	_____	_____	_____
_____	_____	_____	_____
_____	_____	_____	_____
_____	_____	_____	_____
_____	_____	_____	_____

Hospitalizations

Name _____   Date _____   Hospital _____

Address _____   Reason _____

Name _____   Date _____   Hospital _____

Address _____   Reason _____

Name _____   Date _____   Hospital _____

Address _____   Reason _____

Name   Date   Hospital

_____ _____ _____

Address   Reason

_____   _____

Name   Date   Hospital

_____ _____ _____

Address   Reason

_____   _____

Name   Date   Hospital

_____ _____ _____

Address   Reason

_____   _____

Name   Date   Hospital

_____ _____ _____

Address   Reason

_____   _____

Name   Date   Hospital

_____ _____ _____

Address   Reason

_____   _____

Name   Date   Hospital

_____ _____ _____

Address   Reason

_____   _____

Name   Date   Hospital
_____   _____   _____

Address   Reason
_____   _____

Name   Date   Hospital
_____   _____   _____

Address   Reason
_____   _____

Name   Date   Hospital
_____   _____   _____

Address   Reason
_____   _____

Name   Date   Hospital
_____   _____   _____

Address   Reason
_____   _____

Name   Date   Hospital
_____   _____   _____

Address   Reason
_____   _____

Name   Date   Hospital
_____   _____   _____

Address   Reason
_____   _____

358

BOOKS BY THESE AUTHORS

Combs, B. J., D. R. Hales, B. K. Williams, J. F. Fries, and D. M. Vickery. *An Invitation to Health: Your Personal Responsibility*. Menlo Park, Calif.: Benjamin/Cummings Publishing Co., 1979.

Fries, J. F. *Arthritis: A Comprehensive Guide*. Reading, Mass.: Addison-Wesley Publishing Co., 1979.

Fries, J. F., and G. E. Ehrlich. *Prognosis: A Textbook of Medical Prognosis*. Bowie, Md.: The Charles Press Publishers, 1980.

Fries, J. F., and L. Crapo. *Vitality and Aging*. San Francisco, Calif.: W. H. Freeman and Company Publishers, 1981.

Lorig, K., and J. F. Fries. *The Arthritis Helpbook*. Menlo Park, Calif.: Addison-Wesley Publishing Co., 1980.

Pantell, R., J. F. Fries, and D. M. Vickery. *Taking Care of Your Child*. Reading, Mass.: Addison-Wesley Publishing Co., 1977.

Vickery, D. M., and J. F. Fries. *Take Care of Yourself: A Consumer's Guide to Medical Care*. Reading, Mass.: Addison-Wesley Publishing Co., 1977.

Vickery, D. M. *Life Plan for Your Health*. Reading, Mass.: Addison-Wesley Publishing Co., 1978.

ADDITIONAL READING

Books

Bunker, J. P., B. A. Barnes, and F. Mosteller. *Costs, Risks, and Benefits of Surgery.* New York: Oxford University Press, 1977.

Dubos, R. *Mirage of Health: Utopias, Progress, and Biological Change.* New York: Harper & Row Publishers, 1959.

Farquhar, J. W. *The American Way of Life Need Not Be Hazardous to Your Health.* New York: W. W. Norton & Company, 1978.

Ferguson, T. *Medical Self-Care: Access to Health Tools.* New York: Summit Books, 1980.

Frank, J. F. *Persuasion and Healing.* New York: Schocken Books, 1963.

Fuchs, V. R. *Who Shall Live? Health, Economics, and Social Choice.* New York: Basic Books, Inc., Publishers, 1974.

Knowles, J. H. *Doing Better and Feeling Worse: Health in the United States.* New York: W. W. Norton & Company, 1977.

Lowell, S. L., A. H. Katz, E. Holst. *Self-Care: Lay Initiatives in Health.* New York: Prodist, 1979.

McKeown, T. *The Role of Medicine: Dream, Mirage, or Nemesis?* Princeton, N.J.: Princeton University Press, 1979.

Riley, M. W. *Aging from Birth to Death: Interdisciplinary Perspectives.* Boulder, Colo.: Westview Press, 1979.

Silverman, M., and P. R. Lee. *Pills, Profits & Politics.* Berkeley, Calif.: University of California Press, 1974.

Totman, R. *Social Causes of Illness.* New York: Pantheon Books, 1979.

Articles

Addison County Health Council. Take Care of Yourself Distribution Project: A Cost Containment Program. *Final Report*, July 1980, Middlebury, Vt.

American Cancer Society, Inc., The Cancer-Related Health Checkup. 8 February 1980.

Berg, A. O., and J. P. LoGerfo. Potential Effect of Self-Care Algorithms on the Number of Physician Visits. *N. Eng. J. Med.* 300(1979):535–37.

Betz, B. J., and C. B. Thomas. Individual Temperament as a Predictor of Health or Premature Disease. *Johns Hopkins Med. J.*, 144(1979):81–89.

Breslow, L., and A. R. Somers. The Lifetime Health-Monitoring Program. *N. Eng. J. Med.* 296(1977):601–608.

Brody, D. S. The Patient's Role in Clinical Decision Making. *Ann. Intern. Med.* 93(1980):718–22.

Creagan, E. T., et al. Failure of High-Dose Vitamin C (Ascorbic Acid) Therapy to Benefit Patients with Advanced Cancer. *N. Eng. J. Med.* 301(1979):687–90.

Delbanco, T. L., and W. C. Taylor. The Periodic Health Examination: 1980. *Ann. Intern. Med.* 92(1980):251–52.

Dinman, B. D. The Reality and Acceptance of Risk. *JAMA* 244(1980):1226–28.

Eisenberg, L. The Perils of Prevention: A Cautionary Note. *N. Eng. J. Med.* 297(1977):1230–32.

Farquhar, J. W. The Community-Based Model of Life Style Intervention Trials. *Am. J. Epidemiol.* 108(1978):103–111.

Fletcher, S. W., and W. O. Spitzer. Approach of the Canadian Task Force to the Periodic Health Examination. *Ann. Intern. Med.* 92(1980):253.

Franklin, B. A., and M. Rubenfire. Losing Weight Through Exercise. *JAMA* 244(1980):377–79.

Fries, J. F. Aging, Natural Death, and the Compression of Morbidity. *N. Eng. J. Med.* 303(1980):130–35.

Glasgow, R. E., and G. M. Rosen. Behavioral Bibliotherapy: A Review of Self-Help Behavior Therapy Manuals. *Psych. Bull.* 85(1978):1–23.

Hennekens, C. H., W. Willett, et al. Effects of Beer, Wine, and Liquor in Coronary Deaths. *JAMA* 242(1979):1973–74.

Huddleston, A. L., D. Rockwell, et al. Bone Mass in Lifetime Tennis Athletes. *JAMA* 244(1980):1107–09.

Huttenen, J. K., et al. Effect of Moderate Physical Exercise on Serum Lipoproteins. *Circulation* 60:(1979):1220–29.

Kotchen, T. A., and R. J. Havlik. High Blood Pressure in the Young. *Ann. Intern. Med.* 92(1980):254.

LoGerfo, J. P., S. H. Moore, and T. S. Inui. Effect of Self-Care Book. *JAMA* 245(1981):341–42.

Moore, S. H., J. LoGerfo, and T. S. Inui. Effect of a Self-Care Book on Physician Visits. *JAMA* 243(1980):2317–20.

Nash, J. D., and J. W. Farquhar. Community Approaches to Dietary Modification and Obesity. *Psychiatric Clinics of No. Amer.* 1(1978):713–24.

Oppenheim, M. Healers. *N. Eng. J. Med.* 303(1980):1117–20.

Paffenbarger, R. S., and R. T. Hyde. Exercise as Protection Against Heart Attack. *N. Eng. J. Med.* 302(1980):1026–27.

Phelps, C. E. Illness Prevention and Medical Insurance. *J. Human Resources* 13(1978):183–207.

Relman, A. S. The New Medical-Industrial Complex. *N. Eng. J. Med.* 303(1980):963–70.

Rosen, G. M. The Development and Use of Nonprescription Behavior Therapies. *Amer. Psych.* (February 1976):139–41.

Stallones, R. A. The Rise and Fall of Ischemic Heart Disease. *Scientific American* 243(1980):53–59.

Stamler, R., J. Stamler, et al. Weight and Blood Pressure: Findings in Hypertension Screening of 1 Million Americans. *JAMA* 240(1978):1607–10.

Taylor, W. C., and T. L. Delbanco. Looking for Early Cancer. *Ann. Intern. Med.* 93(1980):773–75.

Thomas, C. B., and O. L. McCabe. Precursors of Premature Disease and Death: Habits of Nervous Tension. *Johns Hopkins Med. J.* 147(1980):137–45.

Tibblin, G. Risk Factors for Developing Myocardial Infarction and Other Diseases: The "Men Born in 1913" Study. In *Preventive Cardiology*. New York: John Wiley & Sons, 1972.

Weinstein, M. C. Estrogen Use in Postmenopausal Women—Costs, Risks, and Benefits. *N. Eng. J. Med.* 303(1980):308–316.

White, J. R., and H. F. Froeb. Small-Airways Dysfunction in Nonsmokers Chronically Exposed to Tobacco Smoke. *N. Eng. J. Med.* 302(1980):720–23.

Williams, R. S., et al. Physical Conditioning Augments the Fibrinolytic Response to Venous Occlusion in Healthy Adults *N. Eng. J. Med.* 302(1980):987–91.

Zook, C. J., and F. D. Moore. High-Cost Users of Medical Care. *N. Eng. J. Med.* 302(1980):996–1002.

Index

364

370

ORDER FORM

____ TAKING CARE OF YOUR CHILD, $7.95 paperback

____ TAKING CARE OF YOUR CHILD, $12.95 hardback

____ LIFEPLAN FOR YOUR HEALTH, $7.25 FPT paperback

____ LIFEPLAN FOR YOUR HEALTH, $10.95 hardback

____ ARTHRITIS, $9.30 FPT paperback

____ ARTHRITIS, $11.95 hardback

____ ARTHRITIS HELPBOOK, $8.25 FPT paperback

____ ARTHRITIS HELPBOOK, $11.95 hardback

☐ My check for full payment is enclosed. (Add state and local sales tax when applicable. We will pay postage and handling.)

☐ Bill (or Charge to) my: BankAmericard (Visa) # _____

Expiration date _____

Master Charge # _____

Four digits above name _____

Expiration date _____

(Applicable sales tax and postage will be added.)

Name _____

Street _____

City _____

State _____ Zip Code _____

Send all orders to: **Addison-Wesley Publishing Company**
Reading, Massachusetts 01867

YOU CAN TAKE BETTER CARE OF YOURSELF AND YOUR FAMILY WITH THESE BESTSELLING BOOKS BY DRS. FRIES AND VICKERY:

Taking Care of Your Child, A Parents' Guide to Medical Care, by Dr. Robert Pantell, Dr. James Fries, and Dr. Donald Vickery. Over 120,000 copies in print. Easy-to-read decision charts for ninety-one of the most common medical problems of childhood—from birth through adolescence.

416 pages, 91 charts, $10.95 FPT quality paperback, $12.95 hardback

Lifeplan for Your Health, by Dr. Donald Vickery. You can dramatically increase your life expectancy with the practical advice in this book. You'll find important information on the ten myths of medicine, lifestyle habits that affect your health, the major causes of disability and death, and how to plan for a healthier life.

256 pages, $7.25 FPT quality paperback, $10.95 hardback

Arthritis: A Comprehensive Guide, by Dr. James Fries. You don't have to be a victim of arthritis. With this book you can identify what kind of arthritis you have, find the most effective treatment and medication, and successfully manage everyday problems of pain and getting around.

480 pages, 30 charts, $9.95 FPT quality paperback, $11.95 hardback

The Arthritis Helpbook, What You Can Do For Your Arthritis, by Kate Lorig, R.N., and Dr. James Fries. This complete self-treatment program is the perfect companion volume to *Arthritis,* offering illustrated exercises, relaxation techniques, diet and nutrition information, and much more.

192 pages, b&w illustrations, $8.25 FPT quality paperback, $11.95 hardback